# ANNUAL REVIEW of Gerontology and Geriatrics

Volume 2, 1981

# ANNUAL REVIEW of Gerontology and Geriatrics

Volume 2, 1981


**Carl Eisdorfer, Ph.D., M.D.**
*EDITOR-IN-CHIEF*

**Richard W. Besdine, M.D.**
**Vincent Cristofalo, Ph.D.**
**M. Powell Lawton, Ph.D.**
**George L. Maddox, Ph.D.**
*ASSOCIATE EDITORS*

**Bernard D. Starr, Ph.D.**
*MANAGING EDITOR*



SPRINGER PUBLISHING COMPANY
New York

Springer Publishing Company, Inc.
200 Park Avenue South
New York, New York 10003

81 82 83 84 85 86 / 10 9 8 7 6 5 4 3 2 1

ISSN 0198–8794
ISBN 0–8261–3081–X

Printed in the United States of America

# Contents

# Introduction

The enthusiastic response to the publication of the first volume of the *Annual Review* lends support to our belief that we have introduced an important contribution to gerontology and geriatrics. This second volume continues the format established with Volume 1. It includes critical and intensive review chapters in each of five sections: (1) Biological Sciences; (2) Behavioral and Social Sciences; (3) Health and Clinical Practices; (4) Policy and Planning; and (5) Social and Community Services. In addition, there is a special section with a brief focused review.

While the review chapters encompass diverse areas of interest, several of them address topics that merit special attention at this time. In the section on Health and Clinical Practices, three chapters review drugs and their use and misuse among the aged. The foci of the individual reviews differ, ranging from those of clinical pharmacists to clinicians, and from mechanisms of action to a concern with nonprescribed and illicit drugs. The review of the most commonly used and abused over-the-counter drug, alcohol, is an important chapter since it has been insufficiently addressed in gerontology.

In the section on Behavioral and Social Sciences, a review of behavior therapies emphasizes a nonmedication orientation to treatment of a range of disorders, both behavioral and somatic. It complements the review on the psychodynamic psychotherapies published in Volume 1. In the Biological Sciences section there is an extensive review of another important topic in gerontology—the immune system. Volume 3, currently in process, will contain a review of clinical issues in immunology which will complement this review. This continuity of coverage will provide the opportunity to develop material in sufficient depth to make it of value to the clinician as well as to the scholar in the field.

In the last section, a special brief review of clinical procedures in the management of urinary incontinence is included. This topic, one of major clinical importance to families, patients, and practitioners, is often given relatively little attention in professional and scientific circles. As a result, a mythology prevails concerning the irreversibility of incontinence, and important clinical research findings may not find their way into common practice.

Changes that appear among the aged, their etiologies, and the ways in which these factors interact with other crucial demographic elements such as sex, ethnicity, and income, are key elements for all gerontologists. This interaction, as covered in this volume, shows that gerontology and geriatrics cross boundaries into other scientific and clinical disciplines.

In the section on Social and Community Services, the chapter on well-being is presented to help understand change with age. The impact of profound loss and of long-term care in the overall health planning of the nation have theoretical as well as practical implications as indicated in the reviews in Chapters 5 and 12.

The reviews in Volume 2 have been prepared by distinguished biological and behavioral scientists as well as by clinicians and planners. Their professional backgrounds include nursing, law, surgery, psychology, pharmacy, and social work, among other disciplines. All are gerontologists.

An additional observation seems in order. By the time this volume is examined by our readers, in all likelihood a new economic and social policy will have been initiated by the federal government in the United States. The ramifications of this change will be felt in a reorganization of federal, state, and local service programs for the aging; a revised budget for research, particularly in the behavioral and social sciences; and changed responsibility for emerging medical, psychological and social problems of aging. It is, of course, too early to deal with the impact of the many changes proposed in the federal government's budget and bureaucratic organization. One fact is clear, however. The population shift in the direction of larger numbers of the aged and increasing longevity among older persons will continue to develop. The implications of this population shift remain monumental. The effect upon our economy, our health and social service system, and on the human condition of those older persons, their families and their world will need to be addressed. In short, the problems of the aged will not disappear. Indeed, the increases in the number and proportion of the older part of the population will have great repercussions for the entire population. Solutions to the problems and opportunities to use the resource potential of older persons will challenge us more in the future than they have in the past.

Knowledge, skills, and creativity as well as clinical and programmatic solutions to the problems of the aging will be urgently needed, and research and training will continue. New coalitions of recipients, providers, and scholars will be called upon to make the increased effort to achieve the necessary goals. It is our hope that this review of the latest knowledge and ideas in the field and the suggestions for further knowledge and improved practice will help find some of these solutions. Once again, we paraphrase Pogo and remind ourselves that "we have met the aged and they are us."

A number of changes concerning the editorial board and staff have taken place. Dr. James Birren, a member of the Advisory Board and a founding member of our Associate Editors group, has had to relinquish his duties as Associate Editor of this volume. Jim, whose help in organizing this *Annual Review* series and in planning for the first five years was invaluable, has accepted the position as Chairman of the 1981 White House Conference on Aging's Technical Committee on Research. This, along with his numerous other duties, meant that he needed to limit many of his commitments. He remains an active member of our Advisory Board, and we are most grateful for his continued work with us. At the same time, we are honored that Dr. Warner Schaie, of the University of Southern California, will become an Associate Editor beginning with Volume 3.

Ms. Jean Pasche, our most valued Assistant to the Editor-in-Chief, has accepted a new position at the University of Washington's Institute on Aging, and she will be leaving us with the publication of this volume. Her efforts, beyond the call of duty, will be gratefully remembered.

**Carl Eisdorfer, Ph.D., M.D.**
**April 1981**

# Contributors

**Patricia Archbold, R.N., M.S.**
School of Nursing
University of California
San Francisco, California

**Joseph H. Atkinson, Jr., M.D.**
Department of Psychiatry
University of California,
San Diego
School of Medicine
La Jolla, California

**Susan K. Bettis, Ph.D.**
Center for Gerontology
University of Oregon
Eugene, Oregon

**Stanley J. Brody, J.D., M.S.W.**
Department of Physical Medicine
and Rehabilitation
University of Pennsylvania
School of Medicine
Philadelphia, Pennsylvania

**Robert L. Clark, Ph.D.**
Department of Economics
North Carolina State University
Raleigh, North Carolina

**Caleb E. Finch, Ph.D.**
Ethel Percy Andrus Gerontology
Center
University of Southern California
Los Angeles, California

**Sue B. Foster, R.N., M.S.N., F.A.A.N.**
Nursing Education Programs
Beth Israel Hospital
Boston, Massachusetts

**Donald E. Gelfand, Ph.D.**
School of Social Work and
Community Planning
University of Maryland
Baltimore, Maryland

**Linda K. George, Ph.D.**
Center for the Study of Aging
and Human Development
Duke University
Durham, North Carolina

**Susan R.S. Gottesman, Ph.D.**
Department of Pathology
University of California
School of Medicine
Los Angeles, California

**Roy King, M.D., Ph.D.**
Department of Psychiatry
and Behavioral Science
Stanford University Medical
School
Stanford, California

**Robert J. Krane, M.D.**
Department of Urology
Boston University School of
Medicine
Boston, Massachusetts

**John F. Marshall, Ph.D.**
Department of Psychobiology
University of California
Irvine, California

**Eugenia M. Parron, Ph.D.**
Department of Psychology and
Human Services
Brookdale Community College
Lincroft, New Jersey

**Elmer M. Plein, Ph.D.**
Department of Pharmacy Practice
University of Washington
Seattle, Washington

**Joy B. Plein, Ph.D.**
Department of Pharmacy Practice
University of Washington
Seattle, Washington

**Patrick K. Randall, Ph.D.**
Ethel Percy Andrus Gerontology Center
University of Southern California
Los Angeles, California

**Robert G. Riedel, Ph.D.**
Department of Psychology
Southwest State University
Marshall, Minnesota

**Marc A. Schuckit, M.D.**
Department of Psychiatry
University of California, San Diego
School of Medicine
La Jolla, California

**Frances G. Scott, Ph.D.**
Center for Gerontology
University of Oregon
Eugene, Oregon

**Mike B. Siroky, M.D.**
Department of Urology
Boston University School of Medicine
Boston, Massachusetts

**Saul M. Spivack, M.S.**
Department of Physical Medicine and Rehabilitation
University of Pennsylvania
School of Medicine
Philadelphia, Pennsylvania

**C.F. Tam, Ph.D.**
Department of Pathology
University of California
School of Medicine
Los Angeles, California

**Lillian E. Troll, Ph.D.**
Department of Psychology
Rutgers University
New Brunswick, New Jersey

**Roy L. Walford, M.D.**
Department of Pathology
University of California
School of Medicine
Los Angeles, California

**Richard H. Weindruch, Ph.D.**
Department of Pathology
University of California
School of Medicine
Los Angeles, California

**Jerome Yesavage, M.D.**
Psychiatric Intensive Care Unit
Veteran's Administration Medical Center
Palo Alto, California
Department of Psychiatry and Behavioral Science
Stanford University Medical School
Stanford, California

# Forthcoming

**THE ANNUAL REVIEW OF**
**GERONTOLOGY AND GERIATRICS, Volume 3**

**Tentative Contents**

SECTION I

# Biological Sciences

CHAPTER 1

# Immunopathology of Aging

Roy L. Walford, M.D.
Susan R.S. Gottesman, Ph.D.
Richard H. Weindruch, Ph.D.
C.F. Tam, Ph.D.
Department of Pathology
University of California
School of Medicine
Los Angeles, California

## THE MAIN HISTOCOMPATIBILITY COMPLEX (MHC)

### The MHC and Related Genes as a Life-Support Homeostatic System

The MHC (HLA system in man, H-2 system in mice) controls not only whether a grafted organ will be recognized as "foreign" and so rejected, but essentially all aspects of thymus-dependent immunity. It represents one among a number of multigene families which display close linkage and related overlapping phenotypic functions (Walford, 1979). In association with so-called "minor" histocompatibility loci (non-H-2 but also influencing graft rejection), it may also comprise a multigene system, that is, a system composed of gene families located on different chromosomes and therefore unlinked, but reacting together. Cytotoxic reactions in mice against "minor" histocompatibility loci may, for example, require identity at H-2 (Bevan, 1975). For the present, however, recent developments concerning the MHC at the multigene family level are sufficiently arresting from the standpoint of gerontology that we need not ascend to more complex levels to find potentially important insights.

It was argued some years ago that the MHC might play a significant role in aging (Walford, 1969, 1970). Analyses unrelated to this surmise

The authors' studies have been aided by USPHS grants AG 00424, AG 00790, and AI-10088.

have since been presented, to the effect that aging may be regulated or caused not so much by activity along the whole genome, but by quite small segments of the genome (Walford, 1972; Cutler, 1975; Sacher, 1975). Based on the demonstration of a relationship between maximum life span and H-2 alleles in congenic mice, it was later suggested that the MHC might represent such a small segment (Smith and Walford, 1977). This suggestion is strengthened by recent observations that not only is the MHC related to many aspects of immune function but in addition (1) the structural gene for superoxide dismutase 2[1] is located on the same chromosome in man as in the MHC, albeit at a considerable distance (Smith et al., 1978); (2) a regulatory gene for superoxide dismutase[1] activity in mice is very closely linked to the mouse MHC complex (the H-2 system) (Novak et al., 1980); (3) part of the mixed function oxidase system[1] might possibly be linked to H-2 (Nebert, 1979); (4) the level of cAMP, which is intimately involved in many cell functions and shows marked age-related alterations, at least in lymphocytes (Tam and Walford, 1978, 1980; Tam et al., 1979), may be MHC regulated (Meruelo and Edidin, 1975); and (5) evidence exists of a preliminary nature that the MHC may influence DNA repair capacity (Walford and Bergmann, 1979). Next we note that remarkable similarities have been found between the three-dimensional protein structures of immunoglobulin and the subunits of one form of superoxide dismutase (Richardson et al., 1977). They may well be evolutionarily related. The histocompatibility antigens of the MHC are also in part coded for by genes evolved from a common ancestral immunoglobulin gene. It follows that genes for immunoglobulin, the MHC, and superoxide dismutase may all have derived from the same ancient source. Also, on the same chromosome in mice as the H-2 system is the T/t complex. This gene system regulates some aspects of embryonic differentiation, decreases the crossover frequency between itself and H-2, and controls the expression of an embryonic antigen called F9 (Snell, 1979). The F9 antigen resembles H-2 antigens in molecular weight and subunit structure and might therefore represent a fourth evolutionary derivative.

While the present review will largely concern immunology and aging, the above overall evidence cannot fail to suggest that the MHC and MHC-linked genes may constitute a multigene family exerting multifactorial influence upon the aging process, a family which includes and goes beyond immune function to comprise a major life-support homeostatic system.

[1]These enzymes are involved in oxygen metabolism. Superoxide dismutase in particular converts the highly toxic free radical, superoxide anion ($O_2^-$), formed in the course of normal metabolism, to $H_2O_2$ and $O_2$. Evidence can be cited for a so-called free radical theory of aging (Harman, 1978). Levels of some mixed function oxidases seem to correlate inversely with species life span (Schwartz, 1975).

**Structure and Function of the MHC**

The main histocompatibility complex of genes is located on chromosome #6 in humans and #17 in mice. MHCs have also been described in rats, chickens, dogs, pigs, chimpanzees, monkeys, guinea pigs, and rabbits (Gotze, 1977). Genes within the MHC in man include those of the HLA system, which contains five recognized histocompatibility loci, namely HLA-A, -B, -C, -D and -DR. Analogous genes comprise the H-2 system in mice. Other genes within or close to the MHC include those coding for complement proteins, for certain disease susceptibilities, structural genes for red cell enzymes and antigens, various regulatory genes, and genes for different types of receptor and binding proteins. Antigens determined by MHC genes are implicated in T cell and B cell specific differentiation (Amos and Kostyu, 1980). MHC-linked genes govern the ability to react against foreign or allogeneic material. The complex is clearly involved in cell-to-cell interactions and in recognition (Snell, 1979), including self-recognition (Levy and Shearer, 1980). There may be immune response genes within the MHC coding for autoantigens: for example the alleles H-2k, H-2s, and H-2q are associated with susceptibility to autoimmune thyroiditis, and H-2s to experimental autoimmune encephalomyelitis in mice (Mackay et al., 1977). In man HLA-B8 and DR3 correlate with high titers of anti-acetylcholine receptor antibodies in myasthenia gravis (Naeim et al., 1978). The immune and other responses to corticosteroids may be MHC-influenced (Becker et al., 1976), as are the levels of testosterone and testosterone-binding protein (Ivanyi et al., 1972). HLA-linked genes are known to be involved in iron metabolism (Bomford et al., 1977). Klein (1978) lists 59 traits reported as associated with or linked to the MHC in mice. Amos and Kostyu (1980) give a similar list for humans. The system is highly pleotrophic.

HLA antigens have been found on all human nucleated cells examined, and in saliva, serum, seminal fluid and milk (Amos and Kostyu, 1980). They are transmembrane cell-surface glycoproteins whose movement in the plasma membrane is associated with the movement of intracellular cytoskeletal elements, either microfilaments or microtubules (Portugal, 1979). The HLA-A and HLA-B molecules consist of two non-covalently associated polypeptide chains, the chain carrying the antigenic specificities having a molecular weight of 44,000 while the other subunit, $\beta_2$-microglobulin, which in man is coded for by a gene on the 15th chromosome (Goodfellow et al., 1975), has a molecular weight of 12,000. Biochemical analysis suggests that the HLA molecule may be structured into two domains similar to immunoglobulins and is homologous to immunoglobulins (Parham et al., 1977; Robb et al., 1978). The H-2 K and D regions in mice, and probably the HLA-A and -B regions in humans, are involved in recognition in cell-mediated cytotoxicity (CML), while the HLA-D antigen in humans serves as the stimulator factor required for recognition of non-self in mixed lymphocyte reactions (MLR). (The CML and MLR are the in vitro correlates of graft rejection). Ir or I-region genes in the mouse and probably homologous genes in humans regulate the quantitative level of the antibody response, that is, they determine high or low response to particular antigens (McDevitt and Tyan, 1968; Naeim and Walford, 1980b).

### Influence on Life Span

Studies in congenic mouse strains (genetically identical except at one gene region) have clearly shown that alleles at the MHC influence maximum life span. Among 14 different strains congenic on C57BL/10, C3H and A strain backgrounds, statistically significant differences in tenth deciles of survivorship were found on all backgrounds (Smith and Walford, 1977). Applying multiple regression analysis techniques to these same data, Buckley (1980) reported that H-2 appears to exert a relatively greater effect on the process of aging than on disease susceptibility. Fifty-seven percent of the variation in life-span was considered as due to background differences, and 22 percent to differences within H-2. Separate investigations indicated that these same H-2 alleles influence the age-related rise and decline of immune responses to mitogens (Meredith and Walford, 1977). In general a higher mitogenic response in old age was associated with a longer maximum life span. The B10.F mouse, which carries the H-2n allele and is congenic to the long-lived C57BL/10 strains, displays a greatly shortened life span and an aging pattern suggesting a progeroid syndrome (Popp, 1978). Using a model in which the various hybrid strains to be compared were derived from a DBA/2J mother and B10 background congenic fathers (the $F_1$ hybrid strains thus being genetically identical except for the H-2 haplotype of the father), Williams and co-workers (1980) noted significant differences in survival when the H-2 haplotypes were different.

It might be difficult to demonstrate a meaningful relationship of the MHC to maximum life span in humans because other polygenic effects on life span in such an outbred species could readily obscure any influence of the HLA complex. Reports are conflicting. Several studies have indicated an increased heterozygosity at the HLA-B locus with age (Macurova et al., 1975; Yunis et al., 1976; Converse and Williams, 1978; Hodge and Walford, 1980). Greenberg and Yunis (1978) found a decrease in incidence of HLA-B8 and HLA–A1, -B8 in older females, possibly reflecting the known correlation of the HLA-B8 antigen with autoimmune-susceptibility in man. Absence of the HLA specificity designated Se7 among a dozen centenarians suggested that it may exert a negative influence on longevity (Takata et al., 1980). HLA determinations on 920 inhabitants of five small Dutch islands failed to reveal significant differences in relation to age groups (Hansen et al., 1977), and the authors concluded that while HLA could hardly be neutral with regard to life span, "multiple selective effects associated with the HLA system balance each other out in the population." Macurova and colleagues (1975) reported a significant age-related increase in W10 (now called HLA-Bw40). Yarnell and co-workers (1979) also reported an increase in the frequency of HLA-Bw40 in the over-70 age group, but denied its significance because the frequency did not continue to increase in the older over-70 cohorts. However, only a small number of persons over 85 years of age were included among their older-population sample. At the Eighth Histocompatibility Workshop, 104 Caucasians and 18 Japanese over 90 years of age were HLA typed (Hodge and Walford, 1980). A statistically significant increase in homozygosity for the public antigens HLA-B4 and -B6 was found, possibly in line with an earlier speculation that so-called "hybrid vigor" may not apply in maximum life span expectations (Walford, 1969). Again Bw40 showed some increase although not to a statistically significant degree.

### Disease Relationships

Striking associations are well documented in man and mouse between different alleles of the MHC and susceptibilities to several forms of malignancy and to many autoimmune and other diseases (Dausset and Svejgaard, 1977; Batchelor and Morris, 1978; Amos and Kostyu, 1980; Naeim and Walford, 1980b). In the mouse, different H-2 alleles correlate with susceptibilities to various leukemia viruses (reviewed by Walford et al., 1971). Perhaps more pertinent to a gerontologic inquiry was the demonstration involving 14 different strains of mice congenic at H-2 on three backgrounds that the MHC may profoundly influence susceptibility to spontaneous late-life-occurring lung, liver, lymphoid, and mammary cancers (Smith and Walford, 1978; Walford et al., 1978). A later analysis of tumor data from recombinant mouse strains indicated that genes in the IB region of H-2 determine susceptibility to lung cancer (Faraldo et al., 1979). The particular MHC allele present in cultured rat fibroblasts influenced the replication of endogenous RNA-tumor viruses and determined whether the cultures would follow a pathway of "transformation" or undergo phase III senescent deterioration (Kontermann and Bayreuther, 1979).

In man, attempts to find association between HLA and malignancy have been somewhat disappointing, with good evidence only in Hodgkin's disease, acute lymphatic leukemia, nasopharyngeal carcinoma, and testicular cancer (Walford et al., 1971; Simons et al., 1974; DeWolf et al., 1979). Probably the polygenic nature of susceptibility to most types of cancer obscures the role of individual genes in an outbred strain such as man (Naeim and Walford, 1980b).

Strong positive associations between autoimmune and some inflammatory diseases and the MHC system have been found (Rose et al., 1978). In ankylosing spondylitis from 90 to 100 percent of affected individuals carry the HLA-B27 antigen, in contrast to only 6 percent in the normal population. Of pertinence to our inquiry is the fact that rheumatoid arthritis, whose incidence increases with age, is associated with an increased frequency of HLA-DRw4 (Batchelor and Morris, 1978; Stastny, 1978). HLA associations have also been found with Addison's disease, multiple sclerosis, insulin-dependent diabetes mellitus, chronic active hepatitis, Graves' disease, psoriasis, myasthenia gravis, systemic lupus erythematosus, leprosy, and many other maladies. Some of these will be discussed in detail later in this review. The apparent diversity of HLA-associated diseases indicates that no single mechanism is involved (Dupont et al., 1978). Indeed some HLA-linked genes are not even primarily involved in immune mechanisms but exert other regulatory functions in maintaining homeostasis.

## BIOCHEMICAL CHANGES IN LYMPHOID CELLS WITH AGE

Immune dysfunction with aging is generally manifested by a decline in the responses of lymphoid cells to immunologic stimuli, such as the presentation of alloantigen or mitogen to the cell surface. Characteristically these responses are measured as incorporation of radioactive thymidine into replicating DNA while the stimulated cell undergoes blastogenesis, as antibody production following injection of alloantigen or as release of $Cr^{51}$ from target cells (cell-mediated lymphocytotoxicity). For all these responses many biochemical events must supervene between the initial stimulus and the final response, which is usually measured three to five days later. While much information is available on the biochemistry of lymphocytes from young-adult animals and humans, including both resting and activated cells (Wedner and Parker, 1976; Hadden, 1977), only a few reports concern the effect of age on these parameters; nevertheless, dramatic and interesting changes have already been demonstrated.

**The Cyclic Nucleotide System**

The cyclic nucleotides are critically involved in hormonal regulation, transcription, replication, and differentiation in many cell systems, including effects in diverse life forms from bacteria to plants to man. They form part of the purine salvage pathway and also influence the "energy charge" within the cell. Cyclic nucleotide biochemistry has been the subject of numerous reviews, many of which emphasize the immune system but are restricted to work in adult animals (Goldberg, 1974; Wedner and Parker, 1976; Strom and Carpenter, 1977; Watson, 1977; Parker, 1979).

We have studied age-related alterations of cyclic nucleotides in lymphocytes of young and old mice and humans, and in Down's syndrome, which is known to show many features of accelerated aging (Tam and Walford, 1978, 1980; Tam et al., 1979, 1980a, 1980b). Resting (unstimulated) levels of cAMP and cGMP, the cAMP/cGMP ratio, and the levels of their generating enzymes (adenylate cyclase and guanylate cyclase) in purified splenic T cells of eight-month and 30-month (C57BL/10 × C3H)$F_1$-hybrid mice are shown in Table 1–1. With age, the level of cAMP declined about five-fold, of cGMP increased seven-fold, the cAMP/cGMP ratio declined 50-fold, adenylate cyclase was about 3.5-fold elevated in T cells in old mice, and guanylate cyclase decreased three-fold. Striking age-related changes in cyclic nucleotide responses have also been found in lymphocytes following activation by mitogens (Tam and Walford, 1978). In addition, isopycnic ultracentrifugation studies revealed different patterns of subcellular distribution of cyclic nucleotides and of adenylate and guanylate cyclases in resting splenic T cells from old compared to young mice. Table 1–2 shows that changes in human peripheral T cells with donor age correspond to those reported for isolated mouse splenic T cells, and that alterations in Down's syndrome accord with the view that Down's is a condition of accelerated aging.

Table 1–1
Levels of cAMP, cGMP, Their Ratios, and of the Adenylate and Guanylate Cyclases in Splenic T Cells from Young Adult and Old Mice[a]

| *Age* | *cAMP*[b] | *cGMP*[b] | *cAMP/cGMP* | *Adenylate cyclase*[c] | *Guanylate cyclase*[d] |
|---|---|---|---|---|---|
| 8 mo. | 18.8 | 1.0 | 32 | 1.5 | 4.1 |
| 30 mo. | 3.3 | 7.3 | 0.6 | 5.4 | 1.3 |

[a]Six to 11 mice from each age group were examined.

[b]pmol/$10^7$ cells.

[c]pmol cAMP formed per mg protein in 15 minutes.

[d]pmol cGMP formed per mg protein in 15 minutes.

Source: Adapted from Tam et al. (1980a).

Table 1–2
Levels of cAMP, cGMP, Their Ratios, and the Adenylate and Guanylate Cyclases in Peripheral Blood T Cells of Young Adult and Old Humans and Patients with Down's Syndrome and Systemic Lupus Erythematosus

| *Condition* | *Age*[a] *(years)* | *cAMP*[b] | *cGMP*[b] | *cAMP/* | *Adenylate cyclase*[c] | *Guanylate cyclase*[d] |
|---|---|---|---|---|---|---|
| Normal young adult | 35 | 18.4 | 0.5 | 124.16 | 0.39 | 3.0 |
| Normal old | 87 | 0.7 | 4.7 | 0.14 | 4.15 | 0.32 |
| Down's | 26 | 4.4 | 6.4 | 0.66 | 1.33 | 0.97 |
| SLE | 47 | 1.2 | 8.9 | 0.31 | — | — |

[a]Six to 13 persons were examined from each subject population.

[b]pmol/$10^7$ cells.

[c]pmol cAMP formed per mg protein in 15 minutes.

[d]pmol cGMP formed per mg protein in 15 minutes.

Source: Adapted from Tam and Walford (1980).

A number of factors affect the adenine nucleotide pool. Investigating the purine salvage pathway, Scholar and co-workers (1980) found no age-related change of adenosine deaminase in mouse lymphocytes, but a significant decrease in purine nucleoside phosphorylase by eight months of age. Clinical states in man characterized by a deficiency in this enzyme are accompanied by impairement of T-cell but not B-cell function. This is like what is seen with normal aging. It is noteworthy that T but not B lymphocytes are known to be sensitive to the toxic effects of deoxyguanosine, one of the substrates which accumulates when purine nucleoside phosphorylase is deficient. We have observed an elevated activity of adenosine deaminase in peripheral blood T cells from old humans but no age-related change in energy charge (Tam et al., 1980b, 1980c).

These various changes in cyclic nucleotides and related substances cannot be interpreted merely as alterations in T cell subsets with age (Tam et al., 1980a, b, c), but must represent intrinsic biochemical alterations in lymphoid cells. As the cyclic nucleotide or "second messenger" system is present throughout the animal kingdom, the demonstration therein of marked changes with age might have general significance as a possible fundamental age-related lesion.

The cyclic nucleotide changes with age are somewhat paradoxical. Low cAMP levels are generally thought of as associated with increased proliferative tendency, but clearly in lymphocytes from old donors the reverse is true. However, the precise physiologic roles of cAMP and cGMP related to the many cellular changes associated with mitogen- or antigen-induced lymphocyte stimulation are controversial and unresolved.

Recently Klimpel and colleagues (1979) suggested that the selective activation of cAMP-dependent protein kinase may be important in regulating lymphocyte mitogenesis. The decreased resting levels of cAMP in old T cells might therefore cause inactivation of cAMP-dependent protein kinase, leading to a diminished response of old cells to mitogens. We have suggested a number of possible explanations for the changes in cyclic nucleotide-generating enzymes with age (Tam et al., 1980a, b, c): they might reflect a compensatory mechanism; functional defects in enzymes might lead to overproduction of the enzymes; free radicals, defective export systems such as the purine salvage pathway, or alterations in phosphodiesterase systems might be involved. Altered redox potentials might correlate with our observations of high cGMP levels and altered guanylate cyclase activities in aging T cells. Mittal and Murad (1977) point out that both superoxide dismutase and free radicals can activate guanylate cyclase to produce increased amounts of cGMP. Elevated levels of cGMP induced by altered redox states in aging T cells might in part be responsible for some of the other changes noted in old T cells. The evidence is not inconsistent with the concept that alterations in the cyclic nucleotide system may in part be responsible for the immunodeficiency of aging.

**DNA Repair**

A relation between DNA repair capacity and aging was clearly suggested by the important finding of Hart and Setlow (1974) of a correlation between deoxyribonucleic acid excision repair and maximum life span in a number of mammalian species. This relationship apparently holds not only between widely separate mammalian species, mouse, elephant, and man for example, but also within the primates (Hart and Hall, 1979), and between different mouse strains (Paffenholz, 1978; Walford and Bergmann, 1979).

DNA repair in lymphocytes measured both as repair of UV-induced lesions (Lambert et al., 1977) and as sentitivity to bleomycin (Seshadri et al., 1979) has been reported to decline with age. These findings, which probably reflect altered DNA repair capacities in lymphocytes, might also be attributable to age-related alterations in nucleosomal structure whereby access of, for example, bleomycin to its site of action becomes altered, or access of repair enzymes to DNA is impaired by conformational abnormalities. This might be secondary to increasing compactness or condensation of chromatin with age, possibly due to S-S bond formation (Tas and Walford, 1980; Tas et al., 1980).

Diminished DNA repair capacity in lymphocytes in advanced age might conceivably be secondary to rather than causative of immunologic disturbances. A wide variety of autoantibodies to nuclear antigens have been described (Miyachi et al., 1978) and if any of these penetrated to the nucleus (for which there is no evidence at present), they might restrict access of repair enzymes to nucleosomal structures. Self-tolerance to single-stranded deoxyribonucleic acid is easily lost, at least in vitro (Roder et al., 1978a). Low levels of autoantibody and autoantigen binding cells exist normally in the body (Roder et al., 1978b). It is structurally conceivable that anti-TNP and/or anti-DNP antibodies might cross-react with certain adjacent base pairs on the DNA backbone if access were in fact attained. It is interesting to note the existence of naturally occurring DNP-binding molecules in chordate sera and hemolymph (Marchalonis and Warr, 1978), as well as evidence of H-2 linked genetic control of immune responsiveness to TNP-mouse serum albumin (an altered self-antigen) in mice (Urba and Hildemann, 1978).

Some evidence exists for linkage between alleles at the main histocompatibility complex (MHC) and DNA repair capacity. If substantiated, this might reflect a direct influence of the MHC on, for example, the level of repair enzymes, or be secondary to MHC-regulation of autoantibody production, with effects thereof on DNA repair as suggested briefly above, or to other mechanisms. DNA repair is defective in the lymphocytes of patients with systemic lupus erythematosus (SLE) (Beighlie and Teplitz, 1975), which is both highly HLA linked (reviewed by Walford and Bergmann, 1979) and shows features of accelerated aging (see below, this chapter). The SLE-like disease of (NZB × NZW)$F_1$-hybrid mice is mediated by at least three, possibly four genes (Knight et al., 1977; Adams and Knight, 1980). One from the NZW parent is tightly linked to H-2 and may be an Ir gene. Another (from NZB parent) shows about 30 percent crossover with H-2, and a third lies on chromosome #4 of NZB next to the H-18 "minor" histocompatibility locus. NZB mice manifest defective DNA repair capacity of their cultured fibroblasts (Paffenholz, 1978) and splenic lymphocytes (K. Hall, K. Bergmann, and R. Walford, unpublished observation). A decrease in DNA repair capacity has also been reported in lymphocytes of rheumatoid arthritis patients (Tuschl and Altmann, 1976; Matsura et al., 1978), a highly HLA-linked malady (Stastny, 1978). Aplastic anemia seems associated with DNA repair deficiency as judged by bleomycin sensitivity of lymphocytes (Morley et al., 1978), and Dausset and colleagues (1977) have provided suggestive but inconclusive evidence for a relationship between HLA and aplastic anemia. The most convincing work claiming a relation between HLA and DNA repair was a familial study of xeroderma pigmentosum (Giraldo et al., 1977), but the original analysis of the data has been shown to be statistically invalid (Hodge et al., 1980a). Data accumulated for the Eighth Histocompatibility Workshop did not confirm a relation between HLA and xeroderma pigmentosum (Hodge et al., 1980b). In preliminary studies involving UV-induced unscheduled DNA synthesis and bleomycin sensitivity, we found evidence of differences in DNA repair capacity in lymphocytes from several strains of mice congenic at the H-2 locus (Walford and Bergmann, 1979). It is clear that more work must be done to determine whether a meaningful relationship exists between the MHC and DNA repair capacity.

## Cell Membranes, Mitochondria

Lymphocytes from old rodents show alterations in cell membrane composition and in the mobility and density of cell surface molecules. The density of "antigen B," Ia, and Fc receptors was decreased on the surface of spleen cells from old rats (Woda et al., 1979). Old cells also showed slower capping rates for three membrane proteins and decreases in membrane fluidity and lateral diffusion. Fewer splenic B cells from old than young rats showed a high density of surface immunoglobulin, and capping rates and shedding of cross-linked surface receptors were slower in old cells (Wonda and Feldman, 1979). Colchicine increased capping rates only in cells from young animals. Results with lymphocytes from old mice concur in that plasma membrane viscosity was about 20 percent higher than with cells from young mice, due possibly to an elevation in the cholesterol/phospholipid ratio of the membrane (Rivnay et al., 1979). Naeim and Walford (1980a) showed that the degree of capping and patching membrane proteins on human lymphocyte declines greatly with age and in Down's syndrome. Callard and co-workers (1979) presented evidence suggesting that new or altered determinants are expressed on the surfaces of old lymphocytes.

A possible site for intrinsic lesions in old lymphoid cells is the mitochondrion. There is evidence for decreases in numbers of liver mitochondria in aged mice (Herbener, 1976) and humans (Tauchi and Sato, 1968), along with alterations of respiratory activity in isolated mitochondria from old rat hearts (Hansford, 1978) and livers (Weinbach and Garbus, 1959). We have observed (Weindruch et al., 1980a) that isolated splenic mitochondria from old mice show a decrease in the respiratory control index (a measure of coupling of electron transport to oxidative phosphorylation) for succinate-supported respiration. By contrast, no influence of age on succinate respiration was observed in brain or liver mitochondria.

## IMMUNODEFICIENCY AND AUTOIMMUNITY IN AGING

### Immunodeficiency

Both humoral and cellular immunity decline markedly with age, the thymus-/dependent system manifesting by a considerable margin the greatest decline (Kay and Makinodan, 1976; Anderson et al., 1977; Hirokawa, 1977; Makinodan, 1977; Blankwater, 1978; Kay, 1979; Kay et al., 1979a; Yunis et al., 1979; Meredith and Walford, 1979; Gottesman and Walford, 1980; Weindruch and Walford, 1980). Many of the age-related changes can apparently be accelerated by chronic viral infection (Kay et al., 1979b), and old mice show a diminished response to infectious agents (Gardner and Remington, 1978a, 1978b). In what follows we shall mostly restrict our citation of papers to those appearing within the last four to six years.

The percentage of circulating T lymphocytes has been reported to decline somewhat with age in man (Carosella et al., 1974; Smith et al., 1974; Alexopoulos and Babitis, 1976; Reddy and Goh, 1979), and B lymphocytes to increase (Gajl-Peczalska et al., 1974), but numerous conflicting reports can be cited. Weksler and Hutteroth (1974) found no age-related change in absolute numbers of T lymphocytes, and Adler and Nagel (1980) found both percentages and absolute numbers of both T and B lymphocytes not to vary with age in man. Following the same persons over a ten-year period, Sparrow and co-workers (1980) found no age-related changes in absolute peripheral lymphocyte counts. Hallgren and colleagues (1978) observed an increase in T-cells in the ninth and tenth decades. Kishimoto and colleagues (1978) reported statistically significant but not numerically marked changes with age in the populations of T cell subsets: E-rosette forming cells were decreased and T$\gamma$ cells increased. Gupta and Good (1979) also noted an increase in T$\gamma$ cells with age, and a decrease in T$\mu$ cells. Carosella and co-workers (1974) noted a decrease in rosette-forming cells from 55 percent at 20–29 years of age down to 34 percent by 60–69 years, a trend also noted by Czlonkowska and Korlak (1979). Strelkauskas and colleagues (1980) reported a decrease in the juvenile rheumatoid arthritis (JRA+)-like T cell subset in old subjects having anti-T cell autoantibodies in their sera. Tyan (1977) found evidence for a decrease with age in T cell progenitors in the bone marrow of mice.

The alloantibody response of old mice of long-lived strains to injection of sheep or rat red blood cells (a thymus-dependent response) declines with advanced age to something like 5 to 10 percent of its peak value in youth (Makinodan et al. 1976; Finger et al., 1977; Segre and Segre, 1977; Butenko and Andrianova, 1979), although the secondary response is somewhat less affected (Finger and Emmerling, 1973). The response can be substantially restored in most mouse strains by in vitro or in vivo treatment with 2-mercaptoethanol (Makinodan and Albright, 1979). There is clearly an age-related decline in the number of immunocompetent units capable of making humoral isoantibodies (Heidrick and Makinodan, 1972), perhaps due to defective interaction between helper T and B cells (Goidl et al., 1976; Korgsrud and Perkins, 1977; Callard and Basten, 1978; Friedman and Globerson, 1978a, 1978b). There appear to be age-related qualitative defects in B cells (Goidl et al., 1976; Callard, 1977; Callard and Basten, 1978; Friedman and Globerson, 1978a, 1978b) as well as T cells. Responses to haptens such as DNP and TNP also decrease with age (Kishimoto et al., 1976; Segre and Segre, 1976; Friedman and Gloverson, 1978a). Measuring the haptenic responses to TNP-HRBC (thymus-dependent) and TNP-Ficoll (thymus-independent), Doria and co-workers (1980a, b) found that both declined markedly with age, and also that two types of helper cells in the T-T cell cooperation suffered a reduction in pool size and/or in ability to interact synergistically. The humoral response to the thymic-independent antigens SIII (Callard, 1977), DNP (Friedman and Globerson, 1978a, 1978b), and DAGG-Ficoll (Nordin and Buchholz, 1980) declines with age. Antibody avidity as measured against TNP or DNP determinants declines with age (Goidl et al., 1976; Doria et al., 1978). The low avidity of IgE anti-DNP antibodies in old mice may result from impaired T-helper activity (Fujiwara and Kishimoto, 1979). Evidence exists for a decrease in antigen-reactive cells in old mice, accompanied by an increase in antigen-binding cells (Popp, 1975). Significant changes have been noted with age in antigen handling in the liver, with altered parceling at both cellular and subcellular levels (Garvey et al., 1980).

Immunoglobulin levels reveal age-related changes in both mice and man, although the precise alterations are not agreed upon by the different investigators (Buckley et al., 1974; Riesen et al., 1976; Girard et al., 1977; Haaijman and Hijimans, 1978; Kishimoto et al., 1978; Matsuyama et al., 1978; Harris and Harris, 1979; Hallgren and Yunis, 1980). Antibody to the Forssman tissue antigen is present in 90 percent of normal persons less than 19 years of age and in only 61 percent of individuals 50 to 80 years of age (Levine, 1978).

The mixed lymphocyte reaction (MLR) decreases with age both in humans (Weksler and Hutteroth, 1974; Merhav and Gershon, 1977; Hallgren et al., 1978) and in long-lived mouse strains (Konen et al., 1973; Gerbase-DeLima et al., 1974; Callard, 1978; Gershon et al., 1979). The defect appears not to be due to adherent accessory cells such as macrophages (Callard, 1978). In the MLR, two T cell subpopulations, so-called $T_1$ and $T_2$ cells, may "synergize" to yield a reaction greater than the sum of the two subpopulations measured separately. This ability to "synergize" diminishes with age (Gerbase-DeLima et al., 1974). Studies with T cell subpopulations in the MLR and of mitogen stimulatory ratios (PHA/ConA) of cells from old as compared to young mice suggest that the $T_2$ subpopulation in particular shows an age-related decline in response capacity (Meredith et al., 1975a, 1975b). Natural killer (NK) activity has been reported to decline with age in mice (Herberman et al., 1975; Haller et al., 1977) but not in man (Adler and Nagel, 1980). Antibody-dependent T cell cytotoxicity (ADCC) has been reported to show peak maturity later than PHA responsiveness but to also decline with age (Haffer et al., 1979).

Cell-mediated lymphocytotoxicity (CML) has been less studied as an aging parameter than the MLR, but is known to decline (Goodman and Makinodan, 1975; Shigemoto et al., 1975; Hirano and Nordin, 1976; Bach, 1977, 1979; Becker et al., 1979). Aging may alter one of the T cell subsets playing a major role in the CML, possibly the Ly2,3 subset, or may induce a block in the last steps of T cell differentiation.

The proliferative response to T cell mitogens declines significantly with age in mice (Callard, 1977, 1978; Gershon et al., 1979), rats (Kruisbeek, 1976), and humans (Hallgren et al., 1978; Adler and Nagel, 1980; Hallgren and Yunis, 1980). Nevertheless, one study revealed an actual increase with age in numbers of mouse spleen cells which bind $^{125}$I-PHA (Callard, 1977) and another showed no age-related alteration in degree of binding to lymphoid cells of PHA or several other mitogens (Hung et al., 1975): hence the drop in response with age is probably not due to a decrease in receptor sites. The average decrease in response has been variously attributed to fewer cells entering the proliferative cycle, to an increased time duration of the cell cycle for older lymphocytes (Tice et al., 1979), and to age-induced structural alterations of the lymphocyte chromatin with blockage in the $G_1$ phase of the cell cycle (Preumont et al., 1978).

The proliferative response to B cell mitogens also clearly declines with age in mice (Abraham et al., 1977; Meredith and Walford, 1977; Callard, 1978), albeit considerably less than to T cell mitogens. Whereas there is no apparent decline with age in actual numbers of B cells, the percent which are reactive may decrease (Andersson et al., 1977).

Suppressor cells have received considerable recent attention in immunogerontologic studies, with reference not only to response to foreign antigens but particularly to autoimmunity and tolerance induction (Gershon and Metzler, 1977). A number of laboratories have reported an increase in suppressor cells with aging in long-lived strains of mice (Gerbase-DeLima et al., 1974; Segre and Segre, 1976, 1977; Goidl et al., 1976, 1980; Mitsuoka et al., 1979; Segre et al., 1980) as determined by suppression of the MLR, of antibody response to sheep red blood cells and to DNP-bovine gamma globulin, and of delayed hypersensitivity. It appears to be mainly a nonspecific suppressor cell population (i.e., which suppresses the response to a variety of T-dependent antigens) which increases with age (Roder et al., 1978c; Singhal et al., 1978; Callard et al., 1980), whereas antigen-specific suppressor cells remain in normal quantities (Callard et al., 1980). The increase in suppressor cells in long-lived strains contrasts to an age-related decline in suppressor T cell function reported for NZB (Barthoid et al., 1974; Talal and Steinberg, 1974; Radar et al., 1975) and possibly other strains of autoimmune-susceptible mice (Smith, 1976); however, cyclophosphamide-induced suppressor cells may in fact increase in NZB mice with age (Segre et al., 1980). Old bone marrow seems more susceptible to the action of suppressor cells than young marrow (Tyan, 1980). Compared to youthful controls, Con-A–activated lymphocytes from an aging human population display a variable loss in the ability to suppress the response to mitogens and to allogeneic cells (Hallgren and Yunis, 1977, 1980). This suppressor test seems to have considerable prognostic value for survival. Among 71–99-year-old humans, those who survived an additional two years had a mean Con-A activated suppressor activity of 20.6 percent and nonsurvivors of 0.1 percent (Hallgren and Yunis, 1980). In general, among subjects over 80 years of age, a significantly higher mortality rate over the next two years may be found for those with the most depressed immune function (Mackay, 1977), including immunodeficiency as indicated by immunoglobulin levels (Buckley et al., 1974). Among various immune parameters tested, decline in PHA response with age in Balb/c mice was a good indication for susceptibility to mastocytoma P815 (Perkins and Cacheiro, 1977).

Both peripheral B cells and possibly T cells—but reports here are somewhat conflicting (McIntosh and Segre, 1976; Weksler et al., 1980)—show increased resistance to tolerance induction with old age. Strain differences exist with age in susceptibility to tolerance induction which may not be related to suppressor-cell alterations (Habicht and Jerrard, 1980). Loss of tolerance susceptibility represents one of the earliest changes in age-related immunoresponsiveness, considerably antedating the appearance of spontaneous autoantibodies, and might be instrumental in the spontaneous autoimmunity seen with aging (Habicht and Jerrard, 1980; Weksler et al., 1980).

Factors extrinsic to stem cells may cause them to age, such as humoral or other regulatory and differentiation-inducing factors. The immune deficiency of age may be due in part to developing failure in the proliferative response capacity of individual lymphoid cells (Stoltzner and Makinodan, 1974; Makinodan and Adler, 1975; Kishimoto et al., 1976). Thus, a

Hayflick-type limit, possibly even an induced limit, may well exist not only for cultured fibroblasts but for cellular components of the immune system as well, especially those comprising the thymic axis (Burnet, 1974). The studies of Williamson and Askonas (1972) demonstrating in vivo senescent changes in an antibody-forming cell clone extend this possibility. In preliminary studies of T-lymphocyte cultures in the presence of T cell Growth Factor, we have observed typical phase III senescence phenomena, with the number of final doublings being inversely correlated with the age of the donor (Walford et al., 1980).

## Autoimmunity

As the normal immune response declines, autoimmune manifestations greatly increase (Talal, 1976; Meredith and Walford, 1979; Gottesman and Walford, 1980). Changes in susceptibility to tolerance (for self) may underlie at least some of these alterations (Habicht and Jerrard, 1980; Weksler et al., 1980). Autoimmune responses to receptor sites would presumably require a genetic predisposition to failure of tolerance, for example in myasthenia graevis and Graves' disease (Carnegie and Mackay, 1975). A striking age-related increase in the incidence of demonstrable autoantibodies to T cell subsets similar to those identified by sera from patients with juvenile rheumatoid arthritis has been reported (Strelkauskas et al., 1980). The regulation of autoantibody production due to cross-reactive antigen appears to be under different control than other age-related autoimmune phenomena (Goidl et al., 1980). There is a 3–4× age-related increase in demonstrable autoantibody-secreting B cells inducible by polyclonal activation (Weigle and Parks, 1978; Meredith et al., 1979). The situation appears to involve a type of deregulation rather than an absolute increase in number of anti-self reactive cells. A potentially fundamental change with aging would be a decreasing ability to distinguish self from non-self, with increased cross-reactivity against self even when confronted with allo- or xenoantigens (Naor et al., 1976). Conflicting evidence exists on the question of age-related reactivity to modified self, possibly depending on the assay system (Naor et al., 1976; Doherty, 1977; Gershon et al., 1980).

## Maintenance or Restoration of Immune Response Capacity in Old Animals

This subject has been reviewed elsewhere in some detail (Makinodan, 1979; Weindruch and Walford, 1980). Lowering internal body temperature (in poikilotherms) and caloric undernutrition initiated very early in life are both proven to extend life span. Only the latter technic has been much investigated immunologically. It does lead to the retention of a vigorous immune response in older animals (Gerbase-DeLima et al., 1975) and a significant decrease in the incidence of autoantibodies (Barnett et al., 1980b), with delay in thymic involution (Weindruch and Suffin, 1980). Carefully instituted and gradual but severe restriction beginning in adulthood in mice may lead to an immunologic rejuvenation and possibly some life span extension (Weindruch et al., 1979, 1980b). Caloric restriction generally leads to a marked decrease in tumor incidence and partial amelioration or postponement of the "diseases of aging" (Cheney et al., 1980).

Various hormonal and drug treatments have been reported to ameliorate senescent changes in the immune system (for review see Weindruch and Walford, 1980). These include thyroxine, various thymic extracts, levamisole, 2-mercaptoethanol, free radical inhibitors, synthetic polynucleotides, and coenzyme $Q_{10}$. Hypophysectomy of adult rats followed by appropriate pituitary hormone replacement led to "younger" responses in allograft rejection, in carbon clearance, and to injected SRBC (Scott et al., 1979).

Grafting both young bone marrow and thymus into late-middle-aged and old mice boosted the response to SRBC as well as PHA reactivity in the recipient animals (Hirokawa and Makinodan, 1975; Hirokawa et al., 1976; Blankwater, 1978). The younger the thymus, the better the results (Hirokawa and Sado, 1978). The age of the bone marrow seemed less critical. However, thymic regeneration in lethally irradiated mice grafted with bone marrow was significantly impaired if the marrow donor was age 117 weeks or older, indicating either a decrease in marrow T cell progenitors with age or a decline in their proliferative capacity (Tyan, 1976).

## DISEASES OF AGING, IMMUNE ASPECTS

### Accelerated Aging

*Animal (Mouse) Strains and Experimental Models.* The autoimmune-susceptible strains of mice (NZB, NZB/W, etc.) show features interpretable as accelerated aging. Reviewing the subject elsewhere in great detail, we came to the conclusion that such strains probably serve as accelerated aging models for a subgroup of the normally aging (Gottesman and Walford, 1980). The B10.F mouse, which is congenic to the C57BL/10 strain, has a life span of only about 18 months compared to two to three or more years for other strains congenic on the same background. It displays early graying of hair and depressed immune response, and may well be undergoing accelerated aging (Popp, 1978). Nude mice and hypopituitary dwarf mice show certain features of accelerated aging due to the relative absence of a thymic-dependent immune system. Haaijman and co-workers (1979) contend that as the nude mouse under proper care can live to at least two years of age, the age-related deterioration of the thymic limb of the immune system is not the cause but a consequence of aging.

The chronic graft-versus-host (GVH) reaction [reviewed in relation to aging by Walford (1974) and by Gottesman and Walford (1980)] appears to be the best experimental model of accelerated aging, showing lymphoid depletion and hypoplasia, fibrosis, eosinophilic deposits, an increased number of plasma cells in lymphoid organs, hyaline changes in renal glomeruli, renal atrophy, immune-complex formation, weight loss, arteriosclerosis, changes in skin and hair, thymic atrophy, amyloidosis, decreased responsiveness to isoantigenic stimuli, positive tests for autoantibodies, a decrease in the ratio of soluble to insoluble collagen, disturbances in T and B cell collaboration, and activation of latent viruses (Datta and Schwartz, 1976; Elie and Lapp, 1976; Grebe and Streilein, 1976; Pickel and Hoffmann, 1977; Shand, 1977). Induction of GVH by immunization across the main histocompatibility complex causes autoimmune hemolytic anemia and production of antinuclear antibodies by the host rather than by the injected parental cells (Gleichmann et al., 1976). Cells of old mice induce a GVH reaction when injected into either young or old syngeneic recipients, whereas cells of younger mice do neither (Gozes et al., 1978). It is interesting to note that the central nervous system is a previously unrecognized site of damage in the GVH reaction (Griffin et al., 1978).

*Human Diseases with Features of Accelerated Aging.* A number of human diseases or so-called "experiments of nature" show to variable degrees features of accelerated aging. Since none of these demonstrates all features, they can best be labeled "progeroid syndromes" (Martin, 1978). An incisive analysis of heredofamilial and genetic diseases which represent progeroid syndromes was made by Martin (1978). Most of these are rare, and little is known about them from the standpoint of immune functional capacity. Down's syndrome, diabetes mellitus, and several of the chromosomal instability syndromes show signs of accelerated aging and have been studied immunologically. To these we would add systemic lupus erythematosus, only recently realized to manifest hallmarks of accelerated aging. Pertinent aspects of these diseases will now be reviewed.

**1.** *Down's syndrome (DS).* Past studies of immune function of Down's syndrome (DS) have been somewhat contradictory, as reviewed elsewhere in depth (Barnett et al., 1980a). In part this is due to the emphasis in most studies on the use of institutionalized patients, many of whom have chronic hepatitis or other inflammatory illnesses, but probably largely due to inclusion of subjects younger than the age-related peak of immune response capacity as representing the "younger" population of the cohorts. This creates a maturation artifact in the data (Walford, 1976). Down's syndrome demonstrates a decrease in life span (Smith and Berg, 1976), pathologic changes characteristic of Alzheimer's disease in all subjects 40 years of age or older (Ellis et al., 1974), lesions in microtubules and neurons characteristic of Alzheimer's disease (Heston, 1976), early involutional changes in the thymus (even in newborns) and morphologic features of aging such as pulmonary and endocardial fibrosis, diffuse degenerative changes in endocrine glands (Ellis et al., 1974), increased amount of lipofuscin pigment, premature graying of hair (Emanuel et al., 1972), and decreased replicative capacity of fibroblasts in culture (Schneider and Epstein, 1972). A decreased repair capacity for UV-induced DNA lesions has been reported (Lambert et al., 1977) but not confirmed (Yotti et al., 1980).

Almost all investigators have documented the occurrence in DS of an age-related decrease in responsiveness to PHA sooner than in age-matched controls. Delayed skin reactivity is also markedly decreased (Burgio and Ugazio, 1978). Thyroid antibodies are significantly increased in frequency not only in DS subjects but in their mothers and siblings. Pathologic changes occur early in the thymus gland in DS, including severe lymphocyte depletion and greatly enlarged Hassell's corpuscles (Levin et al., 1979). We have noted striking alterations in lymphocyte cyclic nucleotide biochemistry in DS, including cAMP, cGMP, and adenylate and guanylate cyclases, corresponding to changes also shown to be characteristic of aging in mice or humans of advanced age (Barnett et al., 1980a; Tam and Walford, 1980). A decrease in mobility and in capping of con-A and SmIg receptors was also found, corresponding to changes seen in very old humans (Naeim and Walford, 1980a). The immune functional changes in Down's syndrome are thus quite characteristic of what one would expect for a progeroid syndrome.

**2.** *Diabetes mellitus.* Diabetes shows features interpretable as accelerated aging. There is an increased incidence of autoantibodies to gastric, thyroid, and nuclear antigens, and in young adults with insulin-dependent diabetes of over 20 years' duration an increase in thyrogastric autoimmune disease and vascular disease (Whittingham et al., 1971). In insulin-dependent diabetics less than 40 years of age, the incidence of autoantibodies equals that of a 60-year-old normal population, leading Whittingham and colleagues (1971) to the surmise that on the average insulin-dependent diabetics are physiologically 20 years older than their chronologic age. The cultured fibroblasts of diabetics exhibit only about half the number of population doublings as those from nondiabetics (Vrackro and Benditt, 1975). Alterations in HLA antigens have been found in cultured cells from diabetics as well as from patients with progeria and Werner's syndrome (Goldstein et al., 1975). The rate of digestion of collagen from diabetic patients by collagenase corresponds to that of a chronologically older population (Kohn and Hamlin, 1975). These comparisons lend support to the notion that diabetics show accelerated aging.

It should be emphasized that diabetes is a disorder of enormous genetic heterogeneity. However, there are no established abnormalities in the cellular immune response in well-controlled diabetics (Galbraith, 1979). Insulin-dependent diabetes (which is mostly juvenile diabetes) shows a complex association with the HLA system, there being a significant positive association with the two haplotypes A1-B8-DW3-DRW3 and A2-B15-CW3-DW4-DRW4 (Cudworth et al., 1979), and/or with the closely linked Bf locus (Raum et al., 1979). Two genes closely linked to or within HLA and operating by separate mechanisms may jointly produce pancreatic beta cell damage. Family studies have also provided evidence for associations between insulin-dependent diabetes and HLA (Rubenstein et al., 1976; Cudworth et al., 1979). There is no association between maturity-onset diabetes and specific alleles of the HLA system (Nelson and Pyke, 1975), although some evidence for linkage between HLA and maturity-onset type of hyperglycemia in the young has been suggested by segregation analysis in families (Barbosa et al., 1978).

**3.** *Systemic lupus erythematosus (SLE).* SLE has not been well recognized as showing features of accelerated aging, chiefly because until recently SLE patients did not survive long enough. With modern treatment, however, survival is greatly increased and many features of aging become manifest sooner than normally: loss of hair, skin changes, hypertension, osteoporosis, hypogonadism, diabetes mellitus or characteristic changes in the glucose tolerance curve, degenerative vascular disease including atherosclerosis, decreased pulmonary functions, increased susceptibility to one or more types of neoplasm, and dementia or related central nervous system pathology—these in addition to immunologic changes similar to those seen in (NZB × NZW)$F_1$ mice. As the situation has been reviewed elsewhere (Barnett et al., 1980b; Gottesman and Walford, 1980), we shall not here enumerate the multiple immune complexities of the disease. An increased frequency of death due to heart disease or stroke in SLE individuals surviving more than ten years is noteworthy. Evidence also exists that cells from SLE patients display a decrease in DNA repair capacity (Beighlie and Teplitz, 1975). SLE is one of the first autoimmune diseases documented as being associated with the HLA system (Grumet et al., 1971; Waters et al., 1971) and is strongly associated with HLA types DR3 and 4 (Gibofsky et al., 1978; Reinertsen et al., 1978). SLE afflicts about 500,000 persons in the United States, with up to 50,000 new cases each year (Marx, 1976). A recently defined category, subacute cutaneous lupus erythematosus, shows DR3 in an incidence of 77 percent versus 24 percent in a normal population (Stastny and Gilliam, 1979). The HLA type also influences the severity of the disease (Rigby et al., 1978). It is of course not surprising that SLE might represent a progeroid syndrome in humans since the analogous disease in (NZB × NZW)$F_1$ mice has long been regarded as a model of accelerated aging (see above).

**3.** *Chromosomal instability syndromes.* These are characterized by deficient DNA repair mechanisms and/or chromosomal aberrations of various types.

Werner's syndrome, or adult progeria, is a rare heredofamilial disease inherited as an autosomal recessive trait, with death usually by 40 to 50 years of age, with teenage graying of hair, cataracts, atherosclerosis at an early age in 25 percent of cases, diabetes mellitus in 50 percent, hypogonadism in 80 percent, the development of neoplasia in 10 percent, a decreased life span of fibroblasts in culture, and an increase in the percentage of heat-labile enzymes. Cases of Werner's syndrome have been shown to exhibit a striking decrease in the population of T cells giving high-intensity staining with anti-T cell antisera, corresponding to the situation of lymphocytes from normal subjects over 90 years of age (Goto et al., 1979). Nine of 11 Werner's syndrome patients revealed naturally occurring anti-T cell autoantibodies in their sera, compared to none in controls (Tada et al., 1978). (These antibodies may also be seen in SLE, rheumatoid disease, and juvenile arthritis.) Four patients revealed low titers of antinuclear antibodies, although non had anti-DNA antibodies or rheumatoid factor. Thus, Werner's demonstrates clear-cut immunologic abnormalities, with autoimmune features. There is no evidence for disequilibrium of the HLA system in Werner's syndrome, and in one large family with several affected siblings HLA-typed as part of the Eighth International Histocompatibility Workshop, the malady did not segregate with the HLA system (Hodge and Walford, 1980).

At least four other chromosomal instability syndromes show to variable degrees features of accelerated aging (Table 1–3). The status of the immune system has not yet been well-studied in these maladies. Some information is available on the immune status of xeroderma pigmentosum from reports of Berkel and Kiran (1974) and Dupuy and Laforret (1974). Delayed skin hypersensitivity and the responses of lymphocytes to PHA are both decreased. Ataxia telangiectasia has been fairly well studied immunologically because of its association with IgA deficiency [see Gatti and Walford (1980) for review]. These patients display impaired lymphocyte responses to mitogens and antigens, and their plasma inhibits the responses of normal lymphocytes. Cell mediated cytotoxicity appears depressed. T cells are decreased in numbers. There is an high incidence of malignancy, including leukemia, lymphomas, and cancers of the ovary,

Table 1–3
Signs of Accelerated Aging Found in Patients with Four Chromosomal Instability Syndromes[a]

| | *Ataxia telangiectasia* | *Xeroderma pigmentosum* | *Fanconi's anemia* | *Bloom's syndrome* |
|---|---|---|---|---|
| Increase suscept. to cancer | + | + | + | + |
| Chromosomal aberrations | + | + | + | + |
| Premature graying of hair | + | + | | |
| Dementia | | + | + | |
| Amyloid deposits | | + | | |
| Diabetes mellitus | + | | + | |
| Hypogonadism | + | | + | |
| Autoimmunity | + | | | |
| Degenerative vascular disease | + | + | + | |
| Cataracts | | + | | |
| Regional fibrosis | | + | | |
| Thymic atrophy | + | | | |
| Lymphoid depletion | + | + | + | |

[a]Blank spaces indicate either that the feature in question is not present or that the information not available. In addition, no reliable information is available on degree of lipofuscin deposits, susceptibility to slow viruses, possible osteoporosis, or incidence of hypertension in these conditions.

Source: Adapted from Satti and Walford (1980).

breast, and gallbladder. IgM monoclonal gammopathy may occur in some patients. The basic defect in the immunopathogenesis of ataxia telangiectasia appears to involve impaired thymic function. There is no apparent association with the HLA system (Hodge et al., 1980b). What limited immune information is available regarding Fanconi's anemia and Bloom's syndrome has been reviewed elsewhere (Gatti and Walford, 1980). Some evidence for immune dysfunction exists for Bloom's syndrome, very little for Fanconi's anemia. Except for Down's syndrome and ataxia telangiectasia, the diseases involving chromosomal instability have not been well studied immunologically but on the scant evidence available can be said probably to show distinct changes.

### Diseases of Late "Normal" Life

If the probability of onset of a disease increases rapidly with age, then the proportion of predisposed or susceptible members of a population who have not succumbed to it will decrease. When this proportion becomes small enough, the age-specific incidence with respect to the general population will fail to increase. Thereupon a peak in age-specific incidence followed by a fall will occur. A decline in incidence after, for example, a peak at age 60 to 70 does not necessarily mean that the malady in question cannot be regarded as a "disease of aging." We shall here review a number of the diseases of aging in which immune dysfunction of some type may play a role. Cancer is of course such a malady but for reasons of limited space will not be reviewed. Suffice it to say that in congenic mice the MHC, which regulates immune function, influences the incidence of different forms of spontaneous late-life-occurring malignancy (Smith and Walford, 1978).

1. *Vascular disease.* There is inconclusive but still considerable evidence favoring the involvement of immune mechanisms in the pathogenesis of arteriosclerosis. Arteriosclerosis can be induced experimentally by the synergistic action of immune complex disease and a lipid-rich diet, which produces allergic injury to arteries (Hardin et al., 1973; Poston and Davies, 1974). The development of rabbit arteriosclerosis can be inhibited by immunosuppressive drugs (Poston and Davies, 1974). Immune complexes may promote platelet thrombosis (Poston and Davies, 1974), and an elastase enzyme has been isolated from platelets (Robert and Robert, 1973). Anti-elastin antibodies have been demonstrated in human sera, and immunofluorescent studies have provided evidence for deposition of immunoglobulins at sites of elastin degradation in human atheromatous plaques (Robert and Robert, 1973). Arteriosclerotic lesions in rabbits can be produced by immunization with elastin plus structural glycoproteins of the aorta (Robert and Robert, 1973). Arteries in transplanted organs, such as kidneys, when subjected to chronic or intermittent rejection processes, are prone to develop arteriosclerotic lesions (Mathews et al., 1974; Finn et al., 1976). The Blaiberg case is a striking example in which a young heart subjected for about 18 months to intermittent rejection crises developed severe atherosclerosis leading to death from myocardial infarction. The primary lesion of endothelial damage in homograft rejection leads to an increase in permeability (Blumenthal and Alex, 1975). The work of Benditt and Benditt (1973) to the effect that intimal plaques may arise from a clone of mutated cells may be interpreted to mean that the "not-self" characteristics of these cells provoke an immune reaction leading to arteriosclerosis (Blumenthal and Alex, 1975). Additional evidence for the role of immune reactions in arteriosclerosis has been summarized cogently by Mathews and co-workers (1974): There is concomitant genetic susceptibility to vascular disease and autoimmunity in mice and men; there is an association of autoimmunity with smoking and vascular disease in man; vascular complications are more prevalent in diabetics with autoantibodies than in those without; coronary disease may be associated with autoimmune thyroiditis in the absence of overt hypothyroidism; autoantibodies are more common in obese men who smoke,

and in men with angina. Pandey and colleagues (1978) noted a significant correlation between HLA-B27 and ischemic heart disease, which might indicate either a predisposition or an increased resistance to death following myocardial infarction [those who are B27 (+) having greater chances of surviving an attack, and so to be included in the study]. Certain HLA alleles have been linked to familial hypercholesterolemia, suggesting a possible influence of the HLA system on lipid metabolism (Raffoux et al., 1978).

An association of HLA with other forms of vascular disease might suggest an immune etiology, although it should be added that not all HLA-linked diseases are immunologic in nature (hemochromatosis, for example). Two studies have reported disequilibrium between HLA and essential hypertension; however, different alleles were involved (Gelsthorpe et al., 1975; Low et al., 1975). Temperal arteritis was found to show 9 percent incidence among rest-home inmates—thus a considerably higher incidence than generally recognized (Nosenzo et al., 1967). The clinically manifested form has been reported to be associated with HLA-B14, present in 23 percent of patients as opposed to 9 percent of a normal population (Seignalet et al., 1977).

In various species of vertebrates not prone to develop arteriosclerosis, other forms of vascular disease may be encountered in relation to aging. For example, depending on the strain, up to 20 percent of old rats manifest periarteritis nodosa (Burek, 1978), a form of autoimmune or at least of immunologic disease.

**2.** *Renal disease.* Glomerular deposition of gammaglobulin was found in 38 of 44 aging $BC3F_1$ mice, accompanied by mesangial cell proliferation demonstrable by electron microscopy (Peter, 1973). In a study of strains SA, CBA, and C57Bl/6 mice from two to eight months of age, Linder and co-workers (1972) found evidence by eight months of progressive intercapillary glomerulosclerosis with granular deposits of immunoglobulin and complement along glomerular capillary walls. The renal disease was considered due to immune-complex formation, and the authors commented, "This study suggests that many of the immunopathological hallmarks of the NZB strain are not entirely specific for or distinctive of this strain and may be observed in other strains of mice." Bolton and colleagues (1976) reported the existence of spontaneous glomerulosclerosis associated with noncomplement-fixing mesangial deposits of rat IgM, and a close correlation between aging and glomerular pathology. The lesions were also found, albeit in lesser amounts, in germ-free rats. There was no evidence for a pathogenetic role of IgM deposits (i.e., the IgM did not have anti-rat antibody activity) and the deposition seemed simply secondary to increased basement membrane permeability with age.

**3.** *Rheumatoid arthritis.* More than five million Americans are afflicted with rheumatoid arthritis. The disease shows a greatly increased incidence beyond the age of 45, which keeps rising with age (Cathcart and O'Sullivan, 1970). Immunoglobulin complexes are found in the blood and joint fluids of 70 percent of patients. In these complexes each molecule serves as both antigen and antibody, resulting in a self-association system which continues to aggregate, to enlarge upon itself (Pope et al., 1974). Rheumatoid arthritis is strongly linked to the HLA system, with a greatly increased incidence of HLA-DR4 in the adult form, and D7 and D8 in the juvenile form (Stastny, 1978; Stastny and Fink, 1979).

**4.** *Benign monoclonal gammopathy (idiopathic paraproteinemia).* This malady is said to achieve an incidence approaching 19 percent by the tenth decade of human life, and a strain-dependent incidence of 10 to 70 percent by age 27–30 months in mice (Radl, 1979; Radl et al., 1979). In man the condition does not develop into a malignancy (such as myeloma), and in mice the paraprotein-producing cells die out after three to four in vivo transfers, in contrast to actual B cell malignancies. The disease may represent an age-related cellular defect in cells of reticuloendothelial origin, manifesting as excessive but benign B cell clonal proliferation.

**5.** *Amyloidosis.* Amyloidosis occurs in primary or idiopathic forms, in senile forms, following prolonged immunization, and in association with many diseases. Microscopically it is a hyaline-like eosinophilic material staining positively with congo red, certain fluorescent dyes such as thioflavine-T, and metachromatic dyes. It is a physicochemical, not just a chemical entity, and all forms of amyloid appear to consist of antiparallel beta pleated sheet fibrils (Glenner et al., 1973).

If one includes the senile form, amyloidosis is the commonest single disease of vertebrates. Atherosclerosis has a higher frequency in most human populations but is relatively rare in other vertebrate species (but common also in whales), whereas senile amyloidosis is a high-incidence phenomenon in all higher vertebrates. The incidence reported depends very much on the sensitivity of the staining techniques employed, just as the incidence of autoantibodies depends on the sensitivity of the immunologic techniques used in their detection. With sufficiently sensitive methods, up to 60 percent of humans over 70 years of age will show cerebral amyloid; 37 percent, cardiac amyloid; 50 percent, aortic amyloid; and 30 percent, pancreatic amyloid (Wright et al., 1969). By the eighth decade aortic amyloid reaches an incidence of 95 percent (Iwata et al., 1978). Females have a heightened incidence of senile cardiac amyloid: 56 percent compared with 38 percent in males over 60 years old (Hodkinson and Pomerance, 1977). There is an increase in age-related amyloid in many endocrine glands (Blumenthal, 1973).

Amyloidosis occurs in association with a hyperactive immune system and also with immunodeficiency diseases such as agammaglobulinemia and reveals a significant age-related increase in germ-free mice (Anderson et al., 1977). The etiopathogenesis may have to do with deregulation of the immune system. For example, germ-free mice lower their suppressor cell population sooner than normal mice (Anderson et al., 1977).

There are at least two distinct chemical forms of amyloid. Primary amyloid and that associated with myeloma or macroglobulinemia are structurally related to immunoglobulins, especially to a fragment of the variable region of the light chain (Glenner et al., 1971) [although most antisera to gammaglobulin do not react well with amyloid, perhaps due to the poor immunogenicity of the variable region (Franklin and Zucker-Franklin, 1972)]. When Bence-Jones protein is cleaved by proteolysis, the fragments from split delta light chains precipitate as typical amyloid fibrils as viewed in the electron microscope. The amyloid fibrils related to immunoglobulin types are most frequently associated with plasma cell dyscrasias or may represent primary amyloid, but sometimes associate with secondary amyloid (Glenner et al., 1973). Other cases of secondary amyloidosis contain a major component of material whose amino acid sequence is unrelated to immunoglobulins (Skinner et al., 1975), although immunoglobulins may also often be found in the amyloid in these cases (Glenner et al., 1973).

In view of the lack of particular disease associations, senile amyloidosis is generally thought of as primary amyloidosis with a strong age-related incidence, particularly as senile cerebral amyloid probably does consist in large part of the light chains of immunoglobulins (Ishii and Haga, 1976; Wisniewski and Terry, 1976). However, equating senile amyloid to an age-related primary form may be incorrect in some cases. The SAA or amyloid A-related serum component (non-immunoglobulin) has been reported to be increased with age as well as in a variety of chronic disorders (Rosenthal and Franklin, 1975), although this finding has not been confirmed (Hijmans and Sipe, 1979). Furthermore, age-associated immune diseases such as rheumatoid arthritis, the gammopathies, and certain forms of Hodgkin's disease are associated with increased incidences of amyloidosis, which could not therefore be regarded as primary (Burnet, 1976). Much of the "senile" amyloid in animals is in fact AA protein. The protein of senile cardiac amyloidosis is clearly different from that of protein AA of secondary amyloidosis and from a variety of other amyloid proteins (Westermark et al., 1977).

The etiology of senile amyloidosis remains unknown although it probably relates to immune deregulation. Recent studies in mice indicate that macrophage activation, which tends to occur with normal aging (see Gottesman and Walford, 1980), associated with T cell suppression and followed by B cell proliferation may be involved in both primary and secondary amyloidosis (Scheinberg and Cathcart, 1978). The substance amyloid in whatever form (light chains if immunoglobulin, or AA-type protein if not) is highly insoluble and tends to persist in the body. Some forms may be amenable to treatment with azothioprine and penicillamine (Bryde and Missmahl, 1975). The antioxidants santoquin, bis-hydroxytoluene, and alpha-tocopherol all decrease the degree of (secondary) amyloidosis following prolonged casein innoculation, which has led to the suggestion that amyloidosis might be secondary to increased oxidative degradation of tissue and serum components, the process becoming autocatalytic as the inhibitors of free radical reactions are depleted (Harman et al., 1976).

Clinical symptoms in amyloidosis are determined by amount and distribution of the otherwise inert filtrate. It is a major constituent of senile plaques (Wisniewski and Terry, 1976). Primary cerebral amyloid angiopathy may cause mental deterioration and vascular accidents in the elderly (Okazaki et al., 1979). Its main significance for the present inquiry resides in its testimonial to a considerable degree of immune deregulation with aging, and one showing a significant strain-specific genetic variation in susceptibility. Analysis of ease of induction of amyloid in CBA and A/J inbred strains of mice following casein injection indicates that resistance or susceptibility is greatly influenced by alleles at a single gene locus (Wohlgethan and Cathcart, 1979).

**6.** *Central nervous system pathology (excluding vascular).* Brain reactive antibodies (autoantibodies) increase in incidence with age in the serum of mice and may be responsible for neuronal degeneration in old mice (Nandy et al., 1975; Nandy, 1977). The age-related formation of neuron-reactive antibodies does not seem secondary to neuronal damage or neuronal death from non-immune causes, but from alterations in the immune system itself in old age (Ingram and Blumenthal, 1970). Gammaglobulin components have been found in the sera of about 80 percent of persons 55–70 years of age which bind with human neuronal cytoplasm (Ingram and Blumenthal, 1970; Ingram et al., 1974).

Alzheimer's disease is by far the commonest of the presenile and senile dementias. Both genetic and environmental influences may interact in its pathogenesis. Immunoglobulins are present in the amyloid fibrils of senile plaques (Ishii and Haga, 1976). The morbidity risk among siblings is over four times the risk in the general population. Two independent studies showed an increased frequency of HLA antigens B7 and Cw3 in Alzheimer's disease (Henschke et al., 1978; Cohen et al., 1979). At the recent Eighth International Histocompatibility Workshop this association was confirmed for both factors and a significantly increased frequency ($p < 10^{-5}$) of the B7Cw3 haplotype reported (Walford and Hodge, 1980). As the haplotype B7Cw3 is quite rare in the general population, its increase in Alzheimer's disease appears meaningful. Finally, an extensive multigenerational study of one family with familial Alzheimer's showed the B7Cw3 allele in most of the afflicted members. These findings constitute suggestive evidence for an immunologic component in the pathogenesis of Alzheimer's disease. However, in the single immunologic study of the disease reported thus far (Henschke et al., 1979), the responses of lymphocytes to PHA appeared normal, there was no excess of antinuclear or lymphocytotoxic antibodies, and no antineuronal antibodies were demonstrated.

*Abbreviations used in this review are:*

cAMP, cyclic adenosine 3′, 5-′monophosphate
cGMP, cyclic guanosine 3′, 5′-monophosphate
CML, cell mediated lymphocytotoxicity
Con-A, concanavalin-A
DNP, dinitrophenyl
DS, Down's syndrome
GVH, graft-versus-host
HLA, human leukocyte antigen
JRA, juvenile rheumatoid arthritis
MHC, main histocompatibility complex
MLR, mixed lymphocyte reaction
PHA, phytohemagglutinin
SIII, Salmonella type 3
SLE, systemic lupus erythematosus
SmIg, surface membrane immunoglobulins
TNP, trinitrophenyl
TNP-HRBC, the TNP haptenic group attached to horse red blood cells

## REFERENCES


Abraham, C., Tal, Y., and Gershon, H. Reduced in vitro response to concanavalin A and lipopolysaccharide in senescent mice: a function of reduced number of responding cells. *European Journal of Immunology,* 1977, *7,* 301–304.

Adams, D.D., and Knight, J.G. H gene theory of inherited autoimmune disease. *Lancet,* 1980, *i,* 396–398.

Adler, W.H., and Nagel, J.E. Studies of immune function in a human population. In D. Segre and L. Smith (Eds.), *Immunological Aspects of Aging.* New York: Marcel Dekker Publishing Co., 1980 (in press).

Alexopoulos, C., and Babitis, P. Age dependence of T lymphocytes. *Lancet,* 1976, *i,* 425–427.

Amos, D.B., and Kostyu, D.D. HLA—a central immunological agency of man. *Advances in Human Genetics,* 1980, *10,* 137–208.

Anderson, R.E., Doughty, W.E., and Troup, G.M. Immunological responsiveness and aging phenomena in germfree mice. In T. Makinodan and E. Yunis (Eds.), *Immunology and Aging*. New York: Plenum Press, 1977.

Anderson, J., Coutinho, A., and Melchers, F. Frequencies of mitogen-reactive B cells in the mouse. I. Distribution in different inbred strains of mice at different ages. *Journal of Experimental Medicine,* 1977, *145,* 1511–1520.

Bach, M.-A. Lymphocyte-mediated cytotoxicity: effects of aging, adult thymectomy and thymic factor. *Journal of Immunology,* 1977, *119,* 641–647.

Bach, M.-A. Influence of aging on T-cell subpopulations involved in the *in vitro* generation of allogeneic cytotoxicity. *Clinical Immunology and Immunopathology,* 1979, *13,* 220–230.

Barbosa, J., King, R., Goetz, F.C., Noreen, H., and Yunis, E.J. HLA in maturity-onset type of hyperglycemia in the young. *Archives of Internal Medicine,* 1978, *138,* 92–93.

Barnett, E.V., Chia, D., Fahey, J.L., Gatti, R.A., Gossett, T.C., Grossman, H., Medici, M.A., Mutola, M., Naeim, F., Sparkes, R.S., Spina, C., Tam, C.F., Tomura, T., Van Lancker, J., and Walford, R.L. Immunological and biochemical studies of Down's syndrome as a model for accelerated aging. In D. Segre and L. Smith (Eds.), *Immunological Aspects of Aging.* New York: Marcel Dekker Publishing Co., 1980a (in press).

Barnett, E.V., Chia, D., Knutson, D., Van Lancker, J., Cheney, K., Weindruch, R., and Walford, R.L. SLE, an accelerated form of aging. In D. Segre and L.Smith (Eds.),*Immunological Aspects of Aging.* New York: Marcel Dekker Publishing Co., 1980b (in press).

Barthoid, D.R., Kysela, S., and Steinberg, A.D. Decline in suppressor T cell function with age in female NZB mice. *Journal of Immunology,* 1974, *122,* 9–16.

Batchelor, J.R., and Morris, P.J. HLA and disease. In W.F. Bodner, J.R. Batchelor, J.G. Bodmer, H. Festenstein, and P.J. Morris (Eds.), *Histocompatibility Testing.* Copenhagen: Munksgaard, 1978.

Becker, B., Shin, D.H., Palmberg, P.F., and Waltman, S.R. HLA antigens and corticosteroid response. *Science,* 1976, *194,* 1427–1428.

Becker, M.J., Farkas, R., Schneider, M., Drucker, I., and Klajman, A. Cell-mediated cytotoxicity in humans: age related decline as measured by xenogeneic assay. *Clinical Immunology and Immunopathology,* 1979, *14,* 204–210.

Beighlie, D.J., and Teplitz, R.L. Repair of UV damaged DNA in systemic lupus erythematosus. *Journal of Rheumatology,* 1975, *2,* 149–160.

Benditt, E.P., and Benditt, J.M. Evidence for a monoclonal origin of human atherosclerotic plaques. *Proceedings of the National Academy of Sciences of the United States,* 1973, *70,* 1753–1759.

Berkel, A.I., and Kiran, O. Immunological studies in children with xeroderma pigmentosum. *Turkish Journal of Pediatrics,* 1974, *16,* 43–49.

Bevan, M.J. Interaction antigens detected by cytotoxic T-cells with the major histocompatibility complex as modifier. *Nature,* 1975, *256,* 419–421.

Blankwater, M. Ageing and the humoral immune response in mice. Ph.D. Thesis. Institute of Experimental Gerontology, Rijswijk, The Netherlands, 1978.

Blumenthal, H.T. Age-linked cell-mediated autoimmunity of endocrine glands. *The Gerontologist,* 1973, *13:*49.

Blumenthal, H.T., and Alex, M. Special issue on athero-arteriosclerosis. *Gerontologia,* 1975, *21,* 131–175.

Bolton, W.K., Ridgely Benton, F., Maclay, J.G., and Sturgill, B.C. Spontaneous glomerular sclerosis in aging Sprague-Dawley rats. *American Journal of Pathology,* 1976, *85,* 227–302.

Bomford, A., Eddleston, A.L.W., Kennedy, L.A., Batchelor, J.R., and Williams, R. Histocompatibility antigens as markers of abnormal iron metabolism in patients with idiopathic haemochromatosis and their relatives. *Lancet,* 1977, *i,* 327–329.

Bryde, M., and Missmahl, H.P. Therapie der generalisierten Amyloidosen. *Therapie Woche,* 1975, *25,* 1–8.

Buckley, C.E. Infection in the special host: the aged patient. In A. Nahias and R.J. O'Reilley (Eds.), *Immunology of Human Infection.* New York: Plenum Press, 1980 (in press).

Buckley, C.E. III, Buckley, E.G., and Dorsey, F.C. Longitudinal changes in serum immunoglobin levels in older humans. *Federation Proceedings,* 1974, *33,* 2036–2039.

Burek, J.D. *Pathology of Aging Rats.* Boca Raton, Fla: CRC Press, Inc, 1978.

Burgio, G.R., and Ugazio, A.G. Immunity in Down's syndrome. *European Journal of Pediatrics,* 1978, *127,* 293–294.

Burnet, F.M. Autoimmunity and aging. *Progress in Immunology,* 1974, *5,* 27–52.

Burnet, F.M. *Immunology, Aging and Cancer. Medical Aspects of Mutation and Selection.* San Francisco: W.H. Freeman and Co., 1976.

Butenko, G.M., and Andrianova, L.F. The effect of antigen priming on immunological response regulation in aging. *Experimental Gerontology,* 1979, *14,* 87–93.

Callard, R.E. Changes in mouse lymphocyte activity with age. *Interdisciplinary Topics in Gerontology,* 1977, *11,* 63–69.

Callard, R.E. Immune function in aged mice. III. Role of macrophages and effect of 2-mercaptoethanol in the response of spleen cells from old mice to phytohemagglutinin, lipopolysaccharide and allogeneic cells. *European Journal of Immunology,* 1978, *8,* 697–705.

Callard, R.E., and Basten, A. Immune function in aged mice. IV. Loss of T-cell and B-cell function in thymus-dependent antibody responses. *European Journal of Immunology,* 1978, *8,* 552–558.

Callard, R.E., Blanden, R.V., and Basten, A. Loss of immune competence with age may be due to a qualitative abnormality in lymphocyte membranes. *Nature,* 1979, *281,* 218–220.

Callard, R.E., Groth, B.F. de, St. Basten, A., and McKenzie, I.F.C. Immune function in aged mice. V. Role of suppressor cells. *Journal of Immunology,* 1980, *124,* 52–58.

Carnegie, P.R., and Mackay, I.R. Vulnerability of cell-surface receptors to autoimmune reactions. *Lancet,* 1975, *ii,* 684–687.

Carosella, E.D., Mochanko, K., and Braun, M. Rosette-forming T-cells in human peripheral blood at different ages. *Cellular Immunology,* 1974, *12,* 323–325.

Cathcart, E.S., and O'Sullivan, J.B. Rheumatoid arthritis in a New England town. *New England Journal of Medicine,* 1970, *282,* 421–424.

Cheney, K.E., Liu, R.K., Smith, G.S., Leung, R.E., Mickey, M.R., and Walford, R.L. Survival and disease patterns in C57BL/6J mice subjected to undernutrition. *Experimental Gerontology,* 1980, *15,* 237–258.

Cohen, D., Zeller, E., Eisdorfer, C., and Walford, R.L. Alzheimer's disease and the main histocompatibility complex. *The Gerontologist,* 1979, *19,* part 2, 57.

Converse, P.J., and Williams, D.R.R. Increased HLA-B heterozygosity with age. *Tissue Antigens,* 1978, *12,* 275–278.

Cudworth, A.G. The HLA system, autoimmune endocrinopathies and diabetes mellitus. *European Journal of Clinical Investigation,* 1978, *8,* 355–357.

Cudworth, A.G., Corsuch, A.N., Wolf, E., and Festenstein, H. A new look at HLA genetics with particular reference to type-l diabetes. *Lancet,* 1979, *ii,* 389–391.

Cutler, R.G. Evolution of human longevity and the genetic complexity governing aging rate. *Proceedings of the National Academy of Sciences of the United States,* 1975, *72,* 4664–4668.

Czlonkowska, A., and Korlak, J. The immune response during aging. *Journal of Gerontology,* 1979, *34,* 9–14.

Dausset, J., and Svejgaard, A. (Eds.). *HLA and Disease.* Copenhagen: Munksgaard, 1977.

Dausset, J., Gluckman, E., Lemarchand, F., Nunez-Roldan, A., Contu, L., and Hors, J. Excès d'HLA-A2 et d'homozygotes HLA-A2 parmi les malades atteints d'aplasie médullaire et maladie de Fanconi. *Nouvelle Revue Française d'Hématologie Blood Cells,* 1977, *18,* 315–324.

Datta, S.K., and Schwartz, R.S. Autoimmunization and graft versus host reactions. *Transplantation Reviews,* 1976, *31,* 44–78.

DeWolf, W.C., Lange, P.H., Einarson, M.E., and Yunis, E.J. HLA and testicular cancer. *Nature,* 1979, *277,* 216–217.

Doherty, P.C. Diminished T cell surveillance function in old mice infected with lymphocytic choriomeningitis virus. *Immunology,* 1977, *32,* 751–761.

Doria, G., D'Agostaro, G., and Garavini, M. Age-dependent changes of B-cell reactivity and T cell-T cell interaction in the *in vitro* antibody response. *Cellular Immunology,* 1980a, *53,* 195–206.

Doria, G., D'Agostaro, G., and Garavini, M. *In vitro* antibody response of spleen cells from aging mice. In D. Segre and L. Smith (Eds.), *Immunological Aspects of Aging.* New York: Marcel Dekker Publishing Co., 1980b (in press).

Doria, G., D'Agostaro, G., and Poretti, A. Age-dependent variations of antibody avidity. *Immunology,* 1978, *35,* 601–611.

Dupont, B., O'Neill, G.J., Yang, S.L., Pollack, M.S., and Levine, L.S. Genetic linkage of disease genes to HLA. In N.R. Rose, P.E. Bigazzi, and N.L. Warner (Eds.), *Genetic Control of Autoimmune Disease.* Amsterdam: Elsevier/North Holland, 1978.

Dupuy, J.M., and Laforret, D. A defect of cellular immunity in xeroderma pigmentosum. *Clinical Immunology and Immunopathology,* 1974, *3,* 52–60.

Elie, R., and Lapp, W.S. Apparent T cell function of bone marrow cells from mice experiencing a graft-versus-host reaction. *Cellular Immunology,* 1976, *21,* 185–191.

Ellis, W.G., McColloch, J.R., and Corley, C.L. Presenile dementia in Down's syndrome. Ultrastructural identity with Alzheimer's disease. *Neurology,* 1974, *24,* 101–106.

Emanuel, I., Sever, I.E., Milham, S., Jr., and Thuline, H.C. Accelerated ageing in young mothers of children with Down's syndrome. *Lancet,* 1972, *i,* 361–366.

Faraldo, M.J., Dux, A., Muhlbock, O., and Hart, G. Histocompatibility genes (the H-2 complex) and susceptibility to spontaneous lung tumors in mice. *Immunogenetics,* 1979, *9,* 383–404.

Finger, H., and Emmerling, P. Duration of immunologic memory in mice primed at different ages. *Gerontologia,* 1973, *19,* 23–30.

Finger, H., Heijmer, B., Emmerling, P., and Hof, H. Antibody-forming potential of lymph nodes in aged mice, with special reference to the influence of adjuvant. *Gerontologia,* 1977, *23,* 185–204.

Finn, R., Nichol. F.E., and Coates. P. Immunological factors in accelerated atheroma associated with renal disease. *Lancet,* 1976, ii, 1141–1142.

Franklin, E.C., and Zucker-Franklin, D. Current concepts of amyloid. *Advances in Immunology,* 1972, *15,* 249–304.

Friedman, D., and Globerson, A. Immune reactivity during aging. I. T-helper dependent and independent antibody responses to different antigens, *in vivo* and *in vitro. Mechanisms of Ageing and Development,* 1978a, *7,* 298.

Friedman, D., and Globerson, A. Immune reactivity during aging. II. Analysis of the cellular mechanisms involved in the deficient antibody response in old mice. *Mechanisms of Ageing and Development,* 1978b, *7,* 299–307.

Fujiwara, M., and Kishimoto, S. IgE antibody formation and aging. I. Age-related changes in IgE antibody formation and avidity for the DNP-determinant in mice. *Journal of Immunology,* 1979, *123,* 263–267.

Gajl-Peczalska, K.J., Hallgren, H., Kersey, J.H., Zusman, J., and Yunis, E.J. B lymphocytes during ageing. *Lancet,* 1974, *ii,* 163.

Galbraith, R.M. *Immunological Aspects of Diabetes Mellitus.* Boca Raton, Fla.: CRC Press, Inc., 1979.

Gardner, I.D., and Remington, J.S. Aging and the immune response. I. Antibody formation and chronic infection in toxoplasma gondii-infected mice. *Journal of Immunology,* 1978a, *120,* 939–943.

Gardner, I.D. and Remington, J.S. Aging and the immune response. II. Lymphocyte responsiveness and macrophage activation in toxoplasma gondii-infected mice. *Journal of Immunology,* 1978b, *120,* 944–949b.

Garvey, J.S., Shafer, J.W., and Caperna, T.C. Antigen handling in relation to ageing. *Mechanisms of Ageing and Development,* 1980, *12,* 287–303.

Gatti, R.A., and Walford, R.L. Immune function and features of aging in chromosomal instability syndromes. In D. Segre and L. Smith (Eds.), *Immunological Aspects of Aging.* New York: Marcel Dekker Publishing Co., 1980 (in press).

Gelsthorpe, K., Doughty, R.W., Bing, R.F., O'Malley, B.C., Smith, A.J. HLA antigens in essential hypertension. *Lancet,* 1975, *i,* 1039–1040.

Gerbase-DeLima, M., Meredith, P., and Walford, R.L. Age-related changes including synergy and suppression in the mixed lymphocyte reaction in long-lived mice. *Federation Proceedings,* 1975, *34,* 159–161.

Gershon, H., Merhav, S., and Abraham, C. T-cell division and aging. *Mechanisms of Ageing and Development,* 1979, *9,* 27–83.

Gershon, H.E., Lattime, E.C., and Stutman, O. Host age and H-2 tolerance in chimeric mice: mixed lymphocyte reactivity, cell mediated lympholysis and responses to hapten modified self. *Mechanisms of Ageing and Development,* 1980, *13,* 253–264.

Gershon, R., and Metzler, C. Suppressor cells in aging. In T. Makinodan and E. Yunis (Eds.), *Immunology and Aging.* New York: Plenum Press, 1977.

Gibofsky, A., Winchester, R.J., Patarroyo, M., Fotino, M., and Kunkel, H.G. Disease associations of the Ia-like human alloantigens. Contrasting patterns in rheumatoid arthritis and systemic lypus erythematosus. *Journal of Experimental Medicine,* 1978, *148,* 1728–1732.

Giraldo, G., Degos, L., Beth, E., Gharbi, R.M., Day, M.K., Dastot, H., Hanse,

M., Reboul, M., and Schmid, M. HLA antigens in 16 families with xeroderma pigmentosum. *Tissue Antigens*, 1977, *9*, 167–170.
Girard, J.P., Paychere, M., Cuevas, M., and Fernandes, B. Cell-mediated immunity in an ageing population. *Clinical Experiments in Immunology* 1977, *27*, 85–91.
Gleichmann, E., Gleichmann, H., and Wilke, W. Autoimmunization an lymphomagenesis in parent → $F_1$ combinations differing at the major histocompatibility complex: model for spontaneous disease caused by altered self-antigens? *Transplantation Reviews*, 1976, *31*, 156–224.
Glenner, C.G., Terry, W., Harada, M., Isersky, C., and Page, D. Amyloid fibril proteins: proof of homology with immunoglobulin light chains by sequence analysis. *Science*, 1971, *172*, 1150–1151.
Glenner, C.G., Terry, W.D., and Isersky, C. Amyloidosis: its nature and pathogenesis. *Seminars in Hematology*, 1973, *10*, 65–86.
Goidl, E.A., Innes, J.B., and Weksler, M.C. Immunological studies of aging. II. Loss of IgG and high avidity plaque-forming cells and increased suppressor cell activity in aging mice. *Journal of Experimental Medicine*, 1976, *144*, 1037–1048.
Goidl, E.A., Kim, K.T., and Weksler, M.E. Studies on auto-immunity in aging. In D. Segre and L. Smith (Eds.), *Immunological Aspects of Aging*. New York: Marcel Dekker Publishing Co., 1980 (in press).
Goldberg, N.D. Cyclic nucleotides and cell function. *Hospital Practice*, May 1974, pp. 127–142.
Goldstein, S., Niewiarowski, S., and Singal, D.P. Pathological implications of cell aging in vitro. *Federation Proceedings*, 1975, *34*, 56–63.
Goodfellow, P.N., Jones, E.G., Heyningen, V.V., Solomon, S., Bobrow, M., Miggianon, U., and Bodmer, W.F. The $\beta_2$m gene is on chromosome 15 and not in the HL-A region. *Nature*, 1975, *254*, 267–269.
Goodman, S.A., and Makinodan, T. Effect of age in cell-mediated immunity in long-lived mice. *Clinical and Experimental Immunology*, 1975, *19*, 533–542.
Goto, M., Horiuchi, Y., Okumura, K., Tada, T., Kawata, M., and Ohmori, K. Immunological abnormalities of aging: an analysis of T lymphocyte subpopulations of Werner's syndrome. *Journal of Clinical Investigation*, 1979, *64*, 695–699.
Gottesman, S.R.S., and Walford, R.L. Autoimmunity and aging. In R.C. Adelman and G.S. Roth (Eds.), *Methods in Aging Research, vol. 14: Testing the Theories of Aging*. Boca Raton, Fla.: CRC Press, Inc., 1980 (in press).
Gotze, D. (Ed.). *The Major Histocompatibility System in Man and Animals*. New York: Springer-Verlag, 1977.
Gozes, Y., Umiel, T., Meshorer, A., and Trainin, N. Syngeneic GvH in popliteal lymph nodes by spleen cells of old C57BL/6 mice. *Journal of Immunology*, 1978, *121*, 2199–2204.
Grebe, S.C., and Streilein, J.W. Graft-versus-host reactions: a review. *Advances in Immunology*, 1976, *22*, 120–221.
Greenberg, L.J., and Yunis, E.J. Histocompatibility determinants, immune responsiveness and aging in man. *Federation Proceedings*, 1978, *37*, 1258–1262.
Griffin, W.S.T., Head, J.R., Woodward, D.J., and Carrol, C. Graft-versus-host disease impairs cerebellar growth. *Nature*, 1978, *275*, 315–317.
Grumet, F.C., Conkel, A., Bodmer, J.G., Bodmer, W.F., and McDevitt, H.O. Histocompatibility (HLA) antigens associated with systemic lupus erythe-

matosus. A possible genetic predisposition to disease. *New England Journal of Medicine*, 1971, *285*, 193–196.

Gupta, S., and Good, R.A. Subpopulations of human T lymphocytes. X. Alterations in T, B third population cells and T cells with receptors for immunoglobulin M (Tμ) or G (Tγ) in aging humans. *Journal of Immunology*, 1979, *122*, 1214–1219.

Haaijman, J.J., and Hijmans, W. Influence of age on the immunological activity and capacity of the CBA mouse. *Mechanisms of Ageing and Development*, 1978, *7*, 375–398.

Haaijman, J.J., Slingerland-Teunissen, J., Benner, R., and Gudenaren, A.V. The distribution of cytoplasmic immunoglobulin containing cells over various lymphoid organs of congenitally athymic (nude) mice as a function of age. *Immunology*, 1979, *36*, 271–278.

Habicht, G.S., and Jerrard, D.A. Tolerance to HGG in mice of different age groups. In D. Segre and L. Smith (Eds.), *Immunological Aspects of Aging*. New York: Marcel Dekker Publishing Co., 1980 (in press).

Hadden, J.W. Cyclic nucleotides in lymphocyte proliferation and differentiation. In J.W. Hadden, R.G. Coffey, and F. Spreafico (Eds.), *Comprehensive Immunology, Vol. 3, Immunopharmacology*. New York: Plenum Medical Book, Co., 1977.

Haffer, K., Freeman, M.J., and Watson, R.R. Effects of age on cellular immune responses, in Balb/cJ mice: increase in antibody-dependent T lymphocyte mediated cytotoxicity. *Mechanisms of Ageing and Development*, 1979, *11*, 279–285.

Hallgren, H.M., and Yunis, E.J. Suppressor lymphocytes in young and aged humans. *Journal of Immunology*, 1977, *118*, 2004–2008.

Hallgren, H.M., and Yunis, E.J. Immune function, immune regulation, and survival in an aging human population. In D. Segre and L. Smith (Eds.), *Immunological Aspects of Aging*. New York: Marcel Dekker Publishing Co., 1980 (in press).

Hallgren, H.M., Kersey, J.H., Dubey, D.P., and Yunis, E.J. Lymphocyte subsets and integrated immune function in aged humans. *Clinical Immunology and Immunopathology*, 1978, *10*, 65–78.

Haller, O., Kiessling, R., Orn, A., and Wigzell, H. Generation of natural killer cells: an autonomous function of the bone marrow. *Journal of Experimental Medicine*, 1977, *145*, 1411–1416.

Hansen, H.E., Sparck, J.V., and Larsen, S.O. An examination of HLA frequencies in three age groups. *Tissue Antigens*, 1977, *10*, 49–55.

Hansford, R.G. Lipid oxidation by heart mitochondria from young adult and senescent rats. *Biochemical Journal*, 1978, *170*, 285–295.

Hardin, N.J., Minick, R., and Murphy, G.C. Experimental induction of atheroarteriosclerosis by the syngergy of allergic injury to arteries and lipid-rich diet. *American Journal of Pathology*, 1973, *73*, 301–321.

Harman, D. Free radical theory of aging: nutritional implications. *Age*, 1978, *1*, 143–150.

Harman, D., Eddy, D.E., and Noffsinger, J. Free radical theory of aging: inhibition of amyloidosis in mice by antioxidants; possible mechanism. *Journal of the American Geriatrics Society*, 1976, *24*, 203–210.

Harris, T.N., and Harris, S. Age-related difference by IgG subclass in the response of mice to allogeneic spleen cells. *Immunology*, 1979, *37*, 631–636.

Hart, R.W., and Hall, K.Y. Evaluation of longevity and DNA repair processes in mammals. In H. Orimo, K. Shimada, M. Iriki, and D. Maeda (Eds.), *Recent Advances in Gerontology*. Amsterdam: Excerpta Medica, 1979.

Hart, R.W., and Setlow, R.B. Correlation between deoxyribonucleic acid excision repair and lifespan in a number of mammalian species. *Proceedings of the National Academy of Sciences of the United States*, 1974, *71*, 2169–2173.

Herberman, R., Nunn, M., and Larvin, D. Natural cytotoxic reactivity of mouse lymphoid cells against syngeneic and allogeneic tumors. I. Distribution of reactivity and specificity. *International Journal of Cancer*, 1975, *16*, 216–224.

Heidrick, M.L., and Makinodan, T. Nature of cellular deficiencies in age-related decline of the immune system. *Gerontology*, 1972, *18*, 305–320.

Henschke, P.J., Bell, D.A., and Cape, R.D.T. Alzheimer's disease and HLA. *Tissue Antigens*, 1978, *12*, 132–139.

Henschke, P.J., Bell, D.A., and Cape, R.D.T. Immunologic indices in Alzheimer's dementia. *Journal of Clinical and Experimental Gerontology*, 1979, *1*, 23–38.

Herbener, G.H. A morphometric study of age-dependent changes in mitochondrial populations of mouse liver and heart. *Journal of Gerontology*, 1976, *31*, 8–12.

Heston, L. Alzheimer's disease, Trisomy 21, and myeloproliferative disorders. Associations suggesting a genetic diathesis. *Science*, 1976, *196*, 322–323.

Hijmans, W., and Sipe, J.D. Levels of the serum amyloid A protein (SAA) in normal persons of different age groups. *Clinical and Experimental Immunology*, 1979, *35*, 96–100.

Hirano, T., and Nordin, A.A. Age-associated decline in the *in vitro* development of cytotoxic lymphocytes in NZB mice. *Journal of Immunology*, 1976, *117*, 1093–1098.

Hirokawa, K. The thymus and aging. In T. Makinodan and E. Yunis (Eds.), *Immunology and Aging*. New York: Plenum Medical Book Co., 1977.

Hirokawa, K., and Makinodan, T. Thymic involution: effect of T-cell differentiation. *Journal of Immunology*, 1975, *114*, 1659–1664.

Hirokawa, K., and Sado, T. Early decline of thymic effect on T cell differentiation. *Mechanisms of Ageing and Development*, 1978, *7*, 89–96.

Hirokawa, K., Albright, J.W., and Makinodan, T. Restoration of impaired immune functions in aging animals. I. Effect of syngeneic thymus and bone marrow grafts. *Clinical Immunology and Immunopathology*, 1976, *5*, 371–376.

Hodge, S.E., Berkel, A.I., Boder, E., Gatti, R.A., and Spence, M.A. Ataxia-telangiectasia and xeroderma pigmentosum: no evidence of linkage to HLA. *Tissue Antigens*, 1980a, *15*, 313–317.

Hodge, S., Degos, L., and Walford, R.L. Joint report on four chromosomal instatibility syndromes; Bloom's syndrome, Fanconi's anemia, Werner's syndrome and xeroderma pigmentosum. In P.I. Terasaki (Ed.), *Histocompatibility Testing 1980*. Los Angeles: UCLA Tissue Typing Lab., University of California 1980ab (in press).

Hodge, S., and Walford, R.L. HLA distribution in aged normals. In P.I. Terasaki (Ed.), *Histocompatibility Testing 1980*. Los Angeles: UCLA Tissue Typing Lab., University of California, 1980 (in press).

Hodkinson, H.M., and Pomerance, A. The clinical significance of senile cardiac amyloidosis: a prospective clinico-pathological study. *Journal of Medicine*, 1977, *46*, 381–387.

Hung, C., Perkins, E.H., and Yang, W. Age-related refractoriness of PHA-induced lymphocyte transformation. II. $^{125}$I-PHA binding to spleen cells from young and old mice. *Mechanisms of Ageing and Development,* 1975, *4,* 103–112.

Ingram, C.R., and Blumenthal, H.T. Cerebral autoimmunity and aging. I. Frequency and significance of neuronal binding serum gamma globulin. *The Gerontologist,* 1970, *10,* 17.

Ingram, C.R., Phegan, K.J., and Blumenthal, H.T. Significance of an aging-linked neuron binding gamma globulin fraction of human sera. *Journal of Gerontology,* 1974, *29,* 20–27.

Ishii, T., and Haga, S. Immuno-electron microscopic localization of immunoglobulins in amyloid fibrils of senile plaques. *Acta Neuropathologica,* 1976, *36,* 243–249.

Ivanyi, P., Hampl, R., Starka, L., and Mickova, M. Levels of testosterone and of testosterone-binding protein are H-2 influenced. *Nature (New Biology),* 1972, *238,* 280–281.

Iwata, T., Kamei, T., Uchino, F., Mimaya, H., Yanagaki, T., Etch, H. Pathological study on amyloidosis—relationship of amyloid deposits in the aorta to aging. *Acta Pathologica Japonica,* 1978, *28,* 193–203.

Kay, M.M.B. An overview of immune aging. *Mechanisms of Ageing and Development,* 1979, *9,* 39–60.

Kay, M.M.B., and Makinodan, T. Immunobiology of aging: Evaluation of current status. *Clinical Immunology and Immunopathology,* 1976, *6,* 394–413.

Kay, M.M.B., Mendoza, J., Diven, J., Denton, T., Union, N., and Lajiness, M. Age-related changes in the immune system of mice of eight medium and long-lived strains and hybrids. I. Organ, cellular, and activity changes. *Mechanisms of Ageing and Development,* 1979a, *11,* 295–346.

Kay, M.M.B., Mendoza, J., Hausman, S., and Dorsey, B. Age-related changes in the immune system of mice of eight medium and long-strains and hybrids. II. Short and long-term effects of natural infection with parainfluenza type 1 virus (Sendai). *Mechanisms of Ageing and Development,* 1979b, *11,* 347–362.

Kishimoto, S., Takahama, T., and Mizumachi, H. *In vitro* immune response to the 2,4,6-trinitrophenyl determinant in aged C57BL/6J mice: changes in the humoral immune response to avidity for the TNP determinant and responsiveness to LPS effect with aging. *Journal of Immunology,* 1976, *116,* 294–300.

Kishimoto, S., Tomino, S., Inomata, K., Kotegawa, S., Saito, T., Kuroli, M., Mitsuyo, H., and Hisamitsu, S. Age related changes in the subsets and functions of human T lymphocytes. *Journal of Immunology,* 1978, *121,* 1773–1780.

Klein, J. H-2 mutations; their genetics and effect on immune functions. *Advances of Immunology,* 1978, *26,* 56–146.

Klimpel, G.R., Byus, C.V., Russell, D.H., and Lucas, D.O. Cyclic AMP-dependent protein kinase activation and the induction of ornithine decarboxylase during lymphocyte mitogenesis. *Journal of Immunology,* 1979, *123,* 817–824.

Knight, J.G., and Adams, D.D. Three genes for lupus nephritis in NZB × NZW mice. *Journal of Experimental Medicine,* 1978, *147,* 1653–1660.

Knight, J.G., Adams, D.D., and Purves, H.D. The genetic contribution of the NZB mouse to the renal disease of the NZB × NZW hybrid. *Clinical Experimental Immunology,* 1977, *28,* 352–357.

Kohn, R.R., and Hamlin, C.R. Aging of diabetic human collagen. *10th International Congress of Gerontology,* Jerusalem, 22 June 1975, p. 21.

Konen, T.G., Smith, G.S., and Walford, R.L. Decline in mixed lymphocyte reactivity of spleen cells from aged mice of a long-lived strain. *Journal of Immunology,* 1973, *110,* 1216–1221.

Kontermann, K., and Bayreuther, K. Cellular aging of rat fibroblasts in vitro is a differentiation process. *Gerontology,* 1979, *25,* 261–274.

Krogsrud, R.L., and Perkins, E.H. Age-related changes in T cell function. *Journal of Immunology,* 1977, *118,* 1607–1611.

Kruisbeek, A.M. Age-related changes in Con A and LPS-induced lymphocyte transformation. I. Effect of culture conditions on mitogen responses of blood and spleen lymphocytes from young and aged rats. *Mechanisms of Ageing and Development,* 1976, *5,* 125–138.

Lambert, B., Ringborg, N., and Swanbeck, G. Repair on UV-induced DNA lesions in peripheral lymphocytes from healthy subjects of various ages, individuals with Down's syndrome and patients with actinic keratosis. *Mutation Research,* 1977, *46,* 133–134.

Levin, S., Schlesinger, M., Handzel, Z., Hahn, T., Altman, Y., Czernobilsky, R., and Boss, J. Thymic deficiency in Down's syndrome. *Pediatrics,* 1979, *63,* 80–87.

Levine, P. Self-nonself concept for cancer and diseases previously known as "autoimmune" diseases. *Proceedings of the National Academy of Sciences of the United States,* 1978, *75,* 5697–5701.

Levy, R.B., and Shearer, G.M. Regulation of T-cell mediated lympholysis by the murine major histocompatibility complex. II. Control of cytotoxic responses to trinitrophenyl-k and -D self products by H-2K and H-2D region differences. *Journal of Experimental Medicine,* 1980, *151,* 252–256.

Linder, E., Pasternack, A., and Edgington, T.S. Pathology and immunology of age-associated disease of mice and evidence for an autologous immune complex pathogenesis of the associated renal disease. *Clinical Immunology and Immunopathology,* 1972, *1,* 140–154.

Low, B., Schersten, B., Sartor, G., Thulin, T., and Mitelman, F. HL-A8 and W15 in diabetes mellitus and essential hypertension. *Lancet,* 1975, *i,* 695.

Mackay, I.R. Changes in human lymphocyte activity with age. *Interdisciplinary Topics in Gerontology,* 1977, *11,* 75–80.

Mackay, I.R., Whittingham, S., and Tait, B. Genetic control of immune responsiveness in man. *Vox Sanguinis,* 1977, *32,* 10–19.

Macurova, H., Ivanyi, P., Sajdlova, H., and Trojan, J. HLA antigens in aged persons. *Tissue Antigens,* 1975, *6,* 269–271.

Makinodan, T. Immunity and aging. In C.E. Finch and L. Hayflick (Eds.), *Handbook of the Biology of Aging.* New York: Van Nostrand Reinhold Co., 1977.

Makinodan, T. Control of immunologic abnormalities associated with aging. *Mechanisms of Ageing and Development,* 1979, *9,* 7–17.

Makinodan, T., and Adler, W.H. Effects of aging on the differentiation and proliferation potentials of cells of the immune system. *Federation Proceedings,* 1975, *34,* 153–158.

Makinodan, T., Albright, J.W., Good, P.I., Peter, C.P., and Heidrick, M.L. Reduced humoral immune activity in long-lived old mice: an approach to elucidating its mechanisms. *Immunology,* 1976, *31,* 903–912.

Makinodan, T., and Albright, J.W. Restoration of impaired immune functions in aging animals. III. Effect of mercaptoethanol in enhancing the reduced primary antibody responsiveness *in vivo. Mechanisms of Ageing and Development,* 1979, *11,* 1–8.

Marchalonis, J.J., and Warr, G.W. Phylogenetic origins of immune recognition: naturally occurring DNP-binding molecules in chordate sera and hemolymph. *Developmental and Comparative Immunology,* 1978, *2,* 443–460.

Martin, G.M. Genetic syndromes in man with potential relevance to the pathobiology of aging. In D. Bergsma and D.E. Harrison (Eds.), *Genetic Effects on Aging.* New York: Alan R. Liss Inc., 1978.

Marx, J.L. Autoimmune disease: new evidence about lupus. *Science,* 1976, *192,* 1089–1091.

Mathews, J.D., Whittingham, S., and Mackay, I.R. Autoimmune mechanisms in human vascular disease. *Lancet,* 1974, *ii,* 1423–1426.

Mathews, J.D., Whittingham, S., Hooper, B.M., and Mackay, I.R. Association of autoantibodies with smoking, cardiovascular morbidity, and death in the Busselton population. *Lancet,* 1978, *ii,* 754–758.

Matsura, M., Shimada, H., and Namba, K. Deficient scheduled and unscheduled DNA synthesis in the cultured fibroblasts derived from patients with rheumatoid arthritis (RA). XIth International Congress of Gerontology, August 20–25, 1978, Tokyo, *Abstract,* p. 39.

Matsuyama, S.S., Cohen D., and Jarvik, L.F. Hypodiploidy and serum immunoglobulin concentration in the elderly. *Mechanisms of Ageing and Development,* 1978, *8,* 407–412.

McDevitt, H.O., and Tyan, M.L. Genetic control of the antibody response in inbred mice. Transfer of response by spleen cells and linkage to the major histocompatibility (H-2) locus. *Journal of Experimental Medicine,* 1968, *128,* 1–11.

McIntosh, K.R., and Segre, D. B- and T-cell tolerance induction in young adult and old mice. *Cellular Immunology,* 1976, *27,* 230–239.

Meredith, P., and Walford, R.L. Effect of age on response to T and B cell mitogens in mice congenic at the H-2 region. *Immunogenetics,* 1977, *5,* 109–128.

Meredith, P., and Walford, R.L. Autoimmunity, histocompatibility and aging. *Mechanisms of Ageing and Development,* 1979, *9,* 61–77.

Meredith, P., Gerbase-DeLima, M., and Walford, P.L. Age-related changes in the PHA:Con A stimulatory ratios of cells from spleens of a long-lived mouse strain. *Experimental Gerontology,* 1975a, *10,* 247–250.

Meredith, P., Tittor, W., Gerbase-DeLima, M., and Walford, R.L. Age-related changes in the cellular immune response of lymph node and thymus cells in long-lived mice. *Cellular Immunology,* 1975b, *18,* 324–330.

Meredith, P.J., Kristie, J.A., and Walford, R.L. Aging increases expression of LPS-induced autoantibody-secreting B cells. *Journal of Immunology,* 1979, *123,* 87–91.

Merhav, S., and Gershon, H. The mixed lymphocyte response of senescent mice: sensitivity to alloantigen and cell replication time. *Cellular Immunology,* 1977, *34,* 354–366.

Meruelo, D., and Edidin, M. Association of mouse liver adenosine 3', 5'-cyclic monophosphate (cAMP) levels with histocompatibility-2 genotypes. *Proceedings of the National Academy of Sciences of the United States,* 1975, *72,* 2644–2648.

Mitsuoka, A., Morkawa, S., Baba, M., and Harada, T. Cyclophosphamide eliminates suppressor T cells in age-associated central regulation of delayed hypersensitivity in mice. *Journal of Experimental Medicine,* 1979, *149,* 1018–1028.

Mittal, C.K., and Murad, F. Properties and oxidative regulation of guanylate cyclase. *Journal of Cyclic Nucleotide Research,* 1977, *3,* 381–391.

Miyachi, K., Fritzler, M.J., and Tan, E.M. Autoantibody to a nuclear antigen in proliferating cells. *Journal of Immunology,* 1978, *121,* 2228–2234.

Morley, A., Seshadri, R., Trainor, K., and Sorrell, J. Is aplastic anemia due to abnormality of DNA? *Lancet,* 1978, *ii,* 9–11.

Naeim, F., and Walford, R.L. Disturbance of redistribution of surface membrane receptors on peripheral mononuclear cells of patients with Down's syndrome and of aged individuals. *Journal of Gerontology,* 1980a, *35,* 650–655.

Naeim, F., and Walford, R.L. Human Ia-like alloantigens and their medical significances. In R.A. Reisfeld and S. Ferrone (Eds.), *Current Trends in Histocompatibility.* New York: Plenum Press, 1980b (in press).

Naeim, F., Keesey, J.C., Herrmann, C. Jr., Lindstrom, J., Zeller, E., and Walford, R.L. Association of HLA-B8, DRw3, and anti-acetycholine receptor antibodies in myasthenia gravis. *Tissue Antigens,* 1978, *12,* 381–386.

Nandy, K. Immune reactions in aging brain and senile dementia. In K. Nandy and I. Sherwin (Eds.), *The Aging Brain and Senile Dementia.* New York: Plenum Press, 1977.

Nandy, K., Fritz, R.B., and Threatt, J. Specificity of brain-reactive antibodies in serum of old mice. *Journal of Gerontology,* 1975, *30,* 269–274.

Naor, D., Bonavida, B., and Walford, R.L. Autoimmunity and aging: the age-related response of mice of a long-lived strain to trinitrophenylated syngeneic mouse red blood cells. *Journal of Immunology,* 1976, *117,* 2204–2208.

Nebert, D. Relation of H-2 to mixed function oxidase system. *Molecular Cellular Biochemistry,* 1979, *27,* 27–46.

Nelson, P.G., and Pyke, D.A. Histocompatibility antigens in diabetic identical twins. *Lancet,* 1975, *ii,* 193–194.

Nordin, A.A., and Buchholz, M. The effect of age on the *in vitro* immune response of C57BL/6 mice to a T-independent antigen. In D. Segre and L. Smith (Eds.), *Immunological Aspects of Aging.* New York: Marcel Dekker Publishing Co., 1980 (in press).

Nosenzo, C., Dughera, L., Macchioni, P. L'incidenza dell arterite temperale nelle persone anziane: studio clinicao su 100 ricoverati in gerontocomio. *Acta Gerontologica,* 1967, *17,* 238–245.

Novak, R., Bosze, Z., Matkovics, B., and Fachet, J. Gene affecting superoxide dismutase activity linked to the histocompatibility complex in H-2 congenic mice. *Science,* 1980, *207,* 86–87.

Okazaki, H., Reagan, R.J., Campbell, R.J. Clinicopathologic studies of primary cerebral amyloid angiopathy. *Mayo Clinic Proceedings,* 1979, *54,* 22–31.

Paffenholz, U. Co-relation between DNA repair of embryonic fibroblasts and different lifespan of 3 inbred mouse strains. *Mechanisms of Ageing and Development,* 1978, *7,* 131–150.

Pandey, J.P., Fudenberg, H.H., Root, B., and Loadholt, C.B. Association of HLA antigens, ischaemic heart disease, and serum calcium levels: a preliminary report. *Age,* 1978, *1,* 21–23.

Parham, P., Alpert, B.N., Orr, H.T., and Strominger, J.L. The carbohydrate moiety of HLA antigens: antigenic properties and amino acid sequences around the site of glycosylation. *Journal of Biological Chemistry,* 1977, *252,* 7555–7567.

Parker, C.W. cAMP and lectin-induced mitogenesis in lymphocytes—possible implications for neoplastic cell growth. *Advances in Cyclic Nucleotide Research,* 1979, *9,* 647–660.

Perkins, E.H., and Cacheiro, L.H. A multiple-parameter comparison of immunocompetence and tumor resistance in aged Balb/c mice. *Mechanisms of Ageing and Development,* 1977, *6,* 15–24.

Peter, C.P. Possible immune origin of age-related pathological changes in long-lived mice. *Journal of Gerontology,* 1973, *28,* 265–275.

Pickel, K., and Hoffmann, M.K. Suppressor T cells arising in mice undergoing a graft-vs-host response. *Journal of Immunology,* 1977, *118,* 653–656.

Pope, R.M., Teller, D.C., and Mannik, M. The molecular basis of self association of antibodies to IgT (rheumatoid factors) in rheumatoid arthritis. *Proceedings of the National Academy of Sciences of the United States,* 1974, *71,* 521–571.

Popp, D.M. The effect of age on antigen-sensitive cells. *Mechanisms of Ageing and Development,* 1975, *4,* 221–230.

Popp, D.M. Use of congeneic mice to study the genetic basis of degenerative disease. In D. Bergsma and D.E. Harrison (Eds.), *Genetic Effects on Aging.* New York: Alan R. Liss, Inc., 1978.

Portugal, F.H. Histocompatibility antigens and cytoskeletal elements. *Nature,* 1979, *279,* 102–103.

Poston, R.N., and Davies, D.F. Immunity and inflammation in pathogenesis of atherosclerosis. *Atherosclerosis,* 1974, *19,* 353–367.

Preumont, A.M., Gansen, P.V., and Brachet, J. Cytochemical study of human lymphocytes stimulated by PHA in function of donor age. *Mechanisms of Ageing and Development,* 1978, *7,* 25–32.

Radar, J.C., Bell, D.A., and Singhal, S.K. T cell activation and cellular cooperation in autoimmune NZB/NZW $F_1$ hybrid mice. *Journal of Immunology,* 1975, *115,* 466–472.

Radl, J. Idiopathic paraproteinemia—a consequence of an age-related deficiency in the T immune system. Three-stage development—a hypothesis. *Clinical Immunology and Immunopathology,* 1979, *12,* 251–255.

Radl, J., Glopper, E.D., Schuit, H.R.E., and Zurcker, C. Idiopathic paraproteinemia. II. Transplantation of the paraprotein-producing clone from old to young C57BL/KaLwRig mice. *Journal of Immunology,* 1979, *122,* 609–613.

Raffoux, C., Pointel, J.P., Drouin, P., Streiff, F., Debry, G., and Sauvanet, J.P. Type IIa hyperlipoproteinemia and the HLA system. *Tissue Antigens,* 1978, *11,* 55–58.

Raum, D., Stein, R., Alper, C.A., and Gabbay, K.H. Genetic marker for insulin-dependent diabetes mellitus. *Lancet,* 1979, *ii,* 1208–1210.

Reddy, M.M., and Goh, K. B and T lymphocytes in man. IV. Circulating B, T and "null" lymphocytes in aging population. *Journal of Gerontology,* 1979, *34,* 5–8.

Reinersten, J.L., Klippel, J.H., Johnson, A.A., Steinberg, A.D., Decker, J.L., and Mann, D.L. B-lymphocytes alloantigens associated with systemic lupus erythematosus. *New England Journal of Medicine,* 1978, *299,* 515–517.

Richardson, J.S., Richardson, D.C., and Thomas, K.A. Similarity of three-dimensional structure between the immunoglobulin domain and the copper, zinc superoxide dismutase subunit. *Journal of Molecular Biology,* 1977, *102,* 221–235.

Riesen, W., Keller, H., Skvaril, F., Morell, A., and Barandun, S. Restriction of immunoglobulin heterogeneity, autoimmunity and serum protein levels in aged people. *Clinical Experiments in Immunology,* 1976, *26,* 280–285.

Rigby, R.J., Dawkins, R.L., Wetherall, J.D., and Hawkins, B.R. HLA in systemic lupus erythematosus: influence on severity. *Tissue Antigens,* 1978, *12,* 25–31.

Rivnay, B., Globerson, A., and Shinitzky, M. Viscosity of lymphocyte plasma membrane in aging mice and its possible relation to serum cholesterol. *Mechanisms of Ageing and Development,* 1979, *10,* 71–79.

Robb, R.J., Terhorst, C., and Strominger, J.L. Sequence of the COOH-terminal hydrophilic region of histocompatibility antigens HLA-A2 and HLA-B7. *Journal of Biological Chemistry,* 1978, *253,* 5319–5324.

Robert, L., and Robert, B. Immunology and aging. *Gerontologia,* 1973, *19,* 330–350.

Roder, J.C., Bell, D.A., and Singhal, S.K. Loss of self-tolerance to single-stranded deoxyribonucleic acid (sDNA) *in vitro. Journal of Immunology,* 1978a, *121,* 29–37.

Roder, J.C., Bell, D.A., and Singhal, S.K. Regulation of the autoimmune plaque-forming cell response to single-strand DNA (sDNA) *in vitro. Journal of Immunology,* 1978b, *121,* 38–43.

Roder, J.C., Duwe, A.K., Bell, D.A., and Singhal, S.K. Immunological senescence. I. The role of suppressor cells. *Immunology,* 1978c, *35,* 837–842.

Rose, N.R., Bigazzi, P.E., and Warner, N.L. (Eds.). *Genetic Control of Autoimmune Disease.* Amsterdam: Elsevier/North Holland, 1978.

Rosenthal, C.J., and Franklin, E.C. Variation with age and disease of amyloid A protein-related serum component. *Journal of Clinical Investigation,* 1975, *55,* 746–755.

Rubenstein, P., Suciu-Foca, N., Nicholson, J.F., Fotino, M., Molinaro, A., Harisiadis, L., Hardy, M.A., Reemtsma, K., and Allen, F.H. Jr. The HLA system in the families of patients with juvenile diabetes mellitus. *Journal of Experimental Medicine,* 1976, *143,* 1277–1282.

Sacher, G.A. Maturation and longevity in relation to cranial capacity in hominid evolution. In E. Tuttle (Ed.), *Antecedents of Man and After. Primates: Functional Morphology and Evolution,* vol. 1. The Hague: Mouton, 1975.

Scheinberg, M.A., Cathcart, E.S. New concepts in the pathogenesis of primary and secondary amyloid disease. *Clinical Experimental Immunology,* 1978, *33,* 185–190.

Schneider, E.L., and Epstein, C.J. Replication rate and lifespan of cultured fibroblasts in Down's syndrome. *Proceedings of the Society for Experimental Biology and Medicine,* 1972, *141,* 1092–1094.

Scholar, E.M., Rashidian, M., and Heidrick, M.L. Adenosine deaminase and purine nucleoside phosphorylase activity in spleen cells of aged mice. *Mechanisms of Ageing and Development,* 1980, *12,* 323–329.

Schwartz, A.G. Correlation between species lifespan and capacity to activate 7,12-dimethylbenz-d-anthracane to a form mutagenic to a mammalian cell. *Experimental Cell Research,* 1975, *44,* 445–457.

Scott, M., Bolla, R., and Denckla, W.D. Age-related changes in immune function of rats and the effect of long-term hypophysectomy. *Mechanisms of Ageing and Development,* 1979, *11,* 127–136.

Segre, D., and Segre, M. Humoral immunity in aged mice. II. Increase suppressor T cell activity in immunologically deficient old mice. *Journal of Immunology,* 1976, *116,* 735, 746.

Segre, D., and Segre, M. Age-related changes in B and T lymphocytes and decline of humoral immune responsiveness in aged mice. *Mechanisms of Ageing and Development,* 1977, *6,* 115–130.

Segre, D., Greeley, E.H., and Segre, M. Cyclophosphamide induction of non-T suppressor cells and their possible role in self-tolerance. In D. Segre and L. Smith (Eds.), *Immunological Aspects of Aging.* New York: Marcel Dekker Publishing Co., 1980 (in press).

Seignalet, J., Janbon, C., Sany, J., Janbon, F., Bidet, J.-M., Brunel, M., Jourdan, J., and Bussiere, J.-L. HLA in temporal arteritis. *Tissue Antigens,* 1977, *9,* 69–70.

Seshadri, R.S., Morley, A.A., Trainor, K.J., and Sorrell, J. Sensitivity of human lymphocytes to bleomycin increases with age. *Experientia,* 1979, *35,* 233–234.

Shand, F.L. Characterization of the suppressor cell generated in a murine graft-versus-host reaction (GVHR). *Transplantation Proceedings,* 1977, *9,* 277–279.

Shigemoto, S., Kishimoto, S., and Hamamura, Y. Change of cell-mediated cytotoxicity with age. *Journal of Immunology,* 1975, *115,* 307–309.

Simon, M.J., Wee, G.B., Day, N.E., Morris, P.J., Shanmugaratnam, K., and de-The, G. Immunogenetic aspects of nasopharyngeal carcinoma. I. Differences in HL-A antigen profiles between patients and comparison groups. *International Journal of Cancer,* 1974, *13,* 122–134.

Singhal, S.K., Roder, J.C., and Duwe, A.K. Suppressor cells in immunosenescence. *Federation Proceedings,* 1978, *37,* 1245–1252.

Skinner, M., Benson, M.D., and Cohen, A.S. Amyloid fibril protein related to immunoglobulin λ-chains. *Journal of Immunology,* 1975, *114,* 1433–1435.

Smith, A.M. The effects of age on the immune response to type III pneumosaccharide (SIII) and bacterial lipopolysaccharide (LPS) in Balb/c, SJL/J and C3H mice. *Journal of Immunology,* 1976, *116,* 469–474.

Smith, A.M., Evans, J., and Steel, C.M. Age-related variation in proportion of circulating T cells. *Lancet,* 1974, *ii,* 922–924.

Smith, G.F., and Berg, J.M. *Down's Anomaly.* Edinburgh: Churchill Livingstone, 1976.

Smith, G.S., and Walford, R.L. Influence of the main histocompatibility complex on aging in mice. *Nature,* 1977, *270,* 727–729.

Smith, G.S., and Walford, R.L. Influence of the H-2 and H-2 histocompatibility systems upon lifespan and spontaneous cancer incidence in congenic mice. In D. Bergsma and D.E. Harrison (Eds.), *Genetic Effects on Aging.* New York: Alan R. Liss, Inc., 1978.

Smith, M., Turner, B.M., Tanigaki, N., and Hirschhorn, K. Regional localization of HLA, Mes, and SODm on chromosome 6. *Cytogenetics and Cell Genetics,* 1978, *22,* 428–433.

Snell, G.D. Recent advances in histocompatibility immunogenetics. *Advances in Genetics,* 1979, *20,* 291–355.

Sparrow, D., Silbert, J.E., and Rowe, J.W. The influence of age on peripheral lymphocyte count in men: a cross-sectional and longitudinal study. *Journal of Gerontology,* 1980, *35,* 163–166.

Stastny, P. Association of the B-cell alloantigen DRw4 with rheumatoid arthritis. *New England Journal of Medicine,* 1978, *298,* 869–871.

Stastny, P., and Fink, C.W. Different HLA-D associations in adult and juvenile rheumatoid arthritis. *Journal of Clinical Investigation,* 1979, *63,* 124–130.

Stastny, P., and Gilliam, J.N. HLA-A1, B8, DRw3 in patients with a distinct form of lupus erythematosus. *Transplantation Proceedings,* 1979, *11,* 1869–1870.

Stoltzner, G., and Makinodan, T. Age-dependent decline in proliferation of lymphocytes. *Exploration in Aging: Advances in Experimental Medicine and Biology,* 1974, *61,* 21–37.

Strelkauskas, A.J., Andrew, J.A., and Hallgren, H.M. Autoantibodies to a regulatory T-cell subset in human aging. In D. Segre and L. Smith (Eds.), *Immunological Aspects of Aging.* New York: Marcel Dekker Publishing Co., 1980 (in press).

Strom, T.B., and Carpenter, C.B. Regulation of alloimmunity by cyclic nucleotides. In J.W. Hadden, R.B. Coffey, and F. Spreafico (Eds.), *Comprehensive Immunology, 3. Immunopharmacology.* New York: Plenum Medical Book Co., 1977.

Tada, T., Okumura, K., Ohmori, K., Kawata, M., and Goro, M. Age-associated changes in the function and subpopulations of mouse and human T lymphocytes. XI International Congress on Gerontology, August 20–25, 1978, *Tokyo Symposium Abstracts,* p. 19.

Takata, H., Sekiguchi, S., Hosoda, Y., Amano, H., Ishii, T., Suzuki, M., Hata, Y., Hatano, S., and Iri, H. Is IaSe7(7J) specificity a risk factor of human survival beyond 100 years in Japanese? *Tissue Antigens,* 1981 (in press).

Talal, N. Disordered immunologic regulation and autoimmunity. *Transplantation Reviews,* 1976, *31,* 240–250.

Talal, N., and Steinberg, A.D. The pathogenesis of autoimmunity in New Zealand black mice. *Current Topics in Microbiology and Immunology,* 1974, *64,* 79–103.

Tam, C.F., and Walford, R.L. Cyclic nucleotide levels in resting and mitogen-stimulated cell suspensions from young and old mice. *Mechanisms of Ageing and Development,* 1978, *7,* 309–320.

Tam, C.F., and Walford, R.L. Alterations in cyclic nucleotides and cyclase activities in T-lymphocytes of aging humans and Down's syndrome subjects. *Journal of Immunology,* 1980 (in press).

Tam, C.F., Mock, D.C., and Walford, R.L. Unstimulated splenic and peripheral T-cell cyclic nucleotide levels, activities of adenylate and guanylate cyclases in old and young mice and Down's and control subjects. *The Gerontologist,* 1979, *19,* 5, part 2, 151.

Tam, C.F., Mock, D.C., Bergmann, K., and Walford, R.L. Age-related changes in basal levels, subcellular localization and compartmentalization of cyclic nucleotides and their generating enzymes (adenylate cyclase and guanylate cyclase) in splenic T-cells of mice. *Life Sciences,* 1980a (in press).

Tam, C.F., Mock, D.C., and Walford, R.L. Alterations in cyclic nucleotide metabolism in resting peripheral T-cells from young and old, Down's and SLE subjects. American Association of Clinical Histocompatibility Testing, St. Louis, Sept. 28–30, 1980b.

Tam, C.F., Cheung, M.K., Mock, D.C., Verity, A.M., and Walford, R.L. Energy charge values and adenine nucleotides in resting peripheral T-cells from young, normal aged, SLE and Down's subjects. *The Gerontologist,* 1980c, *20,* 211.

Tas, S., Tam, C.F., and Walford, R.L. Disulfide bonds and the structure of the chromatin complex in relation to aging. *Mechanisms of Ageing and Development,* 1980, *125,* 1665–1670.

Tas, S., and Walford, R.L. Increased condensation of the chromatin complex in lymphocytes during aging and its modulation in live cells by disulfide reducing agents. *Mechanisms of Ageing and Development,* 1981 (in press).

Tauchi, H., and Sato, T. Age changes in size and number of mitochondria of human hepatic cells. *Journal of Gerontology,* 1968, *23,* 454–461.

Tice, R.R., Schneider, E.L., Kram, D., and Thorne, P. Cytokinetic analysis of the impaired proliferative response of peripheral lymphocytes from aged humans to phytohemagglutinins. *Journal of Experimental Medicine,* 1979, *149,* 1029–1041.

Tuschl, H., and Altmann, H. Unscheduled DNA synthesis in lymphocytes of rheumatoid arthritis patients and spleen cells of rats with experimentally induced arthritis. *Medical Biology,* 1976, *54,* 327–333.

Tyan, M.L. Impaired thymic regeneration in lethally irradiated mice given bone marrow from aged donors. *Proceedings of the Society for Experimental Biology and Medicine,* 1976, *152,* 33–35.

Tyan, M.L. Age-related decrease in mouse T cells progenitors. *Journal of Immunology,* 1977, *118,* 846–851.

Tyan, M.L. Age-related changes in mouse CFU-S regulation. In D. Segre and L. Smith (Eds.), *Immunological Aspects of Aging.* New York: Marcel Dekker Publishing Co., New York, 1980 (in press).

Urba, W.J., and Hildemann, W.H. H-2-linked recessive Ir gene regulation of high antibody responsiveness to TNP hapten conjugated to autogenous albumin. *Immunogenetics,* 1978, *6,* 433–445.

Vracko, R., and Benditt, E.P. Restricted replicative life-span of diabetic fibroblasts *in vitro:* its relation to microangiopathy. *Federation Proceedings,* 1975, *34,* 68–70.

Walford, R.L. *The Immunologic Theory of Aging.* Copenhagen: Munksgaard, 1969.

Walford, R.L. Antibody diversity, histocompatibility systems, disease states and aging. *Lancet,* 1970, *ii,* 1226–1229.

Walford, R.L. Introduction to special issue, "Immunology and Aging." *Gerontologia,* 1972, *18,* 243–246.

Walford, R.L. The immunologic theory of aging: current status. *Federation Proceedings,* 1974, *33,* 2020–2027.

Walford, R.L. When is a mouse "old"? *Journal of Immunology,* 1976, *117,* 352–353.

Walford, R.L. Multigene families, histocompatibility systems, transformation, meiosis, stem cells, and DNA repair. *Mechanisms of Aging and Development,* 1979, *9,* 19–26.

Walford, R.L., and Bergmann, K. Influence of genes associated with the main histocompatibility complex on deoxyribonucleic acid excision repair capacity and bleomycin sensitivity in mouse lymphocytes. *Tissue Antigens,* 1979, *14,* 336–342.

Walford, R.L., and Hodge, S.E. HLA distribution in Alzheimer's disease. In P.I. Terasaki (Ed.), *Histocompatibility Testing 1980.* Los Angeles: UCLA Tissue Typing Lab., University of California, 1980 (in press).

Walford, R.L., Jawaid, S., and Naeim, F. *In vitro* senescence of cultured T-lymphocytes. *The Gerontologist,* 1980, *20,* 219.

Walford, R.L., Smith, G.S., Meredith, P.J., and Cheney, K.E. The immunogenetics of aging. In E.L. Schneider (Ed.), *Genetics of Aging.* New York: Plenum Press, 1978.

Walford, R.L., Smith, G.S., and Waters, H. Histocompatibility systems and disease states with particular reference to cancer. *Transplantation Reviews*, 1971, *7*, 78–111.

Waters, H., Konrad, P., and Walford, R.L. The distribution of HL-A histocompatibility factors and genes in patients with systemic lupus erythematosus. *Tissue Antigens*, 1971, *1*, 68–73.

Watson, J. Involvement of cyclic nucleotides as intracellular mediators in the induction of antibody synthesis. In J.W. Hadden, R.G. Coffey, and F. Speafico (Eds.), *Comprehensive Immunology, 3. Immunopharmacology*. New York: Plenum Press, 1977.

Wedner, H.J., and Parker, C.W. Lymphocyte activation. *Progress in Allergy*, 1976, *20*, 195–300.

Weigle, W.O., and Parks, D. Effect of aging on immune and tolerant states. *Federation Proceedings*, 1978, *37*, 1253–1257.

Weinbach, E.C., and Garbus, J. Oxidative phosphorylation in mitochondria from aged rats. *Journal of Biological Chemistry*, 1959, *234*, 412–417.

Weindruch, R.H., Kristie, J.A., Cheney, K.E., and Walford, R.L. Influence of controlled dietary restriction on immune function and aging. *Federation Proceedings*, 1979, *38*, 2007–2016.

Weindruch, R.H., Cheung, M.K., Verity, M.A., and Walford, R.L. Modification of mitochondrial respiration by aging and dietary restriction. *Mechanisms of Ageing and Development*, 1980a, *12*, 375–392.

Weindruch, R.H., Kristie, J.A., and Walford, R.L. Dietary restriction imposed in middle-age in mice: lifespan, disease and immunologic effects. *The Gerontologist*, 1980b, *20*, 223.

Weindruch, R.H., and Suffin, S.C. Quantitative histologic effects in mouse of controlled dietary restriction. *Journal of Gerontology*, 1980, *35*, 525–531.

Weindruch, R.H., and Walford, R.L. Aging and functions of the RES. In N. Cohen (Ed.), *The Ontogeny and Phylogeny of the Reticuloendothelial System*, vol. 5 of *The Reticuloendothelial System, A Comprehensive Treatise*. New York: Plenum Press, 1980 (in press).

Weksler, M.E., Dekruyff, R., Dobken, J., and Siskind, G.W. Ease of tolerance induction in mice of different ages. In D. Segre and L. Smith (Eds.), *Immunological Aspects of Aging*. New York: Marcel Dekker Publishing Co., 1980 (in press).

Weksler, M.R., and Hutteroth, T.H. Impaired lymphocyte function in aged humans. *Journal of Clinical Investigation*, 1974, *53*, 99–104.

Westermark, P., Natvig, J.B., and Johansson, B. Characterization of an amyloid fibril protein from senile cardiac amyloid. *Journal of Experimental Medicine*, 1977, *146*, 631–636.

Whittingham, S., Mathews, J.D., Mackay, I.R., Stocks, A.E., Ungar, B., and Martin, F.I.R. Diabetes mellitus, autoimmunity and ageing. *Lancet*, 1971, *i*, 763–766.

Williams, R.M., Kraus, L.J., Lavin, P.T., Steele, L.L., and Yunis, E.J. Genetics of survival in mice: localization of dominant effects to subregions of the major histocompatibility complex. In D. Segre and L. Smith (Eds.), *Immunological Aspects of Aging*. New York: Marcel Dekker Publishing Co., 1980 (in press).

Williamson, A.R., and Askonas, B.A. Senescence of an antibody-forming cell clone. *Nature*, 1972, *238*, 337–339.

Wisniewski, H.M., and Terry, R.D. Neuropathology of the aging brain. In R.D. Terry and S. Gershon (Eds.), *Neurobiology of Aging*. New York: Raven Press, 1976.

Woda, B.A., and Feldman, J.D. Density of surface immunoglobulin and capping on rat lymphocytes. I. Changes with aging. *Journal of Experimental Medicine,* 1979, *149,* 416–423.

Woda, B.A., Yguerabide, J., and Feldman, J.D. Mobility and density of AgB, "Ia," and Fc receptors on the surface of lymphocytes from young and old rats. *Journal of Immunology,* 1979, *123,* 2162–2167.

Wohlgethan, J.R., and Cathcart, E.S. Amyloid resistance in A/J mice is determined by a single gene. *Nature,* 1979, *278,* 453–454.

Wright, J.R., Calkins, E., Breen, W.J., Stolte, G., and Schultz, R.T. Relationship of amyloid to aging. *Medicine,* 1969, *48,* 39–60.

Yarnell, J.W.G., St. Leger, A.S., Balfour, I.C., and Russell, R.B. The distribution, age effects and disease associations of HLA antigens and other blood group markers in a random sample of our elderly population. *Journal of Chronic Diseases* 1979, *32,* 555–562.

Yotti, L.P., Glober, T.W., Trosko, J.E., and Segal, D.J. Comparative study of X-ray and UV-induced cytotoxicity, DNA repair, and mutagenesis in Down's syndrome and normal fibroblasts. *Pediatric Research,* 1980, *14,* 88–92.

Yunis, E.J., Fernandes, G., and Greenberg, L.J. Tumor immunology, autoimmunity and aging. *Journal of the American Geriatrics Society,* 1976, *24,* 258–263.

Yunis, E.J., Handiverger, B.S., Hallgren, H.M., Good, R.A., and Fernandes, G. Aging and immunity. In S. Cohen, P.A. Ward, and R.T. McCluskey (Eds.), *Mechanisms of Immunopathology.* New York: John Wiley and Sons, 1979.

# CHAPTER 2

# Aging and Basal Gangliar Functions

CALEB E. FINCH, PH.D PATRICK K. RANDALL, PH.D
THE ANDRUS GERONTOLOGY CENTER
UNIVERSITY OF SOUTHERN CALIFORNIA
LOS ANGELES, CALIFORNIA

JOHN F. MARSHALL, PH.D
DEPARTMENT OF PSYCHOBIOLOGY
UNIVERSITY OF CALIFORNIA
IRVINE, CALIFORNIA

## INTRODUCTION

The mammalian basal ganglia are importantly involved in the regulation of movement. After maturity, these brain regions undergo age changes in their structure and neurochemistry which can profoundly affect the behavior and drug responses of aging animals and humans. The structures of the basal ganglia, which include the substantia nigra, caudate-putamen (neostriatum), and globus pallidus, are richly interconnected (Figure 2–1). By virtue of the neocortical information that they receive and their influence on the motor cortex (through the ventral thalamus), the basal ganglia are well situated to process sensory information and modify signals sent to the neurons of the pyramidal tracts. The cell bodies of pyramidal tract neurons are in the motor cortex and send direct pathways to spinal chord motoneurons controlling the skeletal muscles (Truex and Carpenter, 1969; Papeschi, 1972; Lewis, 1976; Ganong, 1977).

Age changes in the basal ganglia are of much current interest because of their suspected involvement in some of the movement disorders of

The research of the authors was supported by the following grants: CEF (NIA, AG-00117, AG-00446); JFM (AG-00538); PR (AG-00133 and AG-00855) and by a grant from the Weingart Foundation to the Andrus Gerontology Center. JFM is an Alfred P. Sloane Foundation Fellow in Neuroscience.

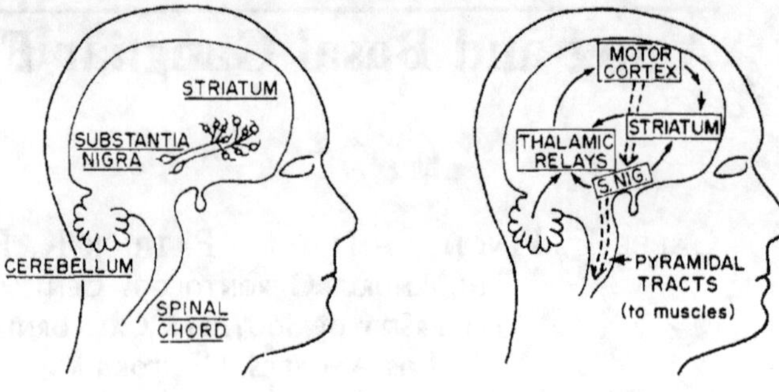


| | Substantia Nigra (pars compacta) | Striatum (caudate-putamen) |
|---|---|---|
| TRANSMITTER | Dopamine | ACh, GABA, Enkephelins, Subst. P |
| HUNTINGTON'S CHOREA | Normal | >50% cell loss |
| PARKINSON'S DISEASE | 80–99% cell loss | Normal |

**Figure 2–1:** Basal gangliar connections and disease-related alterations

advanced age. Elderly individuals tend to take longer to carry out movements, have difficulty compensating for movement errors (Welford, 1977), and show a heightened incidence of involuntary abnormal movements including senile tremors and chorea (Critchley, 1956; Welford, 1977; Krammer and Klawans, 1979; Potvin et al., 1980). In addition, aging brings increased sensitivity to drug-induced Parkinsonism, tardive dyskinesias, and other movement disorders involving the basal ganglia (Ayd, 1961; Crane, 1974; Jus et al., 1976; Simpson et al., 1978 discussed under The Pharmacology and Behavior, below). Recent findings from our laboratories and others describe the use of aging rodents as experimental models for basal ganglia dysfunctions during aging.

Despite extensive study, the physiology and anatomy of the basal ganglia are less well understood than those of cerebellum, hippocampus, or spinal cord, for example. However, the neurochemistry of the basal ganglia is highly developed, and a battery of neuropharmacologic probes is available for manipulating synaptic functions. In addition, two major age-related neurologic diseases consequent to basal ganglia pathology have been extensively documented: Huntington's chorea and Parkinson's disease. We shall briefly describe these diseases of the basal ganglia, indicating how the interaction of clinical neurology with neuropharmacology has set the stage for recent advances in understanding the age-related alterations in this system.

The cardinal symptoms of Parkinsonism are rigidity of the postural and facial muscles, bradykinesia (slowing of movement), and a 4–6 Hz tremor of the limbs which disappears during sleep. The major neural lesion in Parkinson's disease is the massive (80–99 percent) loss of the dopaminergic neurons with cell bodies in the pars compacta of the substantia nigra (Tretiakoff, 1919; Hassler, 1955; Riederer and Wuketich, 1976), which is accompanied by degeneration of the nigroneostriatal dopamine-containing axons and terminals (Hornykiewicz, 1975). There is usually little damage to neurons with cell bodies within the neostriatum, which contain γ-aminobutyric acid (GABA), acetylcholine, substance P, enkephalins, and other putative neurotransmitters. Parkinsonism is rare before 40 years of age, with greatest incidence between 50 and 70 years of age (Ayd, 1961). For many Parkinsonians, most or all of the symptoms may be relieved at least temporarily by L-dopa (Cotzias et al., 1967) or by dopaminergic agonists such as apomorphine (Schwab et al., 1951) or the ergot derivatives (Calne et al., 1978; Lieberman et al., 1979). These compounds are thought to act by stimulating dopaminergic receptors located on neostriatal cells. Dopaminergic antagonists, which may be administered as antipsychotics, generally worsen the rigidity (Freyhan, 1957). In contrast, cholinergic antagonists often relieve the symptoms, whereas cholinergic agonists worsen them (Duvoisin, 1967). These findings have led to the view that there exists a critical balance between the *dopaminergic* and *cholinergic* synapses of the basal ganglia (Barbeau, 1962; Klawans, 1970; Stimmel, 1976); the symptoms of Parkinsonism arise when there is a deficiency of dopaminergic neurotransmission relative to cholinergic activity, that is, a *negative* dopamine balance or tone.

In contrast to Parkinsonism, the involuntary, spasmodic movements in Huntington's chorea (adult onset) are associated with a loss of neostriatal cells that contain acetylcholine and GABA (reviewed in Finch, 1980). The nigro-neostriatal projections are usually undamaged. This autosomal dominant disease is rare before the age of 20 years and has a maximal incidence between 30 and 40 years of age (Burch, 1968). Effective therapy for Huntington's disease includes dopaminergic antagonists (phenothiazines) and cholinergic agonists (Klawans, 1970). Thus, the set of drugs that would exacerbate Parkinsonism palliate Huntington's chorea. These observations gave rise to the view that Huntington's disease involves a deficiency of cholinergic neurotransmission relative to dopaminergic activity, that is, a *positive* dopamine balance or tone. The concept of dopamine–acetylcholine balance, though useful, is doubtless oversimplified, since other neostiatal neurotransmitters are involved in striatal functions, for example, GABA and enkephalins (Perez de la Mora et al., 1979) and glutamate from the cortico-striatal pathway (Spencer, 1976).

## ANATOMIC AND BIOCHEMICAL STUDIES ON THE BASAL GANGLIA DURING AGING

### Neuronal Loss

Neuronal loss during aging is now considered to be selective in most brain regions. Whereas the substantia nigra may lose 30–50 percent of its neurons during the average human life span (McGeer et al., 1977), other brain stem nuclei, such as the inferior olive, may retain their full neuronal complement (Brody, 1976). By comparison, Parkinson's disease is associated with a more than 80 percent loss of nigral neurons (Bernheimer et al., 1973; Hornykiewicz, 1975; Riederer and Wuketich, 1976; McGeer et al., 1977). Because the intersubject variance of neuronal density measurements is considerable at all ages, a much larger sample (probably at least 100 brains) will be required to define the normal extent and limits of age change.

Two little-discussed issues may complicate evaluation of neuronal loss in aging. First the volume of the neuronal nucleolus can decrease by 30 percent or more with age in some human brain regions (Mann and Yates, 1979): if cresyl violet staining were used for RNA with thin sections, geometric considerations (Finch, unpubl.) imply that 15 percent fewer neurons would be recognized in older subjects by the presence of their nucleoli, a common histologic method for counting neurons, which could lead to corresponding overestimates of the neuronal loss.[1] Additionally, the historical trends for increasing brain and body size within the last 100 years (Corsellis, 1978) could overestimate neuronal loss with advancing age, if the young subjects were from more recent cohorts and had more neurons in particular structures corresponding to their larger brains. Although it is not known whether intraspecies variations of brain size result from individual differences in neuronal number, glial number, or cell size, it would seem desirable to match subjects of different ages for similar body size (heights) as young adults.

Preliminary studies suggest that neostriatal neurons may also be lost during normal aging in humans (Bugiani et al., 1978) and in C57BL/6J mice (Mensah, 1979). Over the human life span during normal aging the loss may amount to 30–50 percent (comparable to the losses reported in the substantia nigra), affecting both large and small neostriatal neurons. The loss in mice may be smaller. In Huntington's chorea, small cells tend

[1]Although some types of neurons contain less RNA with increasing age, most rodent brain cells show little if any change in RNA content or sequence complexity of their nuclear or cytoplasmic poly(A)RNA (Colman et al., 1980). The rodent striatum may be exceptional in its age-related decrease (10–20 percent) in RNA concentration; no changes of bulk RNA were detected in other major brain regions (Chaconas and Finch, 1973; Shaskan, 1977).

to be preferentially lost, and the losses are usually very extensive (Forno and Jose, 1973; Klintworth, 1973). It is of interest to compare "normal" age-related losses of neostriatal neurons with those observed in Huntington's chorea: the semiquantitative data available suggest that the range of loss in Huntingtonians (Bernheimer et al., 1973) overlaps at its lower end with the 30–50 percent loss which may subsequently occur normally in old age (Bugiani et al., 1978). The extent of human neostriatal neuronal loss roughly parallels the decrease of caudate volume during normal aging, which may reach 50 percent only after 90 years (Bowen et al., 1976), whereas in Huntington's chorea, the shrinkage is commonly at least 50 percent (Bird and Iversen, 1974; Bowen et al., 1976). Additionally, in a recent study of Parkinsonism, neostriatal neuron losses of 35–50 percent were detected by comparison with age-matched controls (Bugiani et al., 1980). The cell losses during normal aging thus appear to overlap with losses found in Parkinson's as well as in Huntington's disease.

Synapses and neuronal processes (including dendritic spines and axon collaterals) appear to be lost during aging, independently of neuronal loss in at least some brain regions (Machado-Salas et al., 1977; Feldman and Dowd, 1975; Geinisman et al., 1977; Huttenlocher, 1979) and result in a "progressively impoverished neuropile" (Machado-Salas and Scheibel, 1979). Possible losses of neostriatal dopaminergic synaptic complexes during aging are implied from a 20 percent reduction of synaptosomal dopamine uptake from mice more than 18 months old (Jonec and Finch, 1975). Also, an exploratory electron microscopic study suggested that the old rat striatum contained fewer dense vesicles (putative catecholamine storage vesicles) (Sun, 1976).

Impaired axonal flow is implied from peculiar, catecholamine containing aggregates in the nigro-neostriatal pathway in aging C57BL/6J mice (Masuoka et al., 1979). Axonal flow may be slowed in the septal-hippocampal pathway in aging rats (Geinisman et al., 1977), but this issue has not yet been directly investigated for the nigro-neostriatal pathway.

### Neurotransmitter Functions

*Dopamine Metabolism.* In general, neostriatal dopamine concentration tends to decrease with age. In humans, the decrease is progressive with adult age at a rate of about 1 percent per year, resulting in a 30–60 percent loss by the average life span, 75 years (Carlsson and Winblad, 1976; Riederer and Wuketich, 1976; Adolffson et al., 1979). Tyrosine hydroxylase shows a similar trend (Cote and Kremzner, 1974; McGeer and McGeer, 1976; Adolffson et al., 1979). Progressive decreases with age were also detected in the globus pallidus and mesencephalon (Adolfsson et al., 1979). Tyrosine hydroxylase in the human substantia nigra decreases with age according to one report (Cote and Kremzner, 1974) but not another (McGeer and McGeer, 1976): Striatal tyrosine hydroxylase losses might be expected to parallel the 30–50 percent loss of substantia nigra neurons (McGeer et al., 1977), since the loss of neostriatal tyrosine hydroxylase and dopa decarboxylase is proportional to the extent of substantia nigra lesions in experimental studies with young rats (Hefti et al., 1979). In 20-year-old macaque monkeys, substantia nigra cell bodies had markedly reduced dopamine content per cell, as determined by histofluorescence (Sladek and Sladek, 1978). The total age-related loss of dopamine and tyrosine hydroxylase may be greater if calculated per caudate (rather than per gram caudate) because of caudate shrinkage with age in humans (Bowen et al., 1976).

In laboratory rodents, the neostriatal dopamine concentration (from whole, freehand-dissected regions) tends to decrease at later ages, for example, 20–30 percent by the average life span according to some studies (Finch, 1973; Joseph et al., 1978; Demarest et al., 1980); however, decreases were not found in all studies (Ponzio et al, 1978). Measurements in subdivisions of the striatum (obtained from 1 mm diameter "punches" of cryotome coronal sections) showed no age change in 3-, 10-, 17-, and 21-month-old brains of C57BL/6J mice; a trend for decreased dopamine concentration was detected in some samples of mice aged 24–30 months (the average life span of this strain) (Osterburg et al., in press). Small decreases of striatal tyrosine hydroxylase occur in aging rats (McGeer et al., 1971; Reis et al., 1977), but not in CFI mice (Reis et al., 1977). In the substantia nigra of CFI mice, tyrosine hydroxylase did not decrease (Reis et al., 1977). Thus the decrease of neostriatal dopamine is not as progressive or as severe in aging rodents, as compared to humans at similar stages of their life span.

Several studies suggest that metabolism of neostriatal dopamine is slowed in two-year-old or older rodents. A smaller fraction of [$^3$H]L-tyrosine or [$^3$H]-L-dopa (i.p. injected) was converted to [$^3$H]-dopamine in mice (Finch, 1973); similar results were obtained with [$^3$H]-tyrosine delivered intraventricularly to 33-month-old rats (Ponzio et al., 1978). Since the uptake of tyrosine and L-dopa by neostriatal slices was not impaired with age in C57BL/6J mice (Finch et al., 1975), precursor availability may not change significantly. A study of dopamine turnover in C57BL/6J male mice by the α-methyl-*p*-tyrosine technique indicated no age changes before midlife (3 vs. 12 months); turnover was slowed by 24 months (Osterburg et al., in press). Small reductions of striatal dopac are also detected in old rodents (Demarest et al., 1980; Osterburg et al., in press). Taken together, the impairments of neostriatal dopamine synthesis and turnover in old rodents are relatively small ($\leq$30 percent).

Although no direct studies of dopamine turnover have been done in aging humans, it is of interest that levels of the dopamine catabolite, homovanillic acid, did not change with age postmortem in the same brains showing dopamine loss (Adolfsson et al., 1979). However, homovanillic acid in the cerebrospinal fluid tends to *increase* with age (Gottfries et al., 1971). This increase may represent a compensatory increase of dopamine synthesis by the remaining nigro-neostriatal terminals, such as induced in young rodents by experimental lesions (Agid et al., 1974; Demarest, 1980).

*Dopaminergic Receptors*

1. *Age changes in receptor number.* The neostriatal targets of the nigro-striatal projections show relatively greater and earlier deficits compared to the later onset of reduced dopamine levels and turnover in aging rodents. Neostriatal dopamine receptors decrease with age in rodents, as assayed by the "high affinity" binding of butyrophenones such as spiroperidol or haloperidol (dopaminergic antagonists) (Govoni et al., 1978, 1980; Joseph et al., 1978; Makman et al., 1978; Severson and Finch, 1980a); ADTN decreases of binding (a dopaminergic agonist) are even larger (Severson and Finch, 1980a). The kinetics or stereospecificity of ligand binding does not change in most studies. The decrease of binding is progressive throughout adult life and drops by 20–30 percent before 12 months, midlife (Figure 2–2). Recent data suggest that progressive age-related decreases of dopamine receptors also occur in the human caudate, whereas no age changes occur in the putamen (Severson and Finch, 1980b). The loss of caudate ADTN binding sites in humans is about 7.5 percent per decade (Severson et al., in press.) It is not yet established how much of the high-affinity dopaminergic binding sites are on presynaptic versus postsynaptic dopaminergic sites, although present evidence favors a postsynaptic location for most binding sites.

The dopamine-activated adenylate cyclase is impaired by 50 percent or more in old rodents (Walker and Boas-Walker, 1973; Puri and Volicer, 1976; Govoni et al., 1977) with marked changes before midlife (Makman et al., 1978; Schmidt and Thornberry 1978); these changes closely parallel the loss of dopamine receptors. However, the Gpp(NH)p and fluoride-induced adenylate cyclase activity does not change with age. Gpp(NH)p and fluoride are thought to act on the same regulatory subunit of adenylate cyclase (Pfeuffer, 1977) which is distal to ("downstream") and independent of the receptor (Levitzki, 1977). If the Gpp(NH)p and fluoride-stimulated cyclase is in the same cell membrane containing the dopaminergic receptor, the age-related reduction of the dopamine receptor in the postsynaptic membrane could limit or reduce coupling with adenylate cyclase. This could occur independently of striatal neuronal loss. Another possibility is that altered fluidity or other biophysical properties of membranes

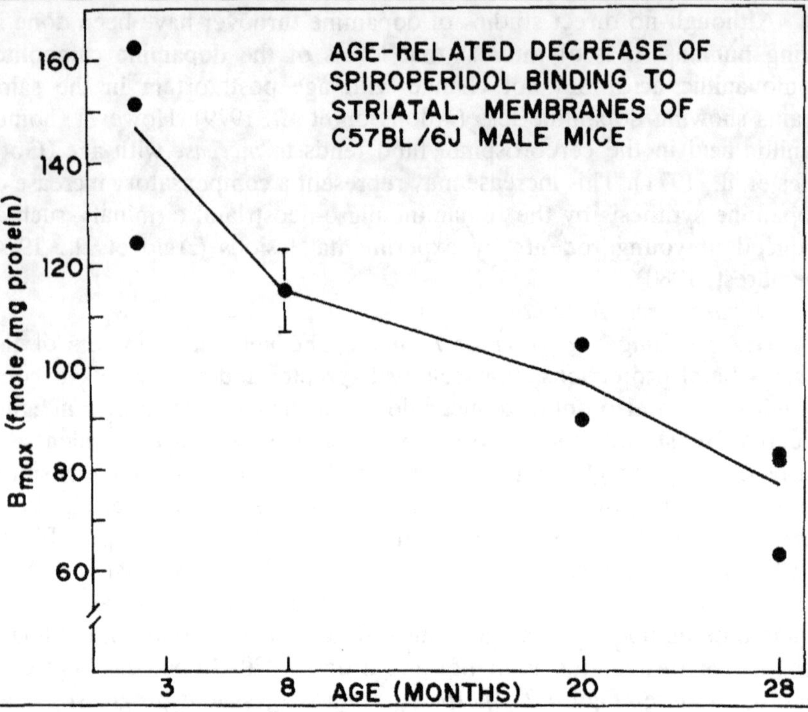


**Figure 2–2:** Decreased dopamine receptors during aging. Relationship between age and specific [3H] spiroperidol binding in striatal membranes from male C57BL/6J mice. Binding isotherms (scatchard analysis) were conducted with 0.1–2nM spiroperidals 10 uM d-butaclalomol was used to estimate non-specific binding. Data are plotted as $B_{max}$ vs. age. Points represent individual experiments (four mice per analysis) except at 8 months, which represents Mean ±SEM of 7 studies. Values for $B_{max}$, other than at 8 months, were normalized for the overall mean of $B_{max}$ at 8 months.
Source: Severson, J.A., and Finch, C.E. Reduced dopaminergic binding during aging in the rodent striatum. *Brain Research,* 1980a, *199,* 147–162. Copyright 1980 by Elsevier North Holland, Inc. Reprinted with permission.

may be a significant phenomenon in aging. Surface lectin binding sites show altered mobility in Deiter's neurons of aging rats (Bennett and Bondareff, 1977). Since receptor-cyclase coupling is influenced by membrane fluidity (Rimon et al., 1978; Hirata et al., 1979), changes in membrane structure during aging could contribute to the reduction of dopamine-activated adenylate cyclase without effecting activation by Gpp(NH)p or fluoride.

The age-related decrease of dopaminergic receptors could result from multiple causes: there may be (1) a decreased density of receptors in each pre- or postsynaptic process or terminal, (2) a loss of presynaptic terminals, or (3) a loss of pre or postsynaptic cells. For example, high-affinity butyrophenone binding sites are associated with neostriatal neurons (Schwarcz et al., 1978). Studies with kainate acid lesions in rodents suggest that small and medium-sized neostriatal neurons contain dopamine receptors, dopamine-activated adenylate cyclase, glutamic acid decarboxylase, and choline acetyltransferase (McGeer et al., 1976; Schwarcz et al., 1978). Kainic acid, a rigid glutamate analogue, when injected locally into the neostriatum, causes a loss of neostriatal neurons and a loss of dopaminergic receptors and other striatal neuronal markers. Loss of neostriatal neurons with age could be a common denominator of age loss in dopaminergic receptors, dopamine-activated adenylate cyclase, and cholinergic parameters (see below).

The decreases of striatal dopamine receptors and dopamine-activated adenylate cyclase which occur before 12 months of age in aging rodents thus appear to precede by 9–12 months the decreases in presynaptic nigro-neostriatal parameters including dopamine levels and turnover. These later changes could be viewed as contributing further to reduced dopaminergic actions at striatal neurons. Mechanisms involving striatonigral feedback may also be involved.

**2.** *Supersensitivity*. An important property of the basal gangliar systems is their capacity to regulate receptor number and behavioral sensitivity. Consider first, the phenomenon of "supersensitivity." Chronic reduction of dopaminergic stimulation of neostriatal cells by denervation (lesions of the nigro-neostriatal pathway) or by chronic treatment with dopamine "receptor" blockers (dopamine *antagonists* such as haloperidol) can induce a "supersensitivity," as monitored by electrical, biochemical, and behavioral responses. For example, unilateral nigral lesions, which reduce neostriatal dopamine, also reduce markedly the threshold dose of apomorphine required for depressing the firing of neostriatal neurons or inducing rotation contralateral to the lesion (Marshall and Ungerstedt, 1977; Schultz and Ungerstedt, 1978). This pharmacologic supersensitivity is correlated with a 30 percent increase in the number of neostriatal dopaminergic receptors (Burt et al., 1977). The comparison of nigral lesions in 6= versus 25-month-old male rats suggested important impairments in the post lesion supersensitivity responses (Joseph et al., 1978). Supersensitivity can also be induced in young rodents by chronic treatment with haloperidol. However, old (24–28 month old) C57BL/6J male mice failed to develope dopaminergic supersensitivity in response to chronic haloperidol; the controls, aged 3 and 12 months, did so as monitored by increased neostriatal dopaminergic binding sites (Figure 2–3) and increased behavioral stereotypic responses to apomorphine (Figure 2–4) (Randall, Severson, and Finch, in press). The apomorphine-induced stereotypic responses, which include sniffing, gnawing, climbing, and arching of the back (Protias

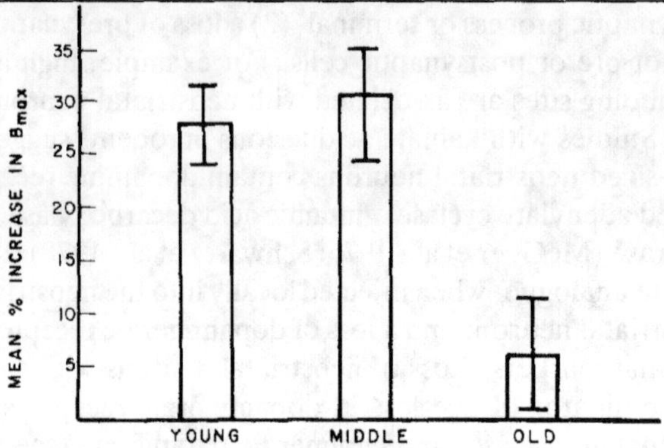


**Figure 2–3:** Haloperidol-induced supersensitivity responses in aging mice: striatal dopamine receptors. The C57BL/6J male mice was treated with haloperidol (1.2 mg/kg/day, i.p. for 21 days). Their striata were assayed for spiroperidol binding sites and showed significant increases of $B_{max}$ in mice aged 4 (young) and 12 months (middle-aged); no changes were detected in mice 24 months (old). For details, see Figure 2–2.

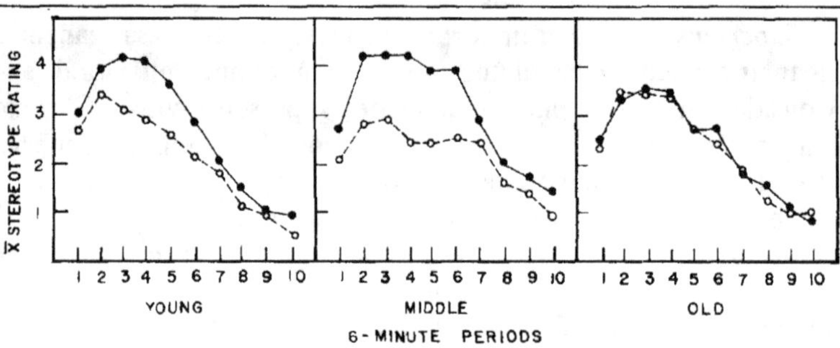


**Figure 2–4:** Haloperidol-induced supersensitivity response in aging mice: apomorphine-induced stereotypic responses. After chronic haloperidol treatment (see Figure 2–3), mice were tested for stereotypic responses to apomorphine (0.5 mg/kg). Curves represent mean stereotype ratings on a 7-point scale (Randall, Severson, and Finch, in prep.). Significant elevation of stereotypic ratings as a result of chronic haloperidol treatment were observed in young and middle-aged mice ($p < 0.05$) but not in old mice. 0—0, control; 0—0 haloperidal treated.

et al., 1976; Randall, Severson, Finch, in press) can also be induced by direct intrastriatal injection of dopaminergic drugs (Ernst and Smelik, 1966; Fog and Pakkenberg, 1971) and are widely used as an index of neostriatal dopaminergic functions. In young CBA mice, which lack the behavioral supersensitivity response to chronic haloperidol, there is also no haloperidol-induced increase of striatal dopaminergic receptors (Severson, et al., 1981). The absence of supersensitivity responses to chronic haloperidol in old C57BL/6J mice 24 months old or older as monitored by dopaminergic receptors and stereotypic behaviors suggests that a specific population of receptors may be lost during aging; possibly the same receptor population is congenitally missing or defective in CBA mice. Alternatively, since supersensitivity-type responses are also lost during aging in the pineal gland, cerebellum, and cerebral cortex of old rats (Greenberg and Weiss, 1979; Weiss et al., 1979), a component of membranes required for the induction of supersensitivity responses in many catacholamine systems may be altered during aging. This possibility was also raised in the preceding discussion of adenylate cyclase changes with age. The behavioral aspects of these studies with chronic haloperidol are discussed under The Pharmacology and Behavior, below. The loss of supersensitivity responses in the aging rodent striatum, cortex, and pineal gland could also be considered as another manifestation of impaired synaptic remodeling, such as observed after surgical lesions in old rats (Cotman and Scheff, 1979). The effects of age on the supersensitivity responses which follow striatal denervation from nigral lesions (Joseph et al., 1978), merit further detailed investigation.

**3.** *Subsensitivity.* The converse of dopaminergic blockade-induced supersensitivity is the reduction in neostriatal dopamine receptor number and behavioral responses following chronic treatment with dopaminergic *agonists* such as bromocriptine. Typically, subsensitive young rodents show a 15–30 percent loss of high-affinity dopaminergic receptors (Mishra et al., 1978; Quik and Iversen, 1978); additionally, corresponding reductions occurred in stereotypic responses to apomorphine (Randall, Severson, and Finch, in press). Two-year-old C57BL/6J male mice showed normal induction of dopaminergic subsensitivity after chronic treatment with bromocryptine, as measured by a reduction of dopaminergic receptors and reduced stereotypic responses to apomorphine (Randall, Severson, and Finch, in press). Correspondingly, CBA/J mice also showed normal subsensitivity responses (Severson et al., 1981). Similarly, the pineal and cortex of old rats showed typical subsensitivity responses (Greenberg and Weiss, 1979; Weiss et al., 1979). In conclusion, select features of neural receptor systems are altered during aging and certain of these may be open to biochemical-genetic investigation with inbred mice and their recombinent inbred strains.

*Acetylcholine*

**1.** *Metabolism.* Choline acetyltransferase (CAT), the key enzyme of acetylcholine synthesis, may undergo small decreases in the aging rat striatum, but does not change much in other brain regions (McGeer et al., 1971; Meek et al., 1977). Similar-sized age changes of CAT were detected in the human striatum in some samples (McGeer and McGeer,

1976), but not in others (Bowen et al., 1976, Reisine et al., 1977; McGeer and McGeer, 1978). Cortical and hippocampal CAT tends to decrease more extensively (McGeer and McGeer, 1975; Davies, 1978).

**2.** *Receptors.* The binding of [3H]-quinuclidinyl benzilate (QNB), a ligand for muscarinic receptors, decreased in striata of 30 month old mice (Strong et al., 1979).

*GABA*

**1.** *Metabolism.* Glutamic acid decarboxylase does not change in the aging rat neostriatum (McGeer et al., 1971), but may decrease by 30 percent during aging in humans (Bowen et al., 1976; McGeer and McGeer, 1976, 1978). The possible trend for greater loss of glutamic acid decarboxylase in aging humans, compared to rodents, may be associated with greater loss of a specific population of neostriatal neurons.

**2.** *Receptors.* Specific GABA binding does not change with age in the rat neostriatum (4 vs. 24–30 months), but appears to decrease by 50 percent in the substantia nigra (Govoni et al., 1980).

*Other Basal Gangliar Neurotransmitters.* In aging humans, serotonin levels decrease with age in the globus pallidus (Adolfsson, unpublished). No information is yet available on age changes in levels of substance P or the opiate-related peptides. Neostriatal opiate receptors, estimated by binding of dihydromorphine, are decreased by about 30 percent in 5- versus 26-month-old rats (R. Messing, et al., personal commun.). Hopefully, details of age-related profiles will soon be available for the other known synaptically active transmitter-like compounds and their receptors in the basal ganglia.

*Bloodflow and Metabolism.* Reductions of metabolism in the neostriatum of aging rats have also been detected by the 2-deoxyglucose technique; the largest age changes occur before midlife (Smith et al., 1980; London et al., in press). Additionally, Kozlowski and Marshall (in prep.) have found reduced uptake of 2-deoxyglucose into the pars reticulata (substantia nigra) of old rats. Regional blood flow in the neostriatum decreases only slightly after 3 months (Ohata et al., in press). Other studies show that cerebral metabolism may decrease more strikingly than blood flow with age in rodents (Le Poncin-Lafitte and Rapin, 1980). Taken together with reductions of neurotransmitters and RNA in aging, these data suggest that many metabolic activities are reduced during aging in the basal ganglia, possibly involving glia as well as neurons. No data are yet available on age changes in electric activities in this region. The expected emergence of a detailed neurophysiologic understanding of the basal ganglia in the next decade may permit detailed hypotheses about cause-effect relationships, for instance, does the early loss of dopamine receptors and dopamine-activated cyclase result from striatal neuron loss; if so, do these changes lead gradually to a later reduction of nigro-striatal activity?

**Basal Gangliar Interactions During Aging and Disease**

Since the losses of nigro-neostriatal functions in some humans by the ninth decade approach the extent of loss during Parkinson's disease, the slow movement and shuffling gait of many elderly persons may represent a pre-Parkinsonian state in association with their nigro-neostriatal impairments (Marshall and Berrios, 1979). It was suggested by Bugiani and co-workers (1978) that the loss of striatal neurons during aging might reduce the incidence of Parkinsonism during aging, since neostriatal interneuronal loss, by reducing cholinergic tone, might reduce and partially ameliorate the negative dopaminergic imbalance. This possibility is testable: in young rodents with nigro-neostriatal lesions, additional kainate lesions to kill neostriatal interneurons might blunt the effects of nigral lesions. Conversely, the age-related loss of nigral afferents may be a factor in the mildness of motor symptoms in late-onset Huntington's chorea, that is, onset in the fifth and sixth decades (Bruyn, 1968). The loss of nigral afferents during normal aging may blunt the impact of the neostriatal neuron loss and reduce the risk of senile chorea (Finch, 1980).

The characteristic age of onset of Huntington's chorea and Parkinson's disease has been considered to result from interactions of the lesions with normal trends in basal gangliar aging (Finch, 1976, 1980). For example, in carriers of the Huntingtonian lesion, a presymptomatic period (commonly from birth to the fourth decade) may prevail until the lesion summates with the general aging trend for neostriatal impairments, for example, the early progressive losses of dopaminergic receptors and dopamine-activated cyclase before midlife in rodents (reviewed above). The possibility of silent neostriatal abnormalities was suggested by the ability of L-dopa to transiently elicit chorea in suspected Huntingtonian carriers, with no such effects on noncarriers (Klawans et al., 1972, 1980). In lesions of the basal ganglia, there appears to be a relatively large margin of safety before abnormalities are manifested (Ranje and Ungerstedt, 1977).

Similar arguments may be made for the late onset of Parkinson's disease. In the postencephalitic variety, the initial damage to the substantia nigra may not be sufficient for producing motor abnormalities until summated with the aging trend. There may also be genetic modifiers of Parkinsonism, suspected in some families (Mjones, 1949). Moreover, relatives of Parkinsonians in two samples had a greater incidence of drug-induced Parkinsonism during treatment with antipsychotic dopaminergic antagonists (Myrianthopoulos et al., 1962, 1969); this sensitivity suggests genetic variations in the "dopaminergic reserve" which might be detected by dopaminergic antagonists. Given the mouse strain differences in dopamine receptor regulation (see above), it seems likely that mammalian populations contain diverse genetic polymorphisms influencing basal gangliar functions and the patterns of basal ganglia aging. The changes observed during aging and in neurologic diseases could therefore represent different components in a spectrum of specific genetic controls over basal gangliar development and aging.

## MOVEMENT DISORDERS OF THE AGING RAT IN RELATION TO THE BASAL GANGLIA

While changes in brain catecholaminergic mechanisms are considered a ubiquitous finding in aged mammals, the consequences of these alterations for the behavioral capacities and psychologic functioning of elderly humans are just beginning to be explored. With advanced age, humans show marked impairments in the ability to learn and remember new information (Talland, 1968) and deficits in motor skills (Welford, 1977). While the alterations at basal ganglia dopaminergic synapses reviewed in the preceding section might contribute to any of these age-related disturbances, a relationship of dopaminergic changes to movement disorders is most directly indicated and, at present, most amenable to experimental analysis.

### Experimental Approaches

The time is ripe for a broadly based experimental program to elucidate the relationship between movement disorders and central dopamine-containing synapses in aging. In this and the subsequent section we present the results obtained using two rodent "models" for basal ganglia movement disorders. These findings demonstrate for the first time that the age-related alterations in neostriatal dopaminergic synaptic activity do contribute to the movement dysfunctions of these species. In addition, the findings suggest possible therapeutic approaches to the control of these motor abnormalities.

Damage to the dopamine-containing neurons of young adult rats leads to dramatic and long-lasting impairments in movement and sensorimotor integration (reviewed by Marshall and Teitelbaum, 1977). Many of these deficits are similar to those occurring in Parkinsonian patients. The dopamine-containing cells that innervate the neostriatum and other forebrain structures can be destroyed by injections of the catecholamine neurotoxin, 6-hydroxydopamine (6-OH-DA) near to the cell bodies or their axons (Ungerstedt, 1968). This procedure leads to a marked depletion of dopamine in the neostriatum, accompanied by a loss of nigral DA-containing cell bodies, whereas non-catecholamine-containing axons passing through the region of the injection are typically spared (Hökfelt and Ungerstedt, 1973). Rats whose nigro-neostriatal neurons have been damaged by bilateral 6-OH-DA injections show diminished spontaneous movement (bradykinesia), rigidity of the limbs, and impairments in orienting their heads toward impinging visual, olfactory, and tactile stimuli (Ungerstedt, 1971; Marshall et al., 1974).

Those rats with virtually complete loss of neostriatal dopamine show extremely severe and apparently permanent deficts in these sensorimotor dysfunctions. Such rats are analogous to the most severely affected Parkinsonian patient, who is incapable of even simple coordinated motor tasks and who must remain in a wheelchair. However, when as little as 10 percent of the neostriatal dopamine content remains after the 6-OH-DA injections, substantial spontaneous recovery from the sensorimotor disorders can occur (Marshall et al., 1974). This recovery begins within the first week postoperatively and continues during at least one month after the brain injury (Marshall, 1979). During recovery the rats show increasingly normal locomotion in their environment, regaining the ability to orient their heads toward objects. These rats are far from normal, however, even months after the surgery. When placed into a deep tank of water, for example, they will swim well for several minutes; but their swim performance declines much more rapidly than does that of neurologically intact animals (Figure 2–5) (Marshall et al., 1976).

### Age-Related Changes in Swimming Movements

Because sustained swimming is a sensitive measure of movement capacities, this task was used to assess how aging affects motor performance. Male Fischer 344 rats 3–4 months or 24–27 months old were put in a cylindrical tank for 15 minutes. At one-minute intervals the observer rated each rat's swim performance by each of two criteria: (1) the *vigor* with which the animal moved its limbs; and, (2) the *success* with which it maintained its head above water.

The young rats swam with vigorous limb movements and effectively maintained their heads above water (Figure 2–6A). Typically, they kept their body axes nearly horizontal to the water surface, moving all four limbs so as to plane across it (Figure 2–7A). Their swim performance declined only gradually during the 15-minute test. In contrast, the old rats swam with vigorous limb movements at the start of the test, but rapidly lost swim vigor after 5 minutes (Figure 2–6A). They kept their heads above water with difficulty during the entire test, lapsing into a more

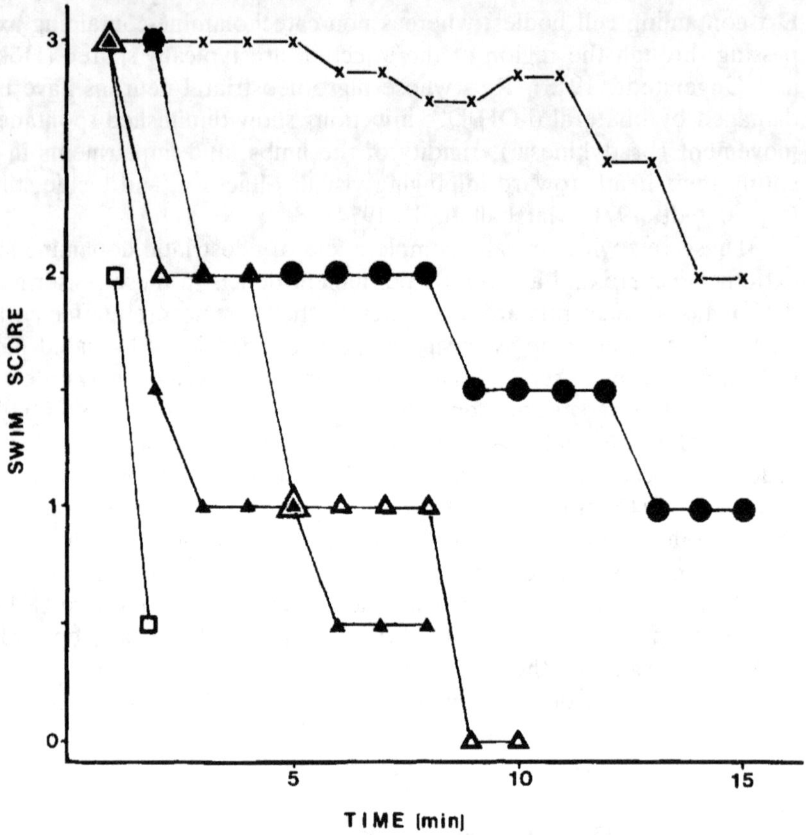


**Figure 2–5:** Recovery from 6-oh-da dopamine lesions in young rats. Swim ratings on representative animals during a 15-minute test. The upper curve (X) represents mean scores for five control young adult rats. The other plots represent individual rats given 6-hydroxydopamine injections (open symbols) or lateral hypothalamic electrolytic lesions (closed symbols) that extensively damage nigroneostriatal dopaminergic neurons. (From Marshall et al., 1976, p. 540.) Three rats were removed from the water before 15 minutes had elapsed to prevent their drowning.

vertical posture soon after the start of the test (Figure 2–7C). After several minutes, most old rats sank repeatedly, intermittently fighting their way back to the surface (Marshall and Berrios, 1979).

## Brain Dopamine and Age-Related Deficits in Swim Performance

In view of the similar impairments in swim performance seen in old rats and in dopamine-deficient young adult animals, it seemed likely that impaired swimming in old rats might be linked to the age-related changes

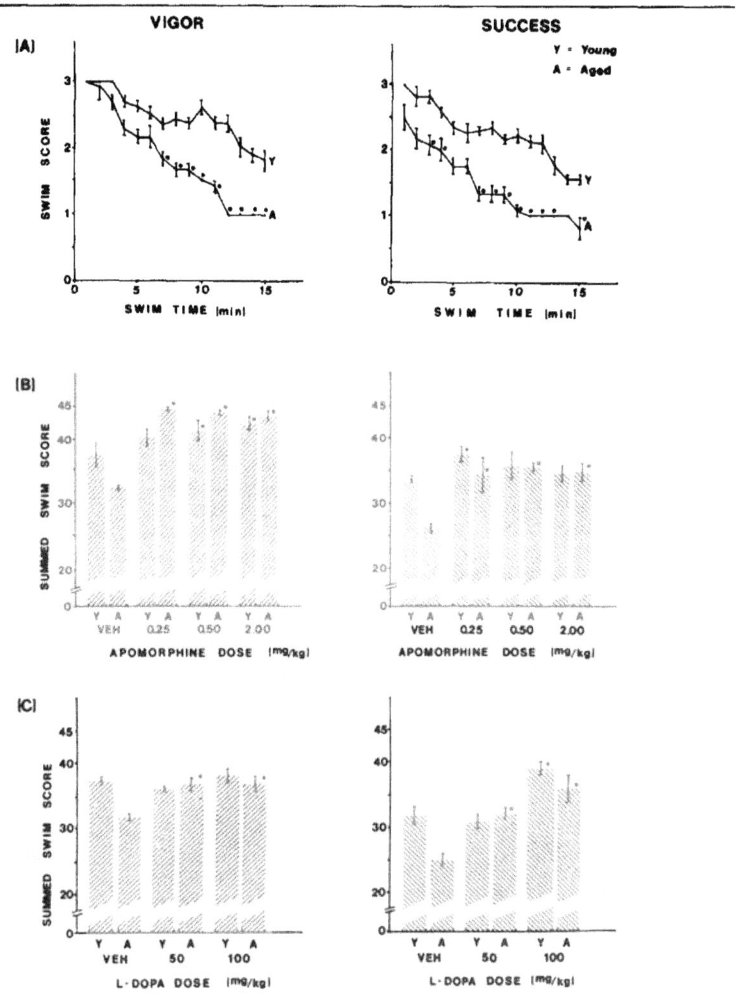


**Figure 2–6:** Swimming in rats—effects of age and response to dopaminegic drugs. Mean (± standard error) swim performance of aged (A, 24–27 months) and young adult (Y, 3–4 months) male Fischer 344 rats that received no drugs (panel A), or were treated with apomorphine (panel B) or L-dopa (panel C). Panel A shows the moment-by-moment swim scores of both age groups. Panels B and C depict the summed swim score for the 15-minute test. In panel A, data indicate significant differences ($p < 0.05$) from young rats. In B and C, dots indicate significant ($p < 0.05$) differences from vehicle (VEH) control group of same age. Each group consisted of 6–25 rats. All drugs were given i.p. The rating scale for *vigor* ranged from 0 (no use of limbs) to 3 (continuous movement of all 4 limbs). The rating scale for success ranged from 0 (rat sank to bottom of tank for ≥ 10 seconds) to 3 (entire head continuously above water).
Source: Marshall, J.F., and Berrios, N. Movement Disorders of aged rats: reversal of dopamine receptor stimulation. *Science*, 1979, *206*, 477–479. Copyright 1979 by the American Association for the Advancement of Science. Reprinted with permission.

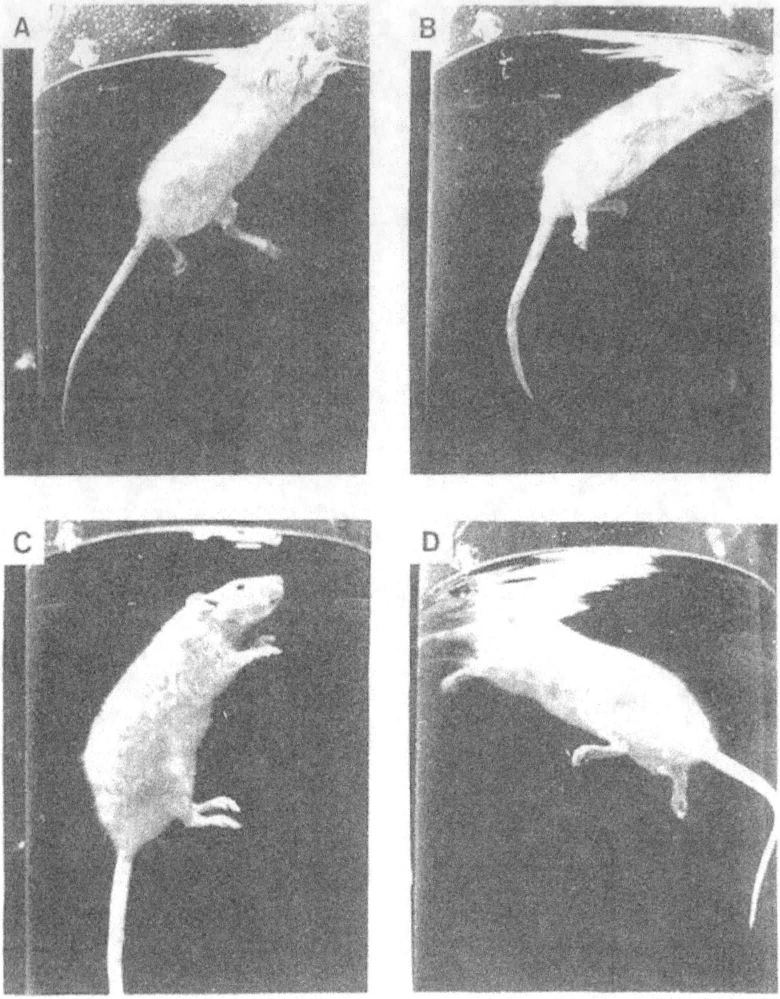


**Figure 2–7:** Effects of age on swimming mechanics in rats. Swimming of young adult (A and B) and old (C and D) rats given apomorphine (0.50 mg/kg) or its vehicle. For description of rats, see Figure 2–6 legend. After apomorphine treatment, the aged animal adopted a more horizontal position (D), similar to that of young adult rats given apomorphine (B) or its vehicle (A).
Source: Marshall, J.F., and Berrios, N. Movement disorders of aged rats: reversal of dopamine receptor stimulation. *Science*, 1979, *206*, 477–479. Copyright 1979 by the American Association for the Advancement of Science. Reprinted with permission.

occurring at brain dopaminergic synapses. If so, then the swimming of old rats should improve following the administration of compounds that enhance brain dopamine receptor stimulation. Prior research demonstrated the efficacy of these drugs in reversing the sensorimotor impairments of young adult rats with brain dopamine depletions (Marshall and Gotthelf, 1979).

Two dopamine agonists have been tested in the aged rats: apomorphine, a dopamine receptor stimulant, and L-dopa, the biosynthetic precursor of catecholamines. When given systemically, L-dopa is decarboxylated to dopamine in the brain (Bartholini et al., 1967). When the old rats were given either of these two compounds, they showed a dramatic rejuvenation of their swim performance, even at very low doses (Figures 2–6B and 2–6C). Their swim performance did not fatigue rapidly, but instead they maintained vigorous and effective swimming for the entire 15 minutes. Like the younger animals, the apomorphine- or L-dopa-treated old rats adopted a more horizontal position (Figure 2–7D), keeping their heads above the water surface for most of the test. Both drugs also produced some improvement in the swimming of the young rats. However, the magnitude of this facilitation was less, and the improvement generally occurred at doses higher than those needed to enhance the swimming of old animals (Marshall and Berrios, 1979).

These pharmacologic experiments provide new evidence that age-related movement disorders are associated with changes in brain dopaminergic synapses. While the poor swim performance of old animals might be attributable to any number of factors (e.g., decreased muscular strength), the finding that this movement disturbance is reversed by centrally acting drugs suggests that the primary deficit is a neurologic one. This conclusion corroborates that reached in studies of motor impairments in aged humans, in which the movement dysfunctions of the elderly are more severe as the psychologic complexity of the task increases (Welford, 1977). Thus, defects in cerebral processing, not of peripheral nerve or muscle, appear to be of overriding importance.

The results suggest the following neurologic model. With advancing age, the neostriatal dopamine synapses undergo progressive neurochemical alterations which affect both the dopamine-containing terminals and their site of action at the postsynaptic membrane. These changes, detailed under Anatomic and Biochemical Studies, above, apparently limit the movement capacities of the old animals by restricting the dopaminergic synaptic activity of the neostriatum. A sudden excess of dopaminergic receptor stimulation, provided either by the dopamine receptor stimulant apomorphine or by the dopamine formed following decarboxylation of L-dopa, would normalize neostriatal dopamine receptor activity, permitting more appropriate sensorimotor functions to occur. The finding that these drugs also slightly enhanced the swim performance in young rats suggests the intriguing possibility that, even in 3–4 month-old rats, the dopamine receptor stimulation is not quite optimal for peak movement capacities to occur. Possibly, young rats maintain a "neurochemical reserve" which is not tapped except in the most extreme emergencies.

### Swimming of Aged Rats and Dopamine-Receptor Blockade

The preceding model predicts that the already fragile dopaminergic synapses of the aging neostriatum should be particularly susceptible to further disruption by administration of drugs that block the action of this neurotransmitter on dopamine receptors. Consequently, the swim performance of the aged rats should be further impaired by dopamine-receptor blocking agents at doses that have little effect on the swim performance of young adult animals. Tests with one such drug, spiroperidol (a potent antagonist of brain dopamine receptors) fully confirmed this expectation and produced a dose-dependent impairment in swimming of aged animals (Figure 2–8). Even at the lowest dose this impairment was obvious. In contrast, young rats showed no impairment in swimming when given the lower doses of spiroperidol. However, young rats swam poorly when given a dose of this drug (O.4 mg/kg) large enough to produce marked catalepsy (Marshall, unpublished).

These findings provide further evidence that age-related movement impairments are associated with a deterioration of neurotransmission at brain dopaminergic synapses. In addition, they suggest a means by which the latent movement problems of aging individuals might be assessed. In elderly subjects who are beginning to display slowness of movements or difficulties in the coordination of complex motor tasks, the extent to which these movement problems are exacerbated by a standard "test dose" of a dopamine-receptor blocking agent might predict the rapidity and/or degree to which these age-related disturbances will increase in later years. Such information might well be used in planning subsequent therapies.

### Neurologic Assessment of the Aged Rat: A Neuropharmacologic Taxonomy

By using swimming as a measure of motor functions, aged rats demonstrate important movement abnormalities that appear related to a hypofunctioning of brain dopaminergic synapses. Swimming is a highly complex act, requiring the coordinated activity of many muscular groups and the appropriate use of sensory information regarding the animal's position in the

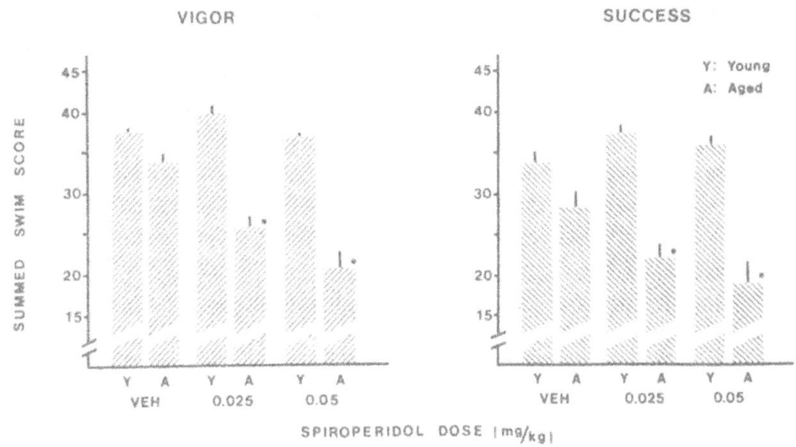


**Figure 2–8:** Effects of spiroperidol (dopamine antagonist) and age on swimming in rats. Mean (± standard error) swim performance of old (A) and young adult (Y) rats that received spiroperidol or its vehicle (VEH). Rats are described in Figure 2–6 legend. Ordinate depicts the summed swim scores for the 15-minute test. Dots indicate significant ($p < 0.05$) differences from vehicle control group of same age.

water and its proximity to the walls of the tank. We are now determining the nature of sensorimotor deficits that afflict the aged rat. To do this, a battery of tests was used to assess the neurologic status of aged and young adult rats. These rodent neurologic tests, adapted from a larger series used on cats and monkeys (Sprague et al., 1963), were previously applied to assessing the neurologic capacities of young rats suffering dopamine-depleting brain injury (see Marshall and Teitelbaum, 1974, for details).

Five classes of sensorimotor capacities are evaluated in this examination.

1. *Limb reflexes:* tactually elicited stepping and proprioceptively evoked placing reactions of the hindlimbs.
2. *Limb tone:* resistance to displacement during passive flexion and extension of all four limbs.
3. *Postural reactions:* latency to remove limbs from an elevated surface, as in the tests for catalepsy (see The Pharmacology and Behavior, below).
4. *Localization of stimuli in space:* extent of head orientation toward olfactory or somatosensory stimuli [light (0.5 g) or moderate (4 g) force applied to different body surfaces] as well as visually elicited limb placing.
5. *Locomotor activity.*

This battery of neurologic examinations has been administered to six aged (30-month-old) and to four young adult (6-month-old) Fischer rats. The old rats were tested twice, once starting 15 minutes after apomorphine (0.5 mg/kg, i.p.) and once after control injection with vehicle. The young adult animals were tested only once, after receiving the vehicle solution. Two comparisons are of interest in this experiment. First, what neurologic functions are different between undrugged aged and young adult animals? Second, which of these age-related neurologic disorders are improved by administration of the dopamine receptor stimulant compound?

The aged control rats showed several neurologic disturbances, when compared with 6-month-old rats (Table 2–1). Marked changes were noted in the tactually elicited placing reflex and proprioceptively elicited lateral stepping reflex of the hindlimbs. The tone of the limbs was also importantly changed, such that the forelimbs showed a spastic flexor reaction when passively extended. The postural reactions studied were normal, as were the measures of exploratory locomotion on a table surface.

The old controls were also deficient in several tests of spatial localization to stimuli. When a light (0.5 g) pressure was applied to their body surface, they oriented less precisely to the contact than did the younger animals. Their orientation to touch of the caudal half of the body surface was particularly impaired. A tendency toward impairment in orientation to odors was also observed. When the animals were moved toward a table surface, they failed to extend their limbs to the sight of the approaching edge.

While the old control rats showed normal locomotor activity in an open field, they typically fell off the table surface at least once during the two-minute test. As they approached the table edge, they would lean over to explore the environment. In contrast to the younger rats, however, the forelimbs would often lose contact with the surface, the old rat would lose balance and fall off. The observed abnormalities in reactions to visual depth (as indicated by the absence of visual placing responses), in limb tone, and in limb reflexes may have contributed to this tendency to fall.

While old rats show a broad spectrum of neurologic deficiencies, only some impairments were reversed by administration of the dopamine-receptor stimulant apomorphine (Table 2–1). The primary effect of apomorphine was to improve the aged rats' localization of odors. Apomorphine also tended to enhance the localization of touch on the body surface ($0.05 < P < 0.1$). However, the visually elicited limb placing reaction was not significantly improved. Neither were these rats' impairments in simple limb reflexes and limb tone affected by this drug.

In conclusion, dopamine agonists markedly enhance the movement capabilities of the aged rat. When the neurologic capacities of the old rat

Table 2–1
Neurologic Examinations
Old (30 mos) v. Young Adult (6 mos) Male Fischer 344 Rats

| | No drug treatment | | Apomorphine |
|---|---|---|---|
| | YOUNG ADULT ($N = 4$) | OLD ($n = 6$) | OLD ($N = 6$) |
| Limb reflexes (% of animals showing normal response in both limbs) | | | |
| Hindlimb tactile placing | 100.0% | 0.0%[a] | 16.7% |
| Hindlimb lateral stepping | 100.0% | 0.0%[a] | 16.7% |
| Limb tone (% of animals showing normal tone in both limbs) | | | |
| Forelimbs | 100.0% | 0.0%[a] | 0.0% |
| Hindlimbs | 100.0% | 83.3% | 50.0% |
| Postural reactions | | | |
| Duration of forelimb catalepsy (sec.) | 6.5 | 4.3 | 5.0 |
| Duration of hindlimb catalepsy (sec.) | 7.2 | 4.8 | 4.3 |
| Open field activity | | | |
| Mean number of squares entered per 2 min. | 5.5 | 11.0 | 6.3 |
| Mean number of upward rears per 2 min. | 1.5 | 1.7 | 1.2 |
| Percentage of rats slipping off surface in 2 min. | 0.0% | 66.7%[a] | 50.0% |
| Localization of stimuli | | | |
| Somatosensory orientation (% of perfect score) | | | |
| Light touch (0.5 g) | 80.4% | 55.7%[a] | 61.4% |
| Moderate touch (4 g) | 84.4% | 70.8% | 68.0% |
| Olfactory orientation (% of perfect score) | 75.0% | 44.0% | 92.0%[b] |
| Visually elicited limb placing (% of animals showing response) | 100.0% | 0.0%[a] | 16.7% |

[a]Significantly different from young adult group, $p < 0.05$.
[b]Significantly different from undrugged old group, $p < 0.05$.

are examined in detail, only certain of their dysfunctions are reversed by this drug treatment. This finding is expected, since the age-related deterioration that occurs in the brains of aged animals and humans involves many other types of synapses and pathways as well as the dopaminergic ones of the basal ganglia. The present findings suggest that the impaired spatial localization of stimuli by aged rats may be linked to age-related disturbances at dopaminergic synapses of the basal ganglia, whereas the alterations in limb tone and limb reflexes may be due to degenerative processes occurring in other, perhaps cortical or spinal neurons (Sant'ambrogio et al., 1961; Feldman and Dowd, 1975; Johnson et al., 1975; Huttenlocher, 1979). These findings provide the basis for a "neuropharamacologic taxonomy" of the sensorimotor disturbances of aging. Perhaps compounds that act directly at noradrenergic, cholinergic, or other central synapses might provide relief for the limb dysfunctions observed.

## THE PHARMACOLOGY AND BEHAVIOR OF BASAL GANGLIA FUNCTIONS IN THE AGING C57BL/6J MOUSE

### Effects of Neuroleptics

The "major tranquilizers," antipsychotics, or neuroleptics are widely used in the elderly as a convenient therapy for various psychotic or behavioral problems (e.g., DeVeaugh-Geiss, 1979). Many of these drugs are also dopamine antagonists, such as the butyrophenones [e.g., haloperidol (Haldol®) and spiroperidol (Spiperone®)] or the phenothiazines (e.g., Thorazine® and chlorpromazine). The number of older patients regularly administered neuroleptics is vast: over 35 percent of the Medicaid prescriptions for the elderly were for tranquilizers and sedatives (Butler, 1976). In view of the diminished dopaminergic functions in the basal ganglia with age, it would be expected that the elderly would be at higher risk for the development of drug-induced movement disorders than the younger population. Children and young adults are more likely to experience transient dystonia (oculogyric crises and abnormal postures of the head and neck) at the onset of neuroleptic therapy (Kramer and Klawans, 1979). However, the elderly have the highest incidence of the more chronic and potentially disabling disorders, including drug-induced Parkinsonism and tardive dyskinesia ("oral-buccal syndrome") which are discussed below. These two disorders are quite distinct and raise basic questions regarding basal ganglia function and aging.

**Drug-induced Parkinsonism**

Drug-induced Parkinsonism (pseudo-Parkinsonism) resulting from neuroleptic treatment may include all the primary symptoms of idiopathic or post-encephalitic Parkinsonism (e.g., tremor, rigidity, and bradykinesia). The most prevalent symptom is bradykinesia, or poverty of movement, which is thought to result from a simple pharmacologic blockade of neostriatal DA receptors by the neuroleptics. Susceptibility to drug-induced Parkinsonism is related to the dose of the neuroleptic, and more importantly increases with the age of the patient (Ayd, 1961; Crane, 1974; Kramer and Klawans, 1979). When this syndrome occurs, symptoms generally arise by three days and spontaneously remit by three months (Hollister, 1972; Klett and Caffey, 1972; Kramer and Klawans, 1979), probably as a result of compensatory mechanisms in the nigro-neostriatal system.

A major animal model for the bradykinetic side effects of drug-induced Parkinsonism is the induction of *catalepsy* in the rodent. Within 20 minutes after administration of neuroleptics, rats and mice placed in an abnormal posture (usually involving a stretching of postural muscles) will remain in that posture for a length of time related to the dose of the drug, often several minutes.

Since elderly humans are more likely to show Parkinsonism during treatment with neuroleptics and since aging rodents show greater motor impairments with these drugs (see above) as well as some similar dopaminergic deficits as humans (see above), it might be expected that the aging rodent would be more sensitive to neuroleptics with respect to catalepsy: that is, the abnormal posture might be held longer in older rodents with the same neuroleptic dose. Surprisingly, in pilot experiments and in control pretests in experiments described below, 24-month-old mice and 16-month-old rats remained in the abnormal posture for *shorter,* rather than longer periods of time than did the 3–5-month-old controls (Randall, unpubl.). Figure 2–9 shows these results in one experiment with three ages of C57BL/6J mice. A progressive *decrease* in immobility time with increasing age is apparent. With increasing exposure, however, the older animals quickly *increase* their immobility time while younger controls developed a moderate tolerance.

These preliminary observations suggest: (1) If an increased sensitivity to haloperidol exists in the older animals, it may be masked by a compensatory process or by an associated counteracting age deficit in some other system. And (2) with increasing exposure to the drug the aging animal's compensatory ability is exhausted and the underlying dopaminergic deficit is exposed.

These hypotheses are not mutually exclusive. In the first case, it is well known that similar cataleptic behavior can be induced by centrally

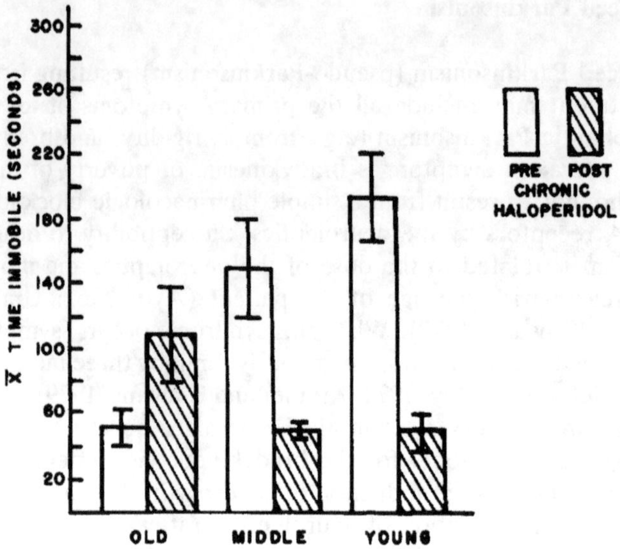


**Figure 2–9:** Haloperidol-induced catalepsy in aging mice. C57BL/6J male mice aged 4 months (young), 12 months (middle-aged), and 24 months (old). Bars represent mean total immobility time across four tests at hourly intervals following injection of 0.6 mg/kg haloperidol, i.p. Testing was conducted by placing mice head-downward on a 45° ramp constructed of 1/4-inch wire mesh and slightly pulling the tail. Movement of all four-paws was used as the criterion for termination of response. The Age × Chronic Drug Treatment interaction (ANOVA) was significant ($p < 0.05$) with significant age effects within both the pre- and post-drug periods. In addition pre- and post-drug differences were significant in all age groups (ANOVA, $p < 0.05$).

acting dopamine blockers or from cholinergic agonists (Timsit, 1966; Zetler, 1968). Furthermore, the cholinergic antagonists scopolamine or atropine block the catalepsy produced by dopaminergic antagonists in young rodents (Costall and Olley, 1971; Baez et al., 1976). These characteristics suggest a mechanism in which dopaminergic antagonists release a cholinergic effector system from inhibition. The integrity of this final cholinergic link is postulated to be a necessary condition for the behavior. Similar relationships appear to hold in Parkinson's disease: cholinergic agonists exacerbate Parkinsonism, while cholinergic antagonists are therapeutic (Duvoisin, 1967; Greenblatt and Shader, 1973). In fact, anticholinergics are often given in combination with neuroleptics to lessen the Parkinsonian side effects of the neuroleptics (Klawans and Rubovits, 1974). A positive cholinergic balance or tone in the striatum tends toward bradykinesia and other Parkinsonian symptoms, whereas a positive dopaminergic tone tends toward choreic movement, dyskinesias, or other uncontrollable motor activity as seen in Huntington's disease or tardive dyskinesia (see Introduction).

If aging rodents have deficient cholinergic effector systems for the cataleptic response, then older mice would be predicted to have a smaller cataleptic response to pilocarpine, a cholinergic stimulant. This prediction is realized: older mice had a shorter immobility after pilocarpine and significantly less catalepsy (Figure 2–10)(Randall, unpubl.).

Age-related deficiencies in cholinergic neostriatal neurons could contribute to the behavioral differences during aging in laboratory rodents. The small decreases of neostriatal choline acetyltransferase tend to support this possibility (see Anatomic and Biochemical Studies, above). However, the anatomic locus of pilocarpine action is much less clear than that of neuroleptic-induced catalepsy. Since cholinergically mediated catalepsy is still inducible following relatively complete surgical removal of the neostriatum in the rat (Costall and Olley, 1971), catalepsy requires the participation of neuronal systems other than those directly controlled

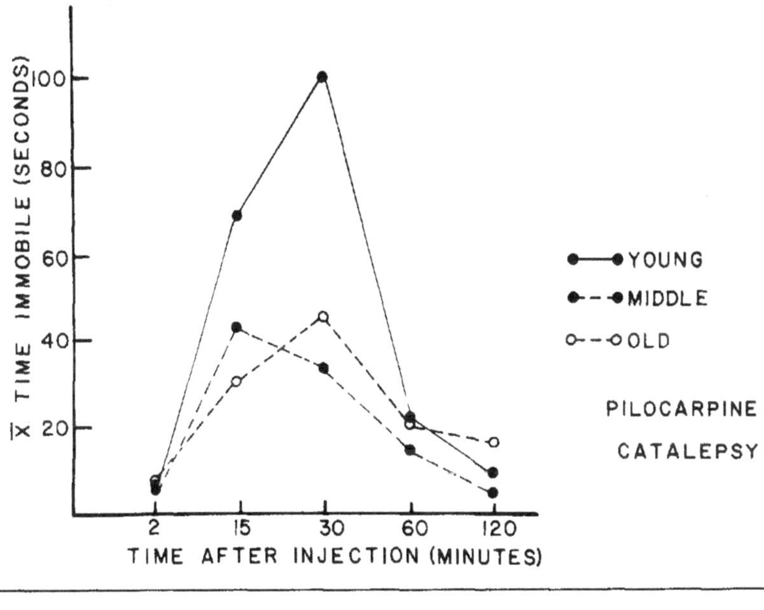


**Figure 2–10:** Pilocarpine-induced catalepsy in aging mice. Mice described in Figure 2–9, legend. Curves represent time immobile at various intervals after injection of 8 mg/kg pilocarpine, i.p. (see Figure 2–9 for testing procedure). The age effect (ANOVA) was significant ($P < 0.05$) with young mice having significantly higher scores ($p < 0.05$) than middle-aged or old mice, which did not differ from each other. Mice were pretreated with methyl-scopolamine (2 mg/kg, i.p.) to protect against peripheral cholinergic effects of pilocarpine.

by the nigrostriatal system. Thus the interaction of age and drugs on catalepsy and swimming responses cannot be simply equated. The swimming deficit caused by very low doses of spiroperidol in old rats (see Anatomic and Biochemical Studies, above) may more directly mirror the status of the nigrostriatal pathway. These data do suggest, however, that in some situations, nigrostriatal deficiencies may be masked by other age-related changes efferent to the dopaminergic synapse (see Dopaminergic Receptors, above).

The second hypothesis, that of decreased compensatory ability in the aging animal, has more direct supporting evidence. Of the several mechanisms which might participate in compensation for nigrostriatal lesions or chronic neuroleptic blockade, one of the most important is thought to be the development of a "denervation" supersensitivity. That is, with decreasing dopaminergic input, certain postsynaptic, neostriatal dopaminergic receptor populations may become more sensitive to the remaining presynaptic dopamine outflow: this compensation could conceivably normalize the functional output of the system as a whole.

It is well-documented that chronic neuroleptic treatment or surgical disruption of the dopamine pathway induces "supersensitivity" to dopaminergic agonists by behavioral, biochemical, and electrophysiologic criteria. Old mice fail to develop dopaminergic supersensitivity responses after chronic treatment with haloperidol (described under Anatomic and Biochemical Studies, above, and Figures 2–3 and 2–4). The increase in dopamine receptors in supersensitivity responses may be partially responsible for the eventual spontaneous disappearance of Parkinsonian symptoms in many patients chronically treated with neuroleptics (Hollister, 1972; Klette and Caffey, 1972). Increased incidence of these disorders in the elderly during neuroleptic treatment then might be a result of a deficiency in the capacity of this mechanism.

An inability to compensate for age-related decreases in presynaptic dopamine may be of importance, not only in the elevated occurrence of drug-induced Parkinsonism in the elderly, but also in the general physiologic importance of those deficits observed with presynaptic biochemical markers. Even very moderate decreases in striatal dopamine outflows might be functionally important if the animal is no longer capable of invoking compensatory mechanisms to counteract them.

Unfortunately, the molecular mechanisms of these age-related deficits of synaptic regulation are extremely obscure. It seems unlikely that aging animals and humans are completely unable to increase dopaminergic receptor number. Tardive dyskinesia, thought to be related to a pathologic dopaminergic supersensitivity, is more common in the elderly population (see below). There is also evidence for increased numbers of dopamine receptors in Parkinson's disease, possibly in association with their massive loss of nigral neurons (Lee et al., 1978), which is observed in patients of slightly younger ages than corresponds to the old mice described above. Additionally, Joseph and co-workers (1978) have observed some turning behavior to apomorphine following unilateral lesions of the substantia nigra in aged rats (this behavior is thought to result from the imbalance occurring with stimulation of dopamine receptors in both striata, one of which is supersensitive). A more potent chronic stimulus than that used in this study may have induced a receptor number elevation. Age-related deficits in receptor synthesis, neural membrane characteristics, or response to the neuroleptic may be involved. In any event, the discovery of the locus of this aging deficit would be extremely significant, not only to the study of aging but to the understanding of the basic striatal function as well.

## Tardive Dyskinesia

Tardive dyskinesia or the "oral-buccal syndrome" is an occasional motoric side effect of neuroleptic treatment which normally occurs much later in the therapeutic regime than does drug-induced Parkinsonism. It is most often marked by uncontrollable and often unconscious movements of the tongue and lower jaw, with occasional involvement of the limbs and trunk in severe cases (Crane and Smeets, 1974; Crane, 1973; Marsden et al., 1975; Jus et al., 1976; Kramer and Klawans, 1979). This disorder is thought to result from a neuroleptic-induced supersensitivity (Klawans, 1973). Several lines of evidence support this contention: (1) the disorder often first appears on discontinuation of the drug; (2) increasing the dose of the neuroleptic will temporarily alleviate the symptoms; and, (3) L-dopa and other dopamine agonists in small doses exacerbate the condition. The presence of uncontrollable oral-buccal movements, rather than bradykinesia, is more suggestive of a dopaminergic *hyper*activity and is consistent with dopaminergic receptor supersensitivity.

However, unlike the drug-induced Parkinsonism, tardive dyskinesia does not usually disappear with withdrawal of neuroleptics, and may even be worsened by withdrawal (Crane, 1968). Some investigators consider the condition permanent. Even in mild cases, it may persist for months or years following drug termination (Degkwitz et al., 1967; Klawans, 1973). Remarkably, even though this effect would seem less likely to occur in an age group associated in C57BL/6J mice with diminished basal receptor number and diminished drug-induced supersensitivity responses, the elderly are more likely to develop this abnormality than are the young (Crane, 1974; Jus et al., 1976; Simpson et al., 1978).

This apparent paradox may derive from the heterogeneity of the dopamine receptors. Various subpopulations of dopamine receptors can be distinguished according to anatomic location (Govani et al., 1978; Minneman et al., 1978; Schwarcz et al., 1978), affinity for pharmacologic ligands (Burt et al., 1976; Beld et al., 1978; Pedigo et al., 1978; Riddall and Levins, 1978; Creese et al., 1979), and degree of coupling with adenylate cyclase (Minneman et al., 1978; Kebabian and Calne, 1979). A critical question regarding the loss of receptors and reduction in receptor supersensitivity in aging is the degree to which these effects are restricted to one or more of the receptor subpopulations. For example, supersensitivity is not restricted to the postsynaptic adenylcyclase coupled receptor. Presynaptic receptors, capable of diminishing the firing rate of nigral neurons or local modulation of dopamine in the synaptic cleft also, are increased in sensitivity (and possibly number) following chronic use of neuroleptics (Gallager et al., 1978). Normally, then, the supersensitivity of the postsynaptic receptor is somewhat counterbalanced by enhanced sensitivity of a negative feedback loop for dopamine release. Major loss during aging of the modulatory receptor change might magnify any slight increase in postsynaptic sensitivity that might occur in elderly subjects. Although highly conjectural at this point, such a mechanism is plausible. For example, dopaminergic cells in the substantia nigra increased, rather than decreased, their firing rate after low doses of apomorphine, i.v. (Lucik et al., 1980). Further electrophysiological studies are now being conducted to characterize the functional output of the nigro-neostriatal system and age–drug interactions (Randall, 1980). It is of interest that some improvement of dyskinesia occurs after low doses of apomorphine (Carroll et al., 1977; Tolosa, 1974); presumably apomorphine selectively stimulates the presynaptic receptor to reduce dopamine outflow.

## CONCLUSIONS

We describe here recent results from our laboratories and elsewhere which demonstrate several types of major changes and dysfunctions during aging in the basal ganglia, at anatomic, biochemical, and behavioral levels. The attrition of the nigro-neostriatal pathway and the impairments of postsynaptic striatal mechanisms during aging are observed to varying extents in laboratory rodents and humans. It thus may be considered that these changes are widely distributed in aging mammals. Even if the roles of neuronal loss and the nature of the cellular dysfunctions is not yet clearly established, effective therapies for the treatment and possibly prevention of basal gangliar disorders with age can still be considered. A remarkable spectrum of dopaminergic, cholinergic, and other interventions is possible through synaptically active drugs and nutrition (Wurtman and Growdon, 1978). The efficacy of apomorphine and L-dopa in ameliorating some problems in old rats indicates that in aging some components of the basal ganglia retain an extensive potential for normal functions, when given appropriate stimuli. Since new approaches can be readily screened in currently available rodent models, a major attack on the basal ganglia dysfunctions with age is now feasible.

## REFERENCES

Adolfsson, R., Gottfries, C.G., Roos, B.E., and Winblad, B. Post-mortem distribution of dopamine and homovanillic acid in human brain, variations related to age, and review of the literature. *Journal of Neural Transmission,* 1979, *45,* 81–105.

Agid, Y., Javoy, F., and Glowinski, J. Chemical or electrolytic lesion of the substantia nigra: early effects on neostriatal dopamine metabolism. *Brain Research,* 1974, *74,* 41–49.

Ayd, F.J. A survey of drug-induced extra-pyramidal reactions. *Journal of the American Medical Association,* 1961, *175,* 1054–1060.

Baez, L.A., Eskridge, N.K., and Shein, R. Postnatal development of dopaminergic and cholinergic catalepsy in the rat. *European Journal of Pharmacology,* 1976, *36,* 155–162.

Barbeau, A. The pathogenesis of Parkinson's disease: A new hypothesis. *Canadian Medical Association Journal,* 1962, *87,* 802–807.

Bartholini, G., Burkard, W.P., Pletscher, A., and Bates, H.M. Increase of cerebral catecholamines caused by 3,4-dihydroxyphenylalanine after inhibition of peripheral decarboxylase. *Nature,* 1967, *215,* 852–853.

Bennett, K.D., and Bondareff, W. Age-related differences in binding of concanavalin A to plasma membranes of isolated neurons. *American Journal of Anatomy,* 1977, *150,* 175–184.

Bernheimer, H., Birkmayer, W., Hornykiewicz, O., Jellinger, K., and Seitilberger, F. Brain dopamine and the syndrome of Parkinson and Huntington. Clinical, morphological and neurochemical correlations. *Journal of Neurological Sciences,* 1973, *20,* 415–455.

Bird, E.D., and Iversen, L.L. Huntington's chorea. Post-mortem measurement of glutamic acid decarboxylase, choline acetyltransferase, and dopamine in basal ganglia. *Brain,* 1974, *97,* 457–472.

Bowen, D.M., Smith, C.B., White, P., and Davison, A.N. Neurotransmitter-related enzymes and indices of hypoxia in senile dementia and other abiotrophies. *Brain,* 1976, *99,* 459–496.

Brody, H. An examination of cerebral cortex and brain stem aging. In R.D. Terry and S. Gershon, (Eds.), *Aging,* vol. 3, *Neurobiology of Aging.* New York: Raven Press, 1976.

Bruyn, G.W. Huntington's chorea. Historical, clinical and laboratory synopsis. In P.J. Vinken and G.W. Bruyn (Eds.), *Handbook of Clinical Neurology,* vol. 6. New York: Wiley, 1968.

Bugiani, O., Salvarani, S., Perdelli, F., Mancardi, G.L., and Leonardi, A. Nerve cell loss with aging in the putamen. *European Neurology*, 1978, *17*, 286–291.

Bugiani, O., Perdelli, F., Salvarini, S., Leonardi, A., and Mancardi, G.L. Loss of striatal neurons in Parkinson's disease: a cytophotometric study. *European Neurology*, 1980, *19*, 339–344.

Burch, P.R.J. Huntington's chorea. Age at onset in relation to etiology and pathogenesis. In P.J. Vinken and G.W. Bruyn (Eds.), *Handbook of Clinical Neurology, Diseases of the Basal Ganglia.* New York: Wiley, 1968.

Burt, D.R., Geese, I., and Snyder, S.H. Anti-schizophrenic drugs: chronic treatment elevates dopamine receptor binding in brain. *Science*, 1977, *196*, 326–328.

Butler, R.N. The overuse of tranquilizers in older patients. *International Journal of Aging Human Development*, 1976, *7*, 185–187.

Calne, D.B., Williams, A.C., Nutt, J.G., Neophytides, A., Eisler, T., and Teychenne, P.F. Ergot derivatives for Parkinsonism. *Medical Journal of Australia*, 1978, Special Suppl. 25–26.

Carlsson, A., and Winblad, B. Influence of age and time interval between death and autopsy on dopamine and 3-methoxytyramine levels in human basal ganglia. *Journal of Neural Transmission*, 1976, *38*, 171–176.

Carroll, B.J., Curtis, G.C., and Kokmen, E. Paradoxical response to dopamine agonists in tardive dyskinesia. *American Journal of Psychiatry*, 1977, *134*, 785–789.

Chaconas, G., and Finch, C.E. The effect of aging on RNA/DNA ratios in brain regions of the C57BL/6J male mouse. *Journal of Neurochemistry*, 1973, *21*, 1469–1473.

Colman, P.D., Kaplan, B.D., Osterburg, H.H., and Finch, C.E. Brain poly(A)RNA during aging: stability of yield and sequence complexity in two rat strains. *Journal of Neurochemistry*, 1980, *34*, 335–345.

Corsellis, J.A.N. From a floor discussion. In R. Katzman, R.D. Terry, and K.L. Bick (Eds.), *Alzheimer's Disease: Senile Dementia and Related Disorders*, vol. 7, *Aging*. New York: Raven Press, 1978.

Costall, B., and Olley, J.E. Cholinergic and neuroleptic-induced catalepsy: modification by lesions in the caudate-putamen. *Neuropharmacology*, 1971, *10*, 297–306.

Cote, L.J., and Kremzner, L.T. Changes in neurotransmitter systems with increasing age in human brain. *Transactions of the American Society for Neurochemistry*, 5th Annual Meeting, New Orleans, 1974, p. 83.

Cotman, C.W., and Scheff, S.W. Compensatory synapse growth in aged animals after neuronal death. *Mechanisms of Ageing and Development*, 1979, *9*, 103–117.

Cotzias, G.C., Van Woert, M.H., and Schiffer, L.M. Aromatic amino acids and modification of Parkinsonism. *New England Journal of Medicine*, 1967, *276*, 374–379.

Crane, G.E. Tardive dyskinesia in patients treated with major neuroleptics. *American Journal of Psychiatry*, 1968, *124*, 40–48.

Crane, G.E. Persistant dyskinesia. *British Journal of Psychiatry*, 1973, *122*, 395–405.

Crane, G.E. Factors predisposing to drug-induced neurologic effects. In F.S. Forrest, C.J. Carr, and E. Usdin (Eds.), *Advances in Biochemical Pharmacology: Phenothiazines and Structurally Related Drugs*, vol. 9. New York: Raven Press, 1974.

Crane, G.E., and Smeets, R.A. Tardive dyskinesia and drug therapy in geriatric patients. *Archives of General Psychiatry*, 1974, *30*, 341–343.

Critchley, M. Neurologic changes in the aged. *Journal of Chronic Diseases*, 1956, *3*, 459–477.

Davies, P. Loss of choline acetyltransferase activity in normal aging and in senile dementia. In C.E. Finch, D. Potter, and A.D. Kenny (Eds.), *Parkinson Disease–II, Aging & Neuroendocrine Relationships*, vol. 113, *Advances in Experimental Medicine and Biology*. New York: Plenum Press, 1978.

Degkwitz, R., Binsack, D.F., Herkert, H., Luxemberger, O., and Wenzel, W. Zum Probleme der persistierenden Hyperkinesien nach langfristiger Anwendung von neuroleptica. *Nervonarzt*, 1967, *38*, 170–174.

De Veaugh-Geiss, S. Neuroleptic drugs: how to reduce the risk of tardive dyskinesia. *Geriatrics*, 1979, *34*, 59–66.

Demarest, K.T., Riegle, G.D., and Moore, K. Characteristics of dopaminergic neurons in the aged male rat. *Neuroendocrinology*, 1980, *31*, 222–227.

Duvoisin, R.C. Cholinergic-anticholinergic antagonism in Parkinsonism. *Archives of Neurology*, 1967, *17*, 124–136.

Ernst, A.M., and Smelik, P.G. Site of action of dopamine and amphetamine on compulsive gnawing in the rat. *Experientia*, 1966, *22*, 837–838.

Feldman, M.L., and Dowd, C. Loss of dendritic spines in aging cerebral cortex. *Anatomy and Embryology*, 1975, *148*, 279–301.

Finch, C.E. Catecholamine metabolism in the brains of aging male mice. *Brain Research*, 1973, *52*, 261–276.

Finch, C.E. The regulation of physiological changes during mammalian aging. *Quarterly Review of Biology*, 1976, *51*, 49–83.

Finch, C.E. The relationships of aging changes in the basal ganglia to manifestations of Huntington's chorea. *Annals of Neurology*, 1980, *7*, 406–411.

Finch, C.E., Jonec, V., Hody, G., Walker, J.P., Morton-Smith, W., Alper, A., and Dougher, G.J. Aging and the passage of L-tyrosine and inulin into mouse brain slices in vitro. *Journal of Gerontology*, 1975, *30*, 33–40.

Fog, R., and Pakkenberg, H. Behavioral effects of dopamine and *p*-hydroxyamphetamine injected into corpus striatum of rats. *Experimental Neurology*, 1971, *31*, 75–86.

Forno, L.S., and Jose, C. Huntington's chorea: a pathological study. *Advances in Neurology*, 1973, *1*, 453–470.

Freyhan, F.A. Psychomotility and parkinsonism in treatment with neuroleptic drugs. *Archives of Pathology* (AMA), 1957, *78*, 465–472.

Gallager, D.W., Pert, A., and Bunney, N.E. Haloperidol-induced presynaptic dopamine supersensitivity is blocked by chronic lithium. *Nature*, 1978, *273*, 309–312.

Ganong, W.F. *The Nervous System*. Los Altos, Calif.: Lange Medical Publishers, 1977.

Geinisman, Y., Bondareff, W., and Telser, A. Diminished axonal transport of glycoproteins in the senescent rat brain. *Mechanisms of Ageing and Development*, 1977, *6*, 363–378.

Gottfries, G.G., Gottfries, I., Johansson, B., Olsson, R., Persson, T., Roos, B.E. and Sjostrom, R. Acid monoamine metabolites in human cerebrospinal fluid and their relations to age and sex. *Neuropharmacology*, 1971, *10*, 665–672.

Govoni, S., Loddo, P., Spano, P.F., and Trabucchi, M. Dopamine receptor sensitivity in brain and retina of rats during aging. *Brain Research*, 1977, *138*, 565–570.

Govoni, S., Memo, M., Saiani, L., Spano, P.F., and Trabucchi, M. Impairment of brain neurotransmitter receptors in aged rats. *Mechanisms of Ageing and Development,* 1980, *12,* 39–46.

Greenblatt, D.J., and Shader, R.I. Anticholinergics. *New England Journal of Medicine,* 1973, *228,* 1215–1219.

Greenberg, L.H., and Weiss, B. Ability of aged rats to alter β-adrenergic receptors of brain in response to repeated administration of reserpine and desmethylimiprimine. *Journal of Pharmacology and Experimental Therapeutics,* 1979, *211,* 309–316.

Hassler, R. The pathological basis of tremor and parkinsonism. *Excerpta Medica,* 1955, Sect. *8*: 769.

Hefti, F., Melamed, E., Liebman, J., and Wurtman, R.J. Decarboxylation of DOPA in the rat striatum after complete and partial unilateral lessions of the nigrostriatal system. Society of Neuroscience, 9th Annual Meeting, *Abstracts,* 1979, *5,* 336.

Hirata, F., Strittmatter, W.J., and Axelrod, J. α-Adrenergic receptors agonists increase phospholipid methylation, membrane fluidity, and α-adrenergic receptor-adenylate cyclase coupling. *Proceedings of the National Academy of Sciences of the United States,* 1979, *76,* 368–372.

Hökfelt, T., and Ungerstedt, U. Specificity of 6-hydroxydopamine-induced degeneration of central monoamine neurones: an electron and fluorescence microscopic study with special reference to intracerebral injection on the nigro-striatal dopamine system. *Brain Research,* 1973, *60,* 269–297.

Hollister, L.E. Mental disorders-antipsychotic and antimanic drugs. *New England Journal of Medicine,* 1972, *286,* 984–987.

Hornykiewicz, O. Commentary: Parkinson's disease and its chemotherapy. *Biochemical Pharmacy,* 1975, *24,* 1061–1065.

Huttenlocher, P.R. Synaptic density in human frontal cortex-development changes and effects of aging. *Brain Research,* 1979, *163,* 195–205.

Johnson, J.E. Jr., Mehler, W.R., and Miquel, J. A fine structural study of degenerative changes in the dorsal column nuclei of aging mice. Lack of protection by Vitamin E. *Journal of Gerontology,* 1975, *30,* 395–411.

Jonec, V.J., and Finch, C.E. Senescence and dopamine uptake by subcellular fractions of the C57BL/6J male mouse brain. *Brain Research,* 1975, *91,* 197–215.

Joseph, J.A., Berger, R.E., Engle, B.T., and Roth, G.S. Age-related changes in the neostriatum: A behavioral and biochemical analysis. *Journal of Gerontology,* 1978, *33,* 643–649.

Jus, A., Pineau, R., Lachance, R., Pelchaut, G., Jus, K., Pires, P., and Villeneuve, R. Epidemiology of tardive dyskinesia. Part I. *Diseases of the Nervous System,* 1976, *37,* 210–214.

Klawans, H.L. A pharmacologic analysis of Huntington's chorea. *European Neurology,* 1970, *4,* 148–163.

Klawans, H.L. The pharmacology of tardive dyskinesia. *American Journal of Psychiatry,* 1973, *130,* 82–86.

Klawans, H.L., and Rubovits, R. Effect of cholinergic and anticholinergic agents on tardive dyskinesia. *Journal of Neurology and Neurosurgery and Psychiatry,* 1977, *27,* 941–947.

Klawans, H.L. Jr., Paulson, G.W., Ringel, S.P., and Barbeau, A. Use of L-DOPA in the detection of presymptomatic Huntington's chorea. *New England Journal of Medicine,* 1972, *286,* 1332–1334.

Klawans, H.L. Jr., Goetz, C.G., and Perlik, S. Presymptomatic and early detection in Huntington's disease. *Annals of Neurology,* 1980, *8,* 343–347.

Klett, C.J., and Caffey, E. Evaluating the long-term need for antiparkinson's drugs by chronic schizophrenics. *Archives of General Psychiatry,* 1972, *26,* 374–379.

Klintworth, G.K. Huntington's chorea—morphologic contributions of a century. *Advances in Neurology,* vol. 1. New York: Raven Press, 1973.

Kramer, J., and Klawans, H.L. Involuntary movement disorders—each has a meaning all its own. *Geriatrics,* 1979, *34,* 63–71.

Le Poncin-Lafitte, M., and Rapin, J.R. Age-associated changes in deoxyglucose uptake in whole brain. *Gerontology,* 1980, *26,* 265–269.

Lee, T., Seeman, P., Rajput, A., Farley, I.J., and Hornykiewicz, O. Receptor basis for dopaminergic supersensitivity in Parkinson's disease. *Nature,* 1978, *273,* 59–60.

Levitzki, A. The role of GTP in the activation of adenylate cyclase. *Biochemical and Biophysical Research Communications,* 1977, *74,* 1154–1159.

Lewis, A.J. *Mechanisms of Neurologic Disease.* Boston: Little, Brown, 1976.

Lieberman, A.N., Kupersmith, M., Gopinathan, G., Goodgold, A., and Goldstein, M. Bromocriptine in Parkinson's diseases. *Neurology,* 1979, *29,* 363–369.

London, E.D., Nespor, S.M., Ohata, M., and Rapoport, S.I. Local cerebral glucose utilization during development and aging of the Fischer–344 rat. *Journal of Neurochemistry,* in press.

Lucik, R.R., Chiodio, L.A., and Caggiula, A.R. Changes in dopamine autoreceptor sensitivity. *Society of Neuroscience Abstracts,* 1980, *6,* 451.

Machado-Salas, J.P., and Scheibel, A.B. Limbic system of the aged mouse. *Experimental Neurology,* 1979, *63,* 347–355.

Machado-Salas, J., Scheibel, M.E., and Scheibel, A.B. Morphologic changes in the hypothalamus of the old mouse. *Experimental Neurology,* 1977, *57,* 102–111.

Makman, M.G., Ahn, H.S., Thal, L.J., Sharpless, N.S., Dvorkin, B., Horowitz, S.G., and Rosenfeld, M. Biogenic amine-stimulated adenylate cyclase and spiroperidol binding sites in rabbit brain: evidence for selective loss of receptors during aging. In C.E. Finch, D.E. Potter, and A.D. Kenny (Eds.), *Parkinson's Disease—II. Aging & Neuroendocrine Relationships,* vol. 113, *Advances in Experimental Medicine and Biology.* New York: Plenum Press, 1978.

Mann, D.M.A., and Yates, P.O. The effects of aging on the pigmented nerve cells of the human locus caeruleus and substantia nigra. Acta *Neuropathologica* (Berlin), 1979, *49,* 93–97.

Marsden, C.D., Tarsy, D., and Baldessarini, R.J. Spontaneous and drug-induced movement disorders in psychiatric patients. In D.F. Benson and D. Blumer (Eds.), *Psychiatric of Aspects Neurological Disease.* New York: Grune & Stratton, 1975.

Marshall, J.F. Somatosensory inattention after dopamine-depleting intracerebral 6-OHDA injections: Spontaneous recovery and pharmacological control. *Brain Research,* 1979, *177,* 311–324.

Marshall, J.F., and Berrios, N. Movement disorders of aged rats: reversal of dopamine receptor stimulation. *Science,* 1979, *206,* 477–479.

Marshall, J.F., and Gotthelf, F. Sensory inattention in rats with 6-hydroxydopamine-induced degeneration of ascending dopaminergic neurons: apomorphine-induced reversal of deficits. *Experimental Neurology*, 1979, *65*, 398–411.

Marshall, J.F., and Teitelbaum, P. Further analysis of sensory inattention following lateral hypothalamic damage in rats. *Journal of Comparative and Physiological Psychology*, 1974, *86*, 375–395.

Marshall, J.F., and Teitelbaum, P. New considerations in the neuropsychology of motivated behavior. In L.L. Iversen, S.D. Iversen, and S.H. Snyder (Eds.), *Handbook of Psychopharmacology*. New York: Plenum Press, 1977.

Marshall, J.F., and Ungerstedt, U. Supersensitivity to apomorphine following destruction of the ascending dopamine neurons: quantification using the rotational model. *European Journal of Pharmacology*, 1977, *41*, 361–367.

Marshall, J.F., Richardson, J.S., and Teitelbaum, P. Nigrostriatal bundle damage and the lateral hypothalamic syndrome. *Journal of Comparative and Physiological Psychology*, 1974, *87*, 808–830.

Marshall, J.F., Levitan, D., and Stricker, E.M. Activation-induced restoration of sensorimotor functions in rats with dopamine-depleting brain lesions. *Journal of Comparative and Physiological Psychology*, 1976, *90*, 536–546.

Masuoka, D.T., Jonsson, G., and Finch, C.E. Aging and unusual catecholamine-containing structures in the mouse brain. *Brain Research*, 1979, *169*, 335–341.

McGeer, E.G., Fibiger, H.C., McGeer, P.L., and Wickson, V. Aging and brain enzymes. *Experimental Gerontology*, 1971, *6*, 391–396.

McGeer, P.L., and McGeer, E.G. The GABA system and functions of the basal ganglia: Huntington's disease. In E. Roberts, T.N. Chase, and D.B. Tower (Eds.), *GABA in Nervous System Function*. New York: Raven Press, 1975.

McGeer, E.G., and McGeer, P.L. Duplication of biochemical changes of Huntington's chorea by intrastriatal injections of glutamic and kainic acids. *Nature* (London), 1976, *263*, 517–519.

McGeer, E.G., Innanen, V.T., and McGeer, P.L. Evidence on the cellular localization of adenyl cyclase in the neostriatum. *Brain Research*, 1976, *118*, 356–358.

McGeer, P.L., McGeer, E.G., and Suzuki, J.S. Aging and extrapyramidal function. *Archives of Neurology*, 1977, *34*, 33–35.

McGeer, P.L., and McGeer, E.G. Aging and neurotransmitter systems. In C.E. Finch, D.E. Potter, and A.D. Kenny (Eds.), *Parkinson's Disease—II Aging & Neuroendocrine Relationships*, vol. 113, *Advances in Experimental Medicine and Biology*. New York: Plenum Press, 1978.

Meek, J.L., Bertilsson, L., Chency, D.L., Zsilla, G., and Costa, E. Aging-induced changes in acetylcholine and serotonin content of discrete brain nuclei. *Journal of Gerontology*, 1977, *32*, 129–131.

Mensah, P.L. The effects of aging on neuron "cell islands" in the mouse neostriatum. Society of Neuroscience, 9th Annual Meeting, *Abstract*, 1979, *5*, 77.

Mishra, R.K., Wong, Y.-W., Varmuza, S.L., and Tuff, L. Chemical lesion and drug induced supersensitivity and subsensitivity of caudate dopamine receptors. *Life Science*, 1978, *23*, 443–446.

Mjones, H. Paralysis agitans. *Acta Psychiatry Neurology*, 1949, Suppl. *54*.

Myrianthopoulos, N.C., Kurland, A.A., and Kurland, L.T. Hereditary predisposition in drug-induced parkinsonism. *Archives of Neurology* (Chicago), 1962, *6*, 19–23.

Myrianthopoulos, N.C., Waldrop, F.N., and Vincent, B.L. A repeat study of hereditary predisposition in drug-induced parkinsonism. In A. Barbeau and J.R. Brunette (Eds.), *Progress in Neuro-Genetics.* Amsterdam:Excerpta Medica, 1969.

Ohata, M., Sundaram, U., Fredericks, W.R., London, E.D., and Rapoport, S.I. Regional cerebral blood flow during development and aging of the rat brain. *Brain,* in press.

Osterburg, H.H., Donahue, H.G., Severson, J.A., and Finch, C.E. Catecholamine levels and turnover during aging in brain regions of male C57BL/6J mice. *Brain Research,* in press.

Papeschi, R. Dopamine, extrapyramidal system and psychomotor function. *Psychiatrie, Neurologie und Neurochiriurgie* (Amsterdam), 1972, *75,* 13–48.

Perez de la Mora, M., Fuxe, K., Anderson, K., Hokfelt, T., Ljungdahl, A., Possani, L., and Tapia, R. Studies on GABA-monoamine and GABA endorphin interactions. In E. Usdin, I.J. Kopin, and J. Barchas (Eds.), *Catecholamines Basic and Clinical Frontiers.* New York: Pergamon Press, 1979.

Pfeuffer, T. GTP-binding proteins in membranes and the control of adenylate cyclase activity. *Journal of Biological Chemistry,* 1977, *252,* 7224–7234.

Ponzio, F., Brunello, N., and Algeri, S. Catecholamine synthesis in brains of aging rats. *Journal of Neurochemistry,* 1978, *30,* 1617–1620.

Potvin, A.R., Syndulko, K., Turtelotte, W., Lemmon, J.A., and Potvin, J.H. Human neurological function and the normal aging process. *Journal of the American Geriatrics Society,* 1980, *28,* 1–9.

Protias, P., Constentin, J., and Schwartz, S.C. Climbing behavior induced by apomorphine in mice: a simple test for the study of dopamine receptors in the striatum. *Psychopharmacology,* 1976, *50,* 1–6.

Puri, S.K., and Volicer, L. Effect of aging on cyclic AMP levels adenylate cyclase, and phosphodiesterase activities in the rat corpus striatum. *Mechanisms of Ageing and Development,* 1976, *6,* 53–58.

Quik, M., and Iversen, L.L. Subsensitivity of the rat striatal dopaminergic system after treatment with bromocriptine: effects on [$^3$H] spiperone binding and dopamine-stimulated cyclic AMP formation Nauyn-Schmiedeberg's. *Archives of Pharmacology,* 1978, *304,* 141–145.

Randall, P.K., Functional aging of the nigro-striatal system. *Peptides,* 1980, *1* (Supp. 1), 177–184.

Randall, P.K., Severson, J.A., and Finch, C.E. Aging and the regulation of striatal dopamine mechanisms in mice. *Journal of Pharmacology and Experimental Therapeutics,* in press.

Ranje, C., and Ungerstedt, U. High correlations between number of dopamine cells and motor performance. *Brain Research,* 1977, *134,* 83–93.

Reis, D.J., Ross, R.A., and Joh, T.H. Changes in the activity and amounts of enzymes synthesizing catecholamines and acetylcholine in brain, adrenal medulla, and sympathetic ganglia of aged rat and mouse. *Brain Research,* 1977, *136,* 465–474.

Reisine, T.D., Fields, J.Z., and Yamamura, H.I. Neurotransmitter receptor alternations in Parkinson's disease. *Life Science,* 1977, *21,* 335–344.

Riederer, P., and Wuketich, S.T. Time course of nigro-striatal degeneration in Parkinson's disease. *Journal of Neural Transmission,* 1976, *38,* 277–301.

Rimon, G., Hanski, E., Braun, S., and Levitzki, A. Mode of coupling between hormone receptors and adenylate cyclase elucidated by modulation of membrane fluidity. *Nature,* 1978, *276,* 394–396.

Sant'ambrogio, G., Frazier, D., and Boyarsky, L.L. Alterations in central latency, motor neurone number and blood volume of spinal cord of the aging rat. *American Journal of Physiology,* 1961, *200,* 927–930.

Schmidt, M.J., and Thornberry, J.F. Cyclic AMP and cyclic GMP accumulation in vitro in brain regions of young, old, and aged rats. *Brain Research,* 1978, *139,* 169–177.

Schwab, R.S., Amador, L.V., and Lettvin, J.Y. Apomorphine in Parkinson's disease. *Transactions of the American Neurological Association,* 1951, *76,* 251–263.

Schwarcz, R., Creese, I., Coyle, J.T., and Snyder, S.H. Dopamine receptors localized on cerebral cortical afferents to rat corpus striatum. *Nature,* 1978, *271,* 766–768.

Schultz, W., and Ungerstedt, U. Striatal cell supersensitivity to apomorphine in dopamine-lesioned rats correlated to behavior. *Neuropharmacology,* 1978, *17,* 349–353.

Severson, J.A., and Finch, C.E. Reduced dopaminergic binding during aging in the rodent striatum. *Brain Research,* 1980a, *199,* 147–162.

Severson, J.A., and Finch, C.E. Age changes in human basal ganglion dopamine receptors. *Federation Proceedings,* 1980b, *39,* 508.

Severson, J.A., Randall, P.R., and Finch, C.E. Genotypic influence on striatal dopaminergic regulation in mice. *Brain Research,* in press.

Shaskan, E.G. Brain region spermidine and spermine levels in relationship to RNA and DNA in aging rat brain. *Journal of Neurochemistry,* 1977, *28,* 504–516.

Simpson, G.M., Varga, E., Lee, J.H., and Zuobok, B. Tardive dyskinesia and psychotropic drug history. *Psychopharmacology,* 1978, *58,* 117–124.

Sladek, J.R., and Sladek, C.D. Relative quantitation of monoamine histofluorescence in young and old non-human primates. In C.E. Finch, D.E. Potter, and A.D. Kenny (Eds.), *Parkinson's Disease—II Aging and Neuroendocrine Relationships,* vol. 113, *Advances in Experimental Medicine and Biology.* New York: Plenum Press, 1978.

Smith, C., Goochee, C., Rapoport, S.I., and Sokoloff, L. Effect of aging on local rates of cerebral glucose utilization in the rat. *Brain,* 1980, *103,* 351–365.

Spencer, H.J. Antagonism of cortical excitation of striatal neurons by glutamic acid diethylester: evidence for glutamic acid as an excitatory transmitter in rat striatum. *Brain Research,* 1976, *102,* 91–101.

Sprague, J.M., Levitt, M., Robson, K., Liu, C.N., Stellar, E., and Chambers, W.W. A neuroanatomical and behavioral analysis of the syndromes resulting from midbrain leminiscal and reticular lesions in the cat. *Archives Italiennes de Biologie,* 1963, *101,* 225–295.

Stimmel, G.L. Neuroleptics and corpus striatum—clinical implications. *Diseases of the Nervous System,* 1976, *37,* 219–224.

Strong, R., Hsu, L., Hickes, P., and Enna, S.J. Age-related decrease in mouse brain cholinergic muscarinic receptor binding. Society for Neuroscience, 9th Annual Meeting, 1979, *Abstracts 5,* 11.

Sun, A.Y. Aging and in vivo norepinephrine-uptake in mammalian brain. *Experimental Aging Research,* 1976, *2,* 207–219.

Talland, G. *Human Aging and Behavior: Recent Advances in Research and Theory,* vol. 1. New York: Academic Press, 1968.

Timsit, J. Sur l'activité cataleptigene de quelques derives de la butyrophenone. *Therapie,* 1966, *21,* 1453–1471.

Tolosa, E.S. Paradoxical suppression of chorea by apomorphine. *Journal of the American Medical Association*, 1974, *229*, 1579–1580.

Tretiakoff, C. Contribution a l'étude de l'anatomie pathologique du locus niger de Soemmering avec quelques deductions relatives à la pathologenie des troubles du tonus musculaire de la maladie de Parkinson. *These de Paris*, 1919, No 293.

Truex, R.O., and Carpenter, M.B. *Human Neuroanatomy*, 6th ed. Baltimore: Williams and Wilkins, 1969.

Ungerstedt, U. 6-Hydroxy-dopamine induced degeneration of central monoamine neurons. *European Journal of Pharmcology*, 1968, *5*, 107–110.

Ungerstedt, U. Adipsia and aphagia after 6-hydroxydopamine induced degeneration of the nigrostriatal dopamine system. *Acta Physiologica Scandinavica*, 1972, Suppl. *397*, 95–122.

Walker, J.P., and Boas-Walker, J. Properties of adenyl cyclase from senescent rat brain. *Brain Research*, 1973, *54*, 391–396.

Weiss, B., Greenberg, H., and Cantor, E. Age-related alterations in the ability of the β-adrenergic receptor-adenylate cyclase complex of brain to develop denervation supersensitivity. *Federation Proceedings*, 1979, *38*, 1815–1921.

Welford, A.T. Motor performance. In J.E. Birren and K.W. Schaie (Eds.), *Handbook of the Psychology of Aging*. New York: Van Nostrand Reinhold, 1977.

Wurtman, R.J., and Growdon, J.H. Dietary enhancement of CNS neurotransmitters. *Hospital Practice*, 1978, *13*, 71–77.

Zetler, G. Cataleptic state and hypothermia in mice, caused by central cholinergic stimulation and antagonized by anticholinergic and antidepressant drugs. *International Journal of Neuropharmacology*, 1968, *7*, 325–335.

SECTION II

# Behavioral and Social Sciences

# CHAPTER 3

# Ethnicity and Aging

DONALD E. GELFAND, PH.D.
SCHOOL OF SOCIAL WORK AND
COMMUNITY PLANNING
UNIVERSITY OF MARYLAND
BALTIMORE, MARYLAND

Researchers delving into the literature on ethnicity face at least two problems: the available research is seriously lacking in completeness and even agreement as to meaning, and the rhetoric surrounding the subject of ethnicity makes it difficult to understand the implications of the substantive data now available. The "new ethnicity" of the 1970s was positive in its revival of interest in the impact of ethnicity on Whites as well as non-Whites. Unfortunately, it also brought a polemical tone to discussions of ethnicity that is negative in its impact on unbiased analyses.

The new ethnicity involved a rejection of the "melting pot" theory and a reassertion of ethnicity identity by many groups, especially White religious and national groups. These groups, such as Jews, Poles, and Italians, are now commonly referred to as "White ethnics" in contrast to the so-called minority grouping of Blacks, Hispanics, Asians and Native-Americans. Some critics have viewed the new ethnicity as a reaction among Whites to the power that non-Whites supposedly obtained during the 1960s. Advocates of the new ethnicity reject this contention. Instead, they proclaim the new ethnicity as a long-awaited recognition of a distinct part of the American heritage in general, and every individual's own personal identity. What these advocates have therefore demanded is a social and political recognition of the importance of ethnicity for Whites as well as for non-Whites.

This review will stay grounded in the literature on ethnicity and assess the relationship between ethnicity and aging. This assessment re-

I am grateful to Judy R. Gelfand and George Maddox for their comments and suggestions on an earlier version of this review.

quires both an historical approach and an ability to move away from a myopic focus on the aged to study younger age cohorts. Understanding the situation of the present ethnic aged requires a grasp of the factors that influenced the development of various ethnic groups in the United States. Understanding future cohorts of ethnic aged requires a focus on middle-aged individuals, the ethnic aged of the next 50 years. Before turning to either of these topics we need to concentrate briefly on the functions of ethnicity for the individual and group.

## THE FUNCTIONS OF ETHNICITY

### Ethnicity and Values

An ethnic group can be defined as a group of individuals with a shared sense of people-hood based on race, religion, or national origin (Gordon, 1964). In this sense, a religious group such as Jews as well as a racial group such as Blacks can be classified as ethnics along with groups whose ethnicity is based on national origin such as Swedes and Russians. Separating out religious, national, and racial influences on many of these groups is a cumbersome and unaccomplished task in social research. This task is vital, however, since the manner in which "ethnicity" is now used does not discriminate among these varied influences. As noted elsewhere (Gelfand and Kutzik, 1979), it is possible that some of these influences are so intermixed that they are separable. Thus, the values of Italian Catholics may not be separable into those that are determined by nationality and those influenced by religious variables. In this sense, the intrinsic importance of the Church in Italian life has resulted in a compound that makes the ethnicity of Italian Catholics very different from that of French Catholics despite the commonalities in religious adherence. In this review, data on ethnicity as it relates specifically to aging will be presented. A variety of implications will be discussed. Unfortunately, the relative importance of religious, national, and racial influences on ethnic patterns will not, and cannot, be resolved at this time.

As Gordon's definition implies, ethnicity provides a mechanism for the transmission of group values. These values can be passed on through discussions and teaching as well as through the socialization of children. Having a reliable mechanism for transmitting values is crucial to the survival of a culture. Ethnic values can also be used as a means of selecting from a pool of possible associates. For individuals strongly imbued with ethnic culture, this may mean a preference for interaction with other members of the same ethnic group. The result is often the formation of ethnic neighborhoods and clubs, or of churches with a particular ethnic focus.

### Ethnicity and Identity

Dashefsky's framework (1973) is helpful in understanding the impact of ethnicity on identity. According to Dashefsky's formulation, there are four major facets of identity: (1) social identity, which is based on major demographic and socioeconomic characteristics including the individual's occupation or age; (2) self-conception, a "cognitive phenomenon which consists of a set of attitudes an individual holds about him- or herself" (p. 6); (3) personal identity, which goes beyond ascribed characteristics to individual traits such as personality and behavior; (4) ego-identity, which involves the core of what the individual feels about him/herself.

The general orientation provided by Dashefsky's theoretical model provides a broad framework for viewing ethnicity. Ethnicity can be important in all four facets of identity. There may be positive or negative consequences for individuals if others define them on the basis of ethnic group membership. Positive or negative consequences may also stem from individuals' feelings about the ethnic group to which they belong. An ethnic groups' values may influence behavior, thus becoming an intrinsic part of personal identity. A conscious decision not to affiliate with ethnic organizations or to abandon traditional forms of behavior or rituals does not necessarily mean that the ethnic culture has not been internalized and become part of a person's ego-identity. Ethnic values can be transmitted by individuals not overtly identifying with the ethnic culture. Greeley (1972) has earmarked child socialization as the most important element in maintaining ethnic culture. Individuals may assert an ethnic identity, belong to ethnic organizations, and transmit ethnic values intergenerationally. Alternatively, individuals may consciously reject identification with ethnic culture but still possess ethnic attitudes and transmit the culture's values intergenerationally.

An overview of ethnicity must include an analysis of how any particular age cohort or class group views its own ethnic culture, how it is viewed by others, the degree to which overt identification with the culture remains the same or has changed, and the continued allegiance to values that have been regarded as traditional to the culture. Before this review can move into grappling wih any of these difficult topics, a historical and sociological framework for examining ethnicity, particularly in the United States, needs to be outlined.

## GROWTH OF ETHNIC CULTURE

### Ethnicity as Historical Roots

A common assumption in ethnic studies is that all ethnic groups, whether in the United States or in other countries, are rooted in their countries of origin. This assumption has been the basis of analyses of both White and non-White groups in the United States.

Cohler and Lieberman's (1979) research attempts to explain the attitudes of Poles, Irish, and Italians in terms of the socioeconomic and status relationships these three groups had in the "old country." Schooler (1976) has utilized a similar historical orientation in his emphasis on the "legacy of serfdom." Schooler argues that for many ethnic groups, especially the "new" immigrants of the late 1800s, the effects of feudalistic society are evident even when differences in social class and religion are controlled. These effects, however, are not permanent. The longer the group is removed from feudalism, the more their value orientations begin to coincide with those associated with industrialized society. According to Schooler (1976) these "industrial" values include a belief in the importance of intelligence, belief in control over one's own life, and assertion of the locus of control as within the individual rather than in any external authority.

Schooler's approach takes into account the fact that ethnic groups are usually unable to transplant their culture into another country without modification. This has been true not only in the United States but in any country where immigrants have arrived as a subordinate group.

### Emergent Ethnicity

Yancey, Eriksen, and Juliani (1976) bring an additional element into the study of ethnicity. Viewing ethnicity as an emergent condition, Yancey, Eriksen, and Juliani argue that the ethnic communities concentrated in inner-city residential areas developed only as large-scale employment in these areas became available. Thus, many of the supposedly traditional institutions and support relationships of these communities can be attributed to

> a selective process which consists of a constantly evolving interaction between the nature of the local community, the available economic opportunities, and the national or religious heritage of a particular group [Yancey et al., 1976, p. 397].

In this analysis, ethnicity is more a dependent than an independent variable. Stressing ethnicity as "emergent" is also important because it focuses our attention on ethnic culture as constantly in flux. This premise is basic to the survival of any culture. A culture unable to change in order to meet new structural conditions must inevitable disappear. Japanese-American culture is thus not the same today as it was in 1900. Among Japanese in the United States, the catastrophe of internment in camps during the 1940s produced major changes in family structures. Among other ethnic groups a more evolutionary process has taken place.

## Class and Ethnic Aged

The major structural changes affecting ethnic culture are those related to social mobility, that is, class and status variables. The available research on ethnicity, especially as it relates to aging, is deficient in sorting out the effect of class on ethnicity. Wilson (1978) has argued that race is becoming less important than class among Blacks. Although class variables do appear to be increasingly important among Black aged, we need more studies of Black aged from higher socioeconomic groups before we can definitively determine the interaction between class and race. As the proportion of non-White and White ethnic aged with higher socioeconomic status grows and better sampling is undertaken, more empirical evidence on class and race should become available. Some preliminary evidence is presented in this review.

It is fortunate for the ethnic aged that many of the class distinctions that characterized 19th-century society have been lessened in 20th-century America. "Old immigrants" who were part of the predominantly northern European immigration into the United States during the 1800s have been better situated on a variety of socioeconomic indicators than later arrivals. Two factors have been assumed to account for this difference: (1) the greater length of time these immigrants have had to acculturate and accommodate themselves to the demands of American society; (2) the fact that these groups came from northern European cultures whose values were close to those transplanted by early Anglo settlers of the United States. In contrast, the languages and cultures of the southern and eastern Europeans who formed the backbone of the "new" immigration of the 1880s produced hostility on the part of settled Americans and a "nativistic" sentiment that culminated in the closing off of immigration in the 1920s (Higham, 1972).

The history of Blacks, Hispanics, and Asians has been characterized by continuous hostility from Whites. The theory that the rural residence of some of these groups slowed down their upward social mobility fails to take into account the overt and covert discrimination that has maintained White and non-White status differentials (Thernstrom, 1973). Discrimination is reflected in the present differences between White and non-White groups. The median educational background of all White males and females over 65 in 1978 was one to three years of high school. In contrast, Black and Hispanic men and women over 65 had only completed a median of five to seven years of school (U.S. Bureau of the Census, 1978). Examining various White groups, Roof (1979) noted that the mean education level among White Catholics of all ages in 1970 ranged from 11 to 12 years of schooling. Jews had the highest educational level of all groups with 13.4 years of education. The median income of White families in 1977 was $16,740 as compared to $9,653 among Black families and $11,421 among Hispanic families (U.S. Bureau of the Census, 1979). Twelve percent of White aged, 34 percent of Black aged and 23 percent of Hispanic aged were still living in poverty during 1979 (Brotman, 1979). Thus despite improvements in recent years, non-White families and non-White aged are still considerably behind Whites in income and education. These differences will continue to be reflected among the older population in the years to come.

The important question is not only the socioeconomic differentials among groups, but the relationship of these differences to the attitudes and behaviors of various ethnic groups. This review will focus on a number of important attitudinal and behavioral variables including:

1. The basic attitudes of ethnic groups toward aging and the life satisfaction of the aged within major ethnic groups.
2. The variations in assistance patterns among ethnic aged.
3. The variations in service utilization among ethnic aged.
4. The differences in values between ethnic aged and younger age cohorts within major ethnic groups.

After examining each of these four topics, the implications of the discussion for policies will be highlighted.

## BASIC ATTITUDES TOWARD AGING

### Ethnic Aged and Personality

We still have little information about major subgroups among the Black population or even about the individual groups that comprise the Hispanic-American population. Research among White ethnics has tried to provide differentiation on a number of dimensions. Cohler and Lieberman's (1979) work is provocative because it attempts to examine personality differences. Studying 386 Italians, Irish, and Poles, age 40–80 years in inner-city Chicago, these two authors attempted to assess the effects of ethnicity and aging upon personality changes.

One of the major differences among the groups was their attitudes toward achievement. Interest in achievement decreased with age among Italian and Polish men but increased among Irish men, a finding inconsistent with any disengagement hypothesis. Among all three groups of women, the orientation toward achievement increased with age. First-generation Italian men had a stronger belief in an "external locus" of control than first-generation Irish or Polish men. The lack of uniform values among these aging populations would appear to indicate the continuing influence of ethnic culture on the aged. As Cohler and Lieberman sum up their work: "The findings of the present study show that personality change across the second half of life is not independent of cultural context and that aging may accentuate differences in modal or ethnic personality" (1979, p. 242).

### Ethnicity and Life Satisfaction

If cultural values are related to personality changes among the elderly, differences in life satisfaction should also emerge across ethnic lines. Differences among White ethnic aged and between White and non-White aged point to an explanation favoring a history rooted not in Africa, Mexico, or Europe but in the United States where non-White groups have been forced into low-status social and economic positions.

Bengtson (1979) and his colleagues encountered manifestations of these historical differences in responses of White, Black, and Hispanic aged in southern California to questions of what they liked about being older. Bengtson remarks that the responses almost seem stereotypic, but the answers may accurately reflect the expectations of these three groups.

The response of Whites stressed their ability to engage in activities not previously possible because of extended work commitments. The major expression of Blacks was happiness at being alive. Primary satisfaction among Hispanics seemed to involve not having to work so hard. If we examine these responses along class lines they do not appear very surprising. Whites, who had higher-status jobs, may now have time to develop avocations which they were not able to indulge in fully before retirement. Hispanics, who have occupied low-paying manual labor jobs in California and the Southwest, may be relieved to be rid of a work obligation despite the loss of income. For Blacks, who possess lower health status and life expectancies than Whites, the fact of being alive may override the disadvantages of being Black and old. The validity of this analysis is indicated by Bengtson's further breakdown of life satisfaction into two elements: tranquility and optimism. While there was little difference among the three groups in tranquility, Mexican-Americans scored significantly lower than either Blacks or Whites on measures of optimism.

The available data remain inconclusive on the factors associated with life satisfaction among each of these three groups. In a recent study of life satisfaction among public housing residents in Cleveland, Black and White elderly stressed different elements of their life as important (Deimling et al., 1979). The major factor in the life satisfaction of White elderly was perceived health status. The major factor in life satisfaction of Black elderly was the maintenance of social relationships. In a Detroit study, perceived health status was the most important determinant of life satisfaction among the Black elderly (Jackson et al., 1977–78). The Detroit researchers also noted that "education, religious attitudes, need affiliation, self-esteem and attitudes towards employment of the aged" were important correlates of life satisfaction (Jackson et al., 1977–78, p. 177).

Since the Detroit study explained 70 percent of the variance and the Cleveland research only 20 percent, it would seem that the comments of the Black elderly in Detroit would be more representative. Statistical comparability, however, is not always as self-evident as it may appear. The Cleveland study utilized low-income Blacks and Whites living in public housing, while the Detroit sample was composed of individuals active in senior centers. Since the latter group was striving to maintain relationships in the community, it could be expected that they would value highly the good health necessary to maintain their current level of activities. The Cleveland sample contains a variety of individuals with varying health statuses, some of whom had only minimal opportunities for involvement in community activities. Developing opportunities for social interaction may be a primary concern of these Black elderly and thus show up more strongly on their life satisfaction scores.

Jackson (1970) and Ward (1979) have noted that Blacks have lower life expectancies, perceive of themselves as being "old" at an earlier age than whites, and are in worse physiologic condition than Whites. Concurrent with the perception of being older may be a more positive attitude toward later life and an unaggressive and undemanding attitude toward this stage of the life cycle (Ward, 1979). As Dancy (1977) argues, the importance of religion in the lives of Blacks also deserves continuing attention as a component in life satisfaction. Older Blacks attend church more frequently than older Whites (Ward, 1979), but there exists little evidence to support the stereotype of Black aged immersing themselves in fundamentalist religious groups.

We must also not forget that Blacks now in their 70s and 80s experienced discrimination restricting their opportunity to enter old age with any income security or a health status comparable to that of their White age peers. As Jackson, Bacon, and Peterson (1977–78) have noted, the limitations placed on Blacks by racism may be a vital factor in lowering their expectations of life in general and of older age in particular:

> It is conceivable that the effects of age discrimination, loss of esteem structures (work, income, status, social contacts) and other attendant consequences of aging in this society, might have different or more negative contrast effects upon such social psychological constructs as life satisfaction for Whites than Blacks. The relative influence of such negative occurrences on the life satisfaction of Blacks might be incrementally less or have different antecedents or correlates due to the omnipresence of discrimination and social inequality in the environment prior to and during the aging period [Jackson et al., 1977–78, p. 177].

Given the negative attitudes toward aging that exist in American society, it would be unreasonable to expect that any ethnic group would have a totally positive attitude toward growing old. While the elderly in many ethnic groups may have occupied positions of power in their countries of origin, there are few indications that these ethnic groups are prepared to accord to the elderly positions of authority in the United States.

Among Japanese families, for example, the reports of Montero (1979) and Kiefer (1974) indicate that the role of the elderly family member may be changing as Nisei (second-generation Americans) and Sansei (third-generation Americans) move closer to "American" values. Wu (1975) examining Chinese Americans in Los Angeles noted a reduction in the social status of the elderly, with children becoming more important than parents in the extended family. The ethnic aged may be able to anticipate respect from their adult children and their grandchildren, but not necessarily any authority comparable to what they might have obtained in the old country.

## Needed Research on Attitudes

Despite the seemingly endless amount of discussion, the variables that account for life satisfaction or even clear distinctions in life satisfaction among the ethnic aged remain only vaguely outlined. Both the factors and differences in life satisfaction require further intensive research. The central questions for this research are becoming evident:

1. Are the types of personality differences found by Cohler and Lieberman (1979) also true of other White ethnic and non-White aged such as Blacks, Hispanics, Asians, and native-Americans?
2. Are these personality differences as distinct among middle-class White and non-White young and old as they are among the lower-class individuals who have been studied?
3. What are the variations in life satisfaction within ethnic subgroups among non-White aged?
4. What variations in life satisfaction are found in urban, suburban, exurban, and rural communities where ethnic aged are residents?
5. What is the extent of interaction between ethnicity and class in determining life satisfaction?

With more carefully undertaken sampling, these questions will begin to be answered. To undertake this larger-scale approach will require greater understanding of the importance of the questions and their answers. Some of these implications will be outlined when we turn to an examination of the ethnic aged and services.

## ETHNICITY AND ASSISTANCE PATTERNS

### Social Networks

The role relationships of the ethnic aged can be divided into an examination of relationships with family members or friends, and relationships that do not involve intimates of any sort. Perhaps the most parsimonious way to examine role relationships is through the utilization of social network approaches.

Social network theorists have distinguished between weak and strong ties. Weak ties are large in number but are low in intensity. Their low intensity does not mean that weak ties are unimportant. Weak ties may be important in locating a job (Granovetter, 1973) or obtaining referral for a variety of services. An individual may thus turn to someone he/she knows only slightly or not at all to recommend a plumber. Seeking employment, the individual may contact a person recommended by another casual acquaintance.

Because of their intensity, strong ties are smaller in number than weak ties. Within the relationships established by strong ties, individuals exchange confidences and personal thoughts that can be shared only with intimates. Through these strong ties individuals develop the confidante relationships that Lowenthal (1968) and others have emphasized as crucial to positive mental health among the elderly.

With the loss of spouse, friends, and casual acquaintances, the number of ties of any kind available to the older person diminishes. The diminution of these ties is naturally accompanied by a diminution of resources. Older individuals thus may become more dependent on persons who remain in their social network. The older adult may utilize weak ties more extensively or attempt to change instrumental weak ties to expressive strong ties. If this strategy is not successful, then individuals who traditionally have the most obligation to provide emotional and social support for the older person, that is, relatives, will be called upon more frequently.

It is important to remember that older adults not only require assistance but also provide assistance. Thus, many strong ties are reciprocal in content. The parent may provide emotional support for an adult child or financial assistance for many years. What differs among ethnic groups is the degree of reciprocity in the relationships. Among Oriental cultures "filial piety," defined by Wu as "the principle that parents should suffer neither want nor sorrow" (1975, p. 274), indicates an ideal that children are beholden to provide a variety of supportive services for parents. Among many White and non-White ethnic groups, younger and older generations are expected to share economic burdens. The sharing of intimate concerns was found to be characteristic of the White ethnics (Jews, Italians, and Slavs) recently studied by Krause (1978).

An important question is not only the type and degree of concerns shared intergenerationally among ethnic groups but whether individuals belonging to various ethnic groups tend to confine their friendships and assistance to other members of the same group. As would be expected, the answer to this query is positive among members of non-White ethnic groups who have been forced by discrimination into segregated housing and segregated occupations. As non-White groups are able to break down barriers of discrimination, each succeeding age cohort may move in the direction of the primary interethnic contacts that Gordon (1964) regards as fundamental to the assimilation process.

### Assistance among White Ethnics

Among White ethnics the patterns of assistance remain unclear. Cohler, Lieberman, and Welch's (1976) examination of 386 middle-aged and elderly Italians, Irish, and Poles indicates that ethnicity does serve as a variable on which individuals make decisions about friends and resources. Italians, who are more likely to live in an ethnic community than Irish or Poles, tend to select their close friends from among other Italians. Poles have fewer contacts with friends than Italians or Irish.

These distinctive ethnic patterns influence the mobilization of friends as resources. If friends from the same ethnic background are available, the members of these three groups tend to rely on them rather than friends from other ethnic groups. Of course the presence of a large number of friends with a common ethnic background is facilitated by living within an ethnic neighborhood, a characteristic most common among Italians in the sample. In New York, intimates of White, Black, and Hispanic elderly tended not to be children or relatives but friends in the neighborhood (Canton, 1979b).

While the Chicago research demonstrates that friendship patterns are drawn along ethnic lines, the same study shows that relatives are usually relied upon to provide a greater amount of assistance than friends. This pattern was also true of New York White, Black, and Hispanic aged except in cases where friends and neighbors were able to compensate for the lack of contact of some elderly with relatives or assist elderly whose children were unable to provide more than limited assistance. Frequent interpersonal contact with relatives was a factor in making needed assistance available to family members. Among the Irish, Italians, and Poles in Chicago, three-fourths of the respondents visited with their adult children at least "a few" times each month. They also visited frequently with their own parents, who usually lived close by or at least an "easy drive" away (Cohler et al., 1976, p. 17). Almost half of the members of each group visited with their siblings at least a few times each month and even more frequent contact was maintained with children.

Cohler, Lieberman, and Welch (1976) also noted that increased contact on the part of the Irish, Italians, and Poles was linked to the use of other relatives or friends as resources. Among Italian men, frequency of contact increased the use of friends as resources. Given equal contact with relatives and friends, Italian men tended to rely on their relatives. The same pattern was found among Polish women. Among women in all three groups, increased contact with adult offspring produced a reliance on children for assistance in problem situations rathern than on other relatives or friends. In cases where adult children were deceased or living at a distance, friends and neighbors played an important role in providing assistance to the elderly.

### Assistance among Whites, Blacks, and Hispanics

Similar patterns of assistance from children to older adults was found in Bengtson's (1979) study of Whites, Blacks, and Hispanics in California and Cantor's research with the same three groups in New York City (1979a, 1979b). These studies indicated the presence of a substantial number of children able to provide assistance to Black and Hispanic aged. This extensive resource may result from a larger number of non-White elderly living with adult children. This residence pattern results not only from the elderly moving in with children, but also from children coming to live with older parents who have larger homes. Mindel (1979) has shown that the number of elderly living in intergenerational households has been consistently declining. Despite this steady decline, 34 percent of males and 32 percent of females over 65 were living with kin in 1977. Unfortunately, Mindel fails to provide a breakdown of these percentages by ethnic background.

Whether White, Black, or Hispanic elderly have more supportive family relationships is as yet unclear. Studies in the early 1970s (Jackson, 1971; Lopata, 1973; Rubenstein, 1971) did not indicate major differentials in visiting patterns among White, Black, or Hispanic elderly. In Cantor's work in New York (1979a, 1979b) Hispanic elderly were found to have a great potential for support due to a large number of children prepared to provide assistance. Hispanic elderly reported a greater sense of closeness with adult children than either of the other two groups. What was most surprising to Cantor was the lack of similar findings among Blacks. As she sums up her data, however:

> Both Black and Hispanic elderly are more likely to be involved in the lives of their children than are the White elderly. This higher level of total assistance probably reflects both the greater presence of the extended family in the Hispanic community and the greater need among low-income minority groups for intergenerational assistance as a means of offsetting the effects of poverty and discrimination [1979a, p. 169].

Cantor's findings have not been shown to be uniformly true in all parts of the United States. Babchuk and Longino's (1979) study of elderly Whites and Blacks in a public housing project found more primary ties among Whites than among Blacks. In southern Virginia, researchers (Kernodle and Kernodle, 1979) found that Blacks had more contacts with children than Whites. The Kernodles interviewed participants in a variety of senior centers and congregate programs. The strongest primary relationships were maintained by the higher-class Blacks in the sample and the weakest by the lower-class Whites.

### Continuity in Ethnic Group Behavior

In addition to the critical issue of whether primary resource networks are available to the ethnic aged living in the community, the data in all of these studies points to a strong continuity in the behavior patterns of the ethnic aged. This continuity of behavior with earlier years is consistent with the previously cited literature on attitudes. Aside from the data on support networks, however, we remain remarkably uninformed about the behavior of the ethnic elderly. In a study of drinking patterns among the elderly, a preliminary unpublished analysis of data from the Normative Aging study of the Veterans Administration fails to indicate a general convergence in drinking behavior among a large number of White and non-White ethnic groups. The evidence that differences in drinking behavior are maintained into old age is striking since drinking has been strongly linked to ethnic culture. The onset of physical and social changes that accompany the aging process produce some similarities among all elderly individuals. There does not appear any evidence, however, that the ethnic group member's "roots" become merely a part of the remembered past when the individual becomes older.

### Needed Research on Assistance Patterns

In order to fill the gaps in our knowledge of assistance patterns among the ethnic aged and their social networks, we need to answer questions that are comparable to those included in the previous section:

1. Are the social networks and assistance patterns the same among subgroups of Black, Hispanic, Asian, and native-American aged?
2. Are there differences in the social networks and resource patterns among various groups of elderly White ethnics?
3. What are the boundaries among ethnic groups and how do these boundaries affect interaction among aged from different ethnic groups?
4. Are there differences by class, health, mental health status, and place of residence in the social networks and resources of White and non-White ethnic aged?
5. What factors are most important in explaining these differences?
6. To what extent are there differences in the social networks and resources of the present cohort of ethnic aged and middle-aged ethnics.

## ETHNICITY, AGING AND SERVICES

If extensive support networks are available, we should not be surprised to find the ethnic aged making only limited use of formal service delivery systems. However, utilization rates do not depend purely on the availability of alternative services. Factors affecting service utilization include awareness, acceptability, and accessibility. There must be a feeling on the older persons' part that they need the services, an awareness of how to get the services, and a generally positive attitude toward making contact with service delivery systems.

### Services and Non-White Aged

Among many Black elderly past experiences have resulted in a low expectation of services (Dancy, 1977). Even if they do not share the common view of many aged that services are charity, contemporary Black elderly, who tend to be a low-income population, often regard services as low quality or not attuned to their cultural needs. The same feelings are also manifest among many other ethnic groups. If these obstacles are overcome, the older person may still be unable to reach a needed service because of transportation problems or may be unable to afford the cost of these services. In many cases middle-income aged may be ineligible for subsidized services but have inadequate resources to pay for expensive private services. Unfortunately, in many ethnic communities, especially non-White areas, we are still at the basic level of attempting to develop adequate services for the aged. This is especially true in rural communities and among groups that remain "ghettoized" and thus invisible to the general population.

One of the most commonly stated reasons for the lack of service utilization on the part of the ethnic aged is their determination and interest in "taking care of their own." In a recent study of Black families now utilizing nursing homes for older relatives and Black community leaders, Schafft (1979) attempted to account for the preference of Blacks for at-home care of the elderly. The reasons Schaftt outlines are:

> a) the elderly are valued participants and have an ongoing role to play in family and community life,
> b) institutional settings are alien to the old person who is used to the spontaneity of family and community life,
> c) blacks are concerned that their elderly will be verbally abused in predominantly white institutions,
> d) blacks find that nursing homes traditionally open to them are often not attractive, not fully staffed or equipped, and overcrowded [Schafft, 1979, p. 3].

In addition, Schafft argues, nursing home care is not available to many Black elderly either because of a shortage of publicly financed beds or the steering of Blacks exclusively to the small number of homes that primarily serve Black elderly. There is also a lack of information in the Black community about the availability of nursing home beds for family members. As the differential mortality rates between Whites and Blacks declines, we can expect that there will be an increasing number of Black elderly with chronic illnesses. The increase in the chronically ill segment of the Black elderly and an increase in the number of middle-income Black families may spur the development and use of both proprietary and nonprofit nursing homes. At this point, however, the use of any formal services among Blacks and other non-White elderly is low.

**Services and White Aged**

The same low rate of service utilization was found by Guttmann (1979) among eight eastern European groups. These groups made practically no use of Meals-on-Wheels, only minimal use of congregate meals programs, limited use of counseling or visiting nurses, and absolutely no use of escort srvices. There were two major differences among the eight ethnic groups: Jewish elderly used services more than any of the other groups, and there was a higher use of church-sponsored services by elderly Greeks, Italians, and Jews.

Among all of these White ethnics, services were utilized more by U.S.-born and "new immigrant" elderly. The U.S.-born elderly and "new immigrants" also had the highest socioeconomic status of all of the respondents in the sample. Selecting from possible service auspices, almost half of the sample indicated a preference for government-sponsored services, an additional 25 percent had no preference, and the final 13 percent preferred services under a combination of public and ethnic agencies. The use of services under church auspices by significant numbers of elderly Greeks, Italians, and Jews indicates a need also to support ethnically oriented churches as potential caregivers for some ethnic groups.

The preference for government-run services has also been noted among Mexican-Americans. Crouch (1972) and Cuellar (1978) have recorded strong feelings among elderly Mexican-Americans that the ultimate obligation for providing for the elderly must rest with the government and not the family, a feeling Cuellar attributes to cultural traditions that stress the older person living independently of children. As Guttmann (1979) argues, government services that take into account the characteristics of the ethnic community and that provide adequate information to the older adult about their availability should be able to increase the low utilization rates now common. Ignoring the feelings toward services among various ethnic groups dooms many services to underutilization. Rosenberg (1979) cites the problems of obtaining participation by elderly Jews in Cleveland in programs not under some form of Jewish auspices. Because of the variations in life experiences and attitudes among White and non-White ethnics, service providers need to consider the effects of ethnically heterogeneous programs on their efforts.

### Needed Research on Service Usage

This brief discussion should indicate the complexity of planning and implementing services to the ethnic elderly, the lack of substantive data on the topic, and the types of questions that need to be raised. These include:

1. What are the attitudes among White and non-White ethnic aged toward services?
2. To what extent are there commonalities in the behaviors and attitudinal responses of ethnic aged toward services?
3. To what extent are these attitudes based on correct information or past experiences with services?
4. Are these attitudes shared by all age cohorts within each ethnic group?
5. What are the service utilization rates among White and non-White ethnic aged?
6. How do these service utilization rates vary by class and generation of immigration?
7. What types of programs can be most effectively delivered to ethnically homogeneous groups?
8. What types of programs can be effectively delivered to groups of aged from a variety of ethnic backgrounds?
9. What specific programming can be developed to increase positive attitudes and utilization of services by the ethnic elderly?
10. What would be the most effective auspices for these programs?

## TRENDS IN ETHNICITY AND AGING

It should already be evident that the research on ethnicity and aging is incomplete. The attitudes, behaviors, and service utilization patterns of the ethnic aged remain only outlined. In part this results from a general lack of attention to ethnicity as a variable in the belief that the "melting pot" had resulted in a disappearance of ethnic distinctiveness. At this point, however, it is possible to focus on trends that may shape the status of the ethnic aged in the 21st century.

The most important trend is the possible dispersal of the ethnic community as a distinct ecological entity. Fandetti (1978) noted that the ethnic community can be a major focus of interaction for individuals from ethnic groups, but the ethnic community can also serve as a locale in which important cultural values are transmitted. The ethnic community thus fulfills a function basic to the sociological definition of culture as learned, shared, and transmitted. A loss of the ethnic community as a place in which culture can be taught, shared, and transmitted to children means that greater reliance has to be placed on other institutions including the family, church, and school.

### Urban and Suburban Elderly

Baroni and Green's (1976) data indicate that there are already major gaps in the age composition of many ethnic communities. Individuals in the 25–44 year age range are prominently absent from these communities. The ethnic communities in many cities have become "older" and may not be able to reproduce their numbers because of the absence of families with children. Golant's (1975) work makes it clear that the movement of older households during the 1960s was not only within the city but also to the suburbs. Between 1965 and 1970 approximately 275,000 elderly moved to the suburbs from the central city, and this trend continued into the 1970s. While the elderly may be moving to escape the crime and pollution they associate with the city, many older people are also moving to be closer to their children, who have previously migrated to the suburbs. The total figures on the elderly suburban population in 1976 indicates that this group will become a significant concern for service providers in the next decades. In the 50 largest Standard Metropolitan Statistical Areas (SMSAs) in the United States in 1976, there were 2,063,000 homeowning heads of household over 65 living in the central city and 2,561,000 living in the suburbs (Gutowski and Field, 1979).

The differences between the central city and suburban population of elderly is larger among renters: 1,711,000 heads of households over 65 renting their homes lived in the center city in 1976 and only 932,000 in suburban communities. These differences in the homeownner and renter data are obviously related to the differential availability of rental units in the inner city and suburbs.

When we examine slightly younger age cohorts (60–64 and 55–59), we find small differences between the central city and suburban renters, but a dramatic difference among homeowing households. There were

400,000 more homeowning heads of households 60–64 years old in suburbia than in the central cities of the 50 largest SMSAs (1,257,000 vs. 803,000). There were also 600,000 more homeowning household heads 55–59 years old in suburbia in 1976 than in the central city (1,573,000 vs. 993,000). As Gutowski and Field (1979) sum up their findings:

> The share of the elderly population living in the suburbs is likely to continue to grow primarily because of the large proportion of preelderly households currently living in the suburbs. These preelderly households can be expected to age in place, contributing to what could be labeled as a suburbanization of the elderly [1979, p. x].

The growth of the suburban elderly should include a significant proportion of "preelderly" or elderly from ethnic backgrounds who have moved to the suburbs. While suburbia has become increasingly expensive, the energy problems that have begun to make the inner city more attractive to younger families have combined with the condominium conversion boom to force the elderly in many inner city neighborhoods to seek new housing. There is no reason to believe that increasing pressures to relocate will not be placed on older ethnic communities located near important downtown commercial districts. Thus, the increase in suburban elderly may be largely among renters, with new rental stock being built to accommodate elderly migrants.

### Ethnic Identification and Suburbia

In Rhode Island, Gabriel (1973) investigated the continuation of strong ethnic identification among successive generations of Providence residents. He focused on ten variables including intermarriage, residence in an ethnic or non-ethnic community, generation, urban or suburban residence, income, education, age, parent's ethnic background, occupational status, and perceived discrimination against the ethnic group. Intermarriage, the ethnic or non-ethnic community, and urban or suburban residence had the strongest statistical relationship to a reduction in ethnic identification. Moving to the suburbs also was found to be more important than moving to another part of the city in reducing ethnic identification. Gabriel concludes that the move to suburbia could result in a loss of the ability to share and reinforce ethnic values, a process common in dense ethnic communities. It is possible that the movers to suburbia have already made a shift in values. In his famous study of Boston in the 1940s Firey commented: "As values cease to be shared, components of the ethnic community splinter off and dispersion occurs" (1947, p. 79). We do not yet know what is entailed in this dispersion, or whether the dispersion that is occurring is not resulting in a redevelopment of an ethnic community in the older inner-ring suburbs.

## Values and Middle-Aged Ethnics

Americans have tended to associate suburban residence with upward social mobility, and until recently this has been true of the ethnic population moving to the suburbs. A recent study in Columbia, Maryland, found that a large number of Italian-American male residents had professional education and high family incomes (Gelfand and Fandetti, 1980). A high percentage of these men were married to non-Italians. Although they favored organizations that could help to transmit Italian culture to their children, the Columbia Italian men objected to any suggestion that they should join a church that was part of an Italian parish, vote for a politician because he/she was Italian, or select friends who were also Italian because they would feel more comfortable with other Italians.

It is thus doubtful that traditional structures such as parochial schools or Italian-oriented churches will continue to play as important a role in the maintenance and transmission of ethnic values for this Columbia group. There will be increased reliance on the family as the maintainer or transmitter of ethnic values. Among Columbia Italians, however, 60 percent lived more than 200 miles away from their parents. Social and geographic mobility may raise questions of whether ethnic values will be maintained in the face of changing living patterns among many ethnic groups.

While Greeley (1977) contends that ethnic values have not proven a hindrance to social mobility, the Columbia data indicate that at some point these socially mobile respondents reduced their identification with "traditional" ethnic values, including parental values and general social orientations. Kessler-Harris and Yans-McLaughlin (1978) emphasize the historical conflict between social mobility and demands of the ethnic family in a comparison of Italians and Jews:

> Although Jewish family loyalties were strong, Jewish emphasis on career success permitted this group to adapt more readily to the geographic mobility frequently attending job improvement in industrial societies. Traditional Jewish culture did not set up such conflict of interest between family needs and individual achievement in the outside world. By the second generation a different pattern emerges. Italians of all classes, for example, still maintained closer family ties than most ethnics, but middle-class Italians showed the same willingness to move away from ethnic neighborhoods as did other middle-class people. Apparently, once second generation Italians achieved

> middle-class status, mobility aspiration superseded extended family traditions of importance [p. 128].

We therefore cannot be sanguine that without support ethnic traditions and values will not undergo major changes as ethnic groups achieve significant social mobility. Changes in these traditions will affect the ability of the older adult to have a significant role in the family, obtain assistance, or even interact on a regular basis with children and grandchildren who may live at a considerable distance.

Social mobility will also affect attitudes toward service usage. In Columbia, Maryland, middle-aged Italian-American men indicated a willingness to use institutional care in caring for seriously ill elderly, an attitude not usually associated with Italians (Gelfand and Fandetti, 1980). These affluent men also expressed an interest in private proprietary services and a negative attitude toward governmentally run programs. The positive attitude toward proprietary services was strongest among the third-generation Americans in the sample. These Italian men in suburbia were more able to pay for formal services and had a strong belief that privately run services would be of the best quality. Upcoming groups of ethnic aged will possess more education, higher incomes, and a more sophisticated knowledge about services. This background should result in a greater willingness to use formal services when they are required.

This comment may apply more to Whites than non-Whites whose social mobility has continued to be retarded by discrimination. In education, for example, it will not be until 2002 that Black elderly will have caught up to the general population in their high school completion rates (Hanushek, 1978). This slower rate of social mobility means that Blacks will continue to enter old age with limited resources and perhaps different attitudes toward service usage. This will also be true among Asian, Hispanic, and native-American elderly. The discrimination that has hampered the ability of older members of non-White ethnic groups to obtain adequate economic and social resources also means that these groups will remain residentially concentrated and reliant on institutions intrinsic to their culture for a longer period of time than White ethnic groups. As social interaction between Whites and non-Whites grows and residential integration and increased intermarriage take place, we can expect a general convergence of values among all ethnic groups.

This does not mean that the distinctiveness of all ethnic groups will disappear. Petersen (1978) has noted the inceased interest of second- and third-generation Asian-Americans in traditional ceremonies while these groups continue to adopt general American values. White and non-White ethnic groups who become more socially and residentially integrated into American society will still continue to adhere to those values and behaviors that they believe represent some of the crucial elements of their culture. Some values and behavior that may be as crucial but are seen as threatening to success in American occupational and social life will be abandoned. How the status and relationships of older ethnics will be affected by these changes over the course of the next few decades remains to be seen.

Whatever the changes that occur, ethnicity will remain a politically sensitive topic, especially since a group designated by the Federal government as a "minority" can apply for a variety of special benefits and programs. In 1980 Hassidic Jews in New York requested designation as an official minority from the Small Business Administration, and an employee in Montgomery County, Maryland, changed his name in an unsuccessful attempt to qualify under a program that gave preference in hiring to individuals with Spanish surnames. Thus, what will determine the number and variety of programs oriented to the ethnic aged may not be the effect of class, culture, and religion on ethnicity but the assertiveness of various ethnic groups in lobbying for programs to benefit their own constituencies.

### Needed Research on Trends in Ethnicity

In order to be able to assess the direction of trends in ethnicity, we need to focus on a number of important questions:

1. What are the important trends in residence patterns of the ethnic aged?
2. What is the extent of ethnic identification and allegiance to ethnic values among younger age cohorts?
3. What are the attitudes of younger age cohorts of ethnic groups toward aging and assistance to their aged relatives?
4. What variations are there in these attitudes among White and non-White ethnic groups in different socioeconomic statuses?

## SOCIAL POLICY AND THE ETHNIC AGED

It is easy to recommend an "ethnically conscious policy" (Trela and Sokolovsky, 1979) for the field of aging. However, this assertion is not very useful unless it provides some guidelines for practitioners and policymakers. This last section discusses eight recommendations that stem from the data now available on ethnicity and aging. The recommendations do not promote specific legislative initiatives, but they are useful approaches in critically thinking through policies toward the ethnic aged that may be viable.

**1.** An ethnically conscious policy in the field of aging must be implemented at a sophisticated level, recognizing that the terms now used to denote ethnic groups are sweeping and hide a variety of differences. For example, there must be recognition of the major differences among native-American tribes and an attempt made to assess critically these differences. Policies must be developed that will benefit the aged of different tribes. The same is true among Blacks and the multifaceted groups we label "Hispanics" or "Spanish-speaking." An ethnically conscious policy must also recognize the differences among Poles, Italians, Jews, Irish, and other White ethnic groups. Attention must be paid to the importance of these differences for policy development.

**2.** Policymakers must recognize that attempts to integrate ethnic groups in aging programs may be unsuccessful or result in hostility and resistance among groups of ethnic aged. Attempts to develop aging programs that combine White and non-White ethnic aged or even different groups of White ethnic aged may result in the failure of these programs to achieve maximum effectiveness or even to be used at all. A widely discussed process such as life review may not be carried out by ethnic aged uncomfortable with the ethnic mix in a community facility.

**3.** As is true of all groups, the ethnic aged prefer to utilize facilities run under auspices with which they feel comfortable. As recent studies have shown, these auspices may include church and ethnic groups. An understanding of the ethnic group and any ethnic community structure that exists is required in planning services for the ethnic aged.

**4.** Ethnic culture is constantly changing due to endogenous and exogenous influences. The ethnic culture that we observe in 1980 may be different from ethnic culture in 2030. The ability to adapt to changes in the social structure is a requirement if cultures are to maintain their viability. Any policy discussions concerning the ethnic aged must maintain an awareness of the structural conditions influencing the attitudes, behaviors, and living patterns of various age cohorts. These discussions should also attempt to estimate the effects alterations in the socioeconomic structure are likely to have on ethnic groups.

**5.** Ethnic groups have had differential success in achieving upward social mobility in the United States. Low rates of social mobility may make the later years difficult for many ethnic aged whose economic and social resources are limited. On the other hand, upward social mobility may correlate with alterations in the important beliefs of many ethnic groups. Social mobility may affect the general culture of ethnic groups and place demands on family structures. An ethnically conscious policy must examine these social mobility patterns and see what changes are being produced in relationships, informal assistance patterns, and roles of the aged in ethnic culture.

**6.** Policymakers must be careful not to romanticize ethnic groups. While ethnic group members may be interested in their roots, it is doubtful that what they are seeking is a return to the living conditions that earlier generations of their ethnic group tolerated. Policymakers need to distinguish between the search for roots that may relate to adoption of ethnic names, dress, foods, or genealogies and the living patterns that affect the status and roles of the ethnic aged in the community.

**7.** Important demographic changes are ongoing among ethnic groups in the United States including the movement of Whites and non-Whites to the suburbs. Efforts to develop policies for the ethnic aged must recognize that these elderly are not only living in dense ethnic communities but may also be scattered within large heterogeneous suburban and rural areas throughout the United States. Critically observing these trends is important if policies are to avoid becoming only reactive in nature.

**8.** The diversity of feeling among ethnic elderly and preelderly must be recognized by policymakers and practitioners. In the same manner that arguments are made for recognition of ethnic differences and the need for acceptance of an individual's ethnic background, policies must also recognize the right of older adults to abandon much of their ethnic heritage. It should thus not be assumed that all Irish will respond equally to a program directed toward Irish heritage.

Older individuals have tended to be defined in terms of physical or mental health problems. Too often we lose sight of their membership in other societal groups. Ethnicity is one important aspect of the older person's life. This review has not intended to imply that it is the most important characteristic of the older adult. Based on the fragmented literature now available, any assertion of this kind would be invalid. What can be said without any hesitation is that ethnicity is deserving of increased attention as well as a research and policy stance that maximizes the visibility of ethnicity as a major attribute of the aged in American society.

It is worthwhile noting that policymakers who take the above suggestions seriously will quickly find themselves embroiled with ambiguous definitions, a lack of conceptual clarity, and volatile groups concerned about the ramifications of political decisions for their own ethnic group. Unfortunately, attempting to avoid the issue of ethnicity may be more disastrous for policymakers and planners working with older people than attempting to confront the complexities of the ethnic heritage of older Americans.

## REFERENCES

Babchuk, N., and Longino, C. Aging and primary relations: racial differentials. Paper presented at the meeting of the Gerontological Society, Washington, D.C., November 1979.

Baroni, G., and Green, G. Who's left in the neighborhoods. Washington, D.C.: National Center for Urban Ethnic Affairs, 1976.

Bengtson, V. Ethnicity and aging: problems and issues in current social science inquiry. In D. Gelfand and A. Kutzik (Eds.), *Ethnicity and Aging: Theory, Research, and Policy*. New York: Springer Publishing Co., 1979.

Brotman, H. Every ninth American. In U.S. Senate Special Committee on Aging, *Developments in Aging: 1979*. Washington, D.C.: U.S. Government Printing Office, 1979.

Cantor, M. The informal support system of New York's inner city elderly: is ethnicity a factor? In D. Gelfand and A. Kutzik (Eds.), *Ethnicity and Aging: Theory, Research, and Policy*. New York: Springer Publishing Co., 1979a.

Cantor, M. Life space and social support. In T. Byerts, S. Howell, and L. Pastalan (Eds.), *Environmental Context of Aging*. New York: Garland STP Press, 1979b.

Cohler, B., and Lieberman, M. Personality change across the second half of life: Findings from a study of Irish, Italian, and Polish-American men and women. In D. Gelfand and A. Kutzik (Eds.), *Ethnicity and Aging: Theory, Research, and Policy*. New York: Springer Publishing Co., 1979.

Cohler, B., Lieberman, M., and Welch, L. Social relations and interpersonal relations among middle-aged and older Irish, Italian and Polish-American men and women. Unpublished paper, 1976.

Crouch, B. Age and institutional support: perceptions of older Mexican-Americans. *Journal of Gerontology*, 1972, *27*, 524–529.

Cuellar, J. El senior citizens club: the older Mexican-American in the voluntary association. In B. Meyerhoff and A. Simic (Eds.), *Life's Career—Aging*. Beverly Hills, Calif.: Sage Publications, 1978.

Dancy, J. *The Black Elderly*. Ann Arbor, Mich.: Institute of Gerontology, 1977.

Dashefsky, A. *Ethnic Identity in Society*. Chicago: Rand-McNally, 1973.

Deimling, G., Noelker, L., and Beckman, A. The impact of race on the resources and well-being of aged public housing residents. Paper presented at the meeting of the Gerontological Society, Washington, D.C., November 1979.

Fandetti, D. Ethnicity and neighborhood services. In D. Thurz and J. Vigilante (Eds.), *Reaching People: The Structure of Neighborhood Services*. Beverly Hills, Calif.: Sage Publications, 1978.

Firey, W. Land use in central Boston. Cambridge, Mass.: Harvard University Press, 1947.

Gabriel, R. Ethnic factor in the urban polity. New York: MSS Information Corp., 1973.

Gelfand D., and Fandetti, D. Suburban and urban white ethnics: attitudes towards care of the aged. *Gerontologist*, 1980, *20*, 588–594.

Gelfand, D., and Kutzik, A. (Eds.). *Ethnicity and Aging: Theory, Research, and Policy*. New York: Springer Publishing Co., 1979.

Golant, S. Residential concentrations of future elderly. *Gerontologist*, 1975, *15*(1), Part II, 15–23.

Gordon, M. *Assimilation in American Life*. New York: Oxford University Press, 1964.

Granovetter, M. The strength of weak ties. *American Journal of Sociology*, 1973, *78*, 1360–1378.

Greeley, A. *That Most Distressful Nation.* Chicago: Quadrangle Books, 1972.

Greeley, A. *The American Catholic.* New York: Basic Books, 1977.

Gutowski, M., and Field, T. *The Graying of Suburbia.* Washington, D.C: The Urban Institute, 1979.

Guttmann, D. Use of informal and formal supports by the ethnic aged. In D. Gelfand and A. Kutzik (Eds.), *Ethnicity and Aging: Theory, Research, and Policy.* New York: Springer Publishing Co., 1979.

Hanushek E. Ethnic income variations: magnitudes and explanations. In T. Sowell (Ed.), *Essays and Data on American Ethnic Groups.* Washington, D.C.: The Urban Institute, 1978.

Higham, J. *Strangers in the land: patterns of American nativism, 1860–1925.* New York: Atheneum, 1972.

Jackson, J. J. Aged Negroes and their cultural departures from statistical stereotypes and rural-urban differences. *Gerontologist,* 1970, *10,* 140–145.

Jackson, J. J. Sex and social class variation in Black aged parent-adult relationships. *Aging and Human Development,* 1971, *2,* 96–107.

Jackson, J., Bacon, J., and Peterson, J. Life satisfaction among Black urban elderly. *International Journal of Aging and Human Development,* 1977–78, *8,* 169–180.

Kernodle, R. W., and Kernodle, R. A comparison of the social networks of Blacks and Whites in a sample of elderly in a southern border state. Paper presented at the meeting of the Gerontological Society, Washington, D.C., November 1979.

Kessler-Harris, A., and Yans-McLaughlin, V. European immigrant groups. In T. Sowell, (Ed.), *Essays and Data on American Ethnic Groups.* Washington, D.C.: The Urban Institute, 1978.

Kiefer, C. *Changing cultures, changing lives.* San Francisco: Jossey-Bass, 1974.

Krause, C. *Grandmothers, Mothers and Daughters.* New York: Institute on Pluralism and Group Identity, 1978.

Lopata, H. Social relationships of Black and White women in a northern metropolis. *American Journal of Sociology,* 1973, *78,* 1003–1100.

Lowenthal, M. Social isolation and mental illness in old age. In B. Neugarten (Ed.), *Middle Age and Aging.* Chicago: University of Chicago Press, 1968.

Mindel, C. Multigenerational family households: recent trends and implications for the future. *Gerontologist,* 1979, *19,* 456–464.

Montero, D. Disengagement and aging among the Issei. In D. Gelfand and A. Kutzik (Eds.), *Ethnicity and Aging: Theory, Research, and Policy.* New York: Springer Publishing Co., 1979.

Petersen, W. Chinese Americans and Japanese Americans. In T. Sowell (Ed.), *Essays and Data on American Ethnic Groups.* Washington, D.C.: The Urban Institute, 1978.

Roof, W. Socioeconomic differentials among white socioreligious groups in the United States. *Social Forces,* 1979, *58,* 280–289.

Rosenberg, M. Ethnicity and social welfare: some policy perspectives. Paper presented at the consultation on Civil Rights Issues of Euro-Ethnic Americans in the United States, Chicago, Ill., December 1979.

Rubenstein, D. An examination of social participaton of Black and White elderly. *Aging and Human Development,* 1971, *2,* 172–188.

Schafft, G. Nursing homes and the Black elderly. Paper presented at the meeting of the Gerontological Society, Washington, D.C., November 1979.
Schooler, C. Serfdom's legacy: an ethnic continuum. *American Journal of Sociology,* 1976, *81,* 1265–1285.
Thernstrom, S. *The Other Bostonians: Poverty and Progress in the American Metropolis, 1880–1970.* Cambridge, Mass.: Harvard University Press, 1973.
Trela, J., and Sokolovsky, J. Culture, ethnicity, and policy for the aged. In D. Gelfand and A. Kutzik (Eds.), *Ethnicity and Aging: Theory, Research, and Policy.* New York: Springer Publishing Co., 1979.
U.S. Bureau of the Census. *Statistical Abstract of the United States: 1979.* Washington, D.C.: U.S. Government Printing Office, 1979.
Ward, R. Minority aging: double jeopardy or leveling? Paper presented at the meeting of the Gerontological Society, Washington, D.C., November 1979.
Wilson, W. *The Declining Significance of Race.* Chicago: University of Chicago Press, 1978.
Wu, F. Mandarin-speaking aged Chinese in the Los Angeles area. *Gerontologist,* 1975, *15,* 271–275.
Yancey, W., Ericksen, E. and Juliani, R. Emergent ethnicity: a review and reformulation. *American Sociological Review,* 1976, *41,* 391–403.

CHAPTER 4

# Age Changes in Sex Roles amid Changing Sex Roles: The Double Shift

LILLIAN E. TROLL, PH.D.
DEPARTMENT OF PSYCHOLOGY
RUTGERS UNIVERSITY
NEW BRUNSWICK, NEW JERSEY

EUGENIA M. PARRON, PH.D.
DEPARTMENT OF PSYCHOLOGY AND HUMAN SERVICES
BROOKDALE COMMUNITY COLLEGE
LINCROFT, NEW JERSEY

Identifying sex-role shifts from middle adulthood through old age is like trying to walk through quicksand. Definitions of sex roles are more inconsistent in the literature on adult development than they are in the literature on child development or that of the psychology of women. Some writers refer to norms, others to behavior, some to overt behavior, others to covert. There is remarkably little coordination of these different bodies of literature despite the potential value of such cross-fertilization.

A fundamental problem is presented by the differences in norms and behaviors from the oldest living generations to the somewhat younger generations whom we also call old (i.e., cohort differences). Allied to this cohort shift is the probability that the oldest generations have been confronted with progressively more deviant norms—from their perspective—over their lifetime. They have lived through a period of such marked social change that definitions of what is proper male and proper female behavior could seem to be inverted. An illustration of these differing baselines is provided by the literature on midlife, which often seems to be referring to a different culture from that on post-retirement. When we consider the effects of reciprocal socialization (see Bengtson and Troll, 1978), we would have to take into account the fact that present-day middle-aged parents of young adults start from a different point than did their own parents. While both parents and grandparents would be influenced by the new sex-role norms of youth, they would probably incorporate respectively different attributes from the new arrays of options, given their differing initial perspectives. Finally, not only do we have to consider cohort effects, but also sex. Patterns of aging for men tend to be very different from those for women, and we must assume that men will respond to changing norms differently than women.

At least four fundamental questions must be addressed, most of them related in some way to the current prominence of the "midlife crisis" concept:

1. Do individuals really experience sex-role changes during their adult years?
2. Are any sex-role behaviors lost or added at some point in aging?
3. If there are sex-role transformations or reorganizations in midlife, what causes them?
4. What would be the consequences in coping or mental health for later life?

In the following review, we shall first sketch in background, which involves economics, biology, and socialization. Following this introduction, we shall review the existing literature on sex-role differences themselves, relating to the questions just posed.

## BACKGROUND

### Economic-Historical

Our prevailing sex-role definitions evolved, according to Hareven (1978), from industrialization processes of the 19th century. These redefined family and work into privatized family life and diversified economic roles. While earlier it was necessary and expected that all members of the family contribute economically, only some family members—men—were needed to supply income, leaving women and children free from income-producing roles outside the home. This, of course, referred primarily to the middle class.

By the middle of the 19th century, few married women in the United States were employed outside the home. In 1893 only 5 percent of all women were employed, and these were mainly from the slum districts—blacks and immigrants.

By the middle of the 20th century, sex division of work changed again. In 1948 it was not uncommon for unmarried women to maintain a job, but atypical for married women (22 percent). By 1969, however, many more married women (40 percent) had jobs: over 29 million American women were in the labor force (Women's Bureau, 1969a,b). Thirty-seven percent of all workers were women, and the rate of increase in women working was almost twice that for men. The increase is attributed to a combination of demographic, economic, and social developments. The ratio of women to men increased progressively. The economy became increasingly an urban, service-dominated one in which physical strength was no longer a significant factor in job performance. Homemaking became easier and fewer children were reared, for a shorter period of time. Now, at least nine out of ten women work outside their home at some time in their lives, and at any given time, at least one-half of the working population consists of women. The extent to which such changes have affected sex-role definitions and attitudes will be discussed later.

The most spectacular development in recent years has been the rise in employment of women over age 30, mostly wives and mothers (Lopata, 1971). By the 1960s, more women in their 40s were working than younger women—a reversal of a long-standing trend. And these middle-aged women who were returning to work were often the same women who, ten years earlier, claimed that they had no interest in jobs or careers (Troll, 1975).

Whereas fewer men continue to work as they get older (from age 44 on), more women work between 45 and 54 than at younger ages—or older. This shift in proportion working is particularly interesting in view of the shift in age of the American population. There are more older people available for employment than ever before. Perhaps their return to the labor force feels like a new start on life. Perhaps also women are cheaper to employ, or more efficient employees. Or perhaps their health is better than men their age. The rise in employment among 40-year-old women may be as much a historical change as an age change. That is, perhaps these women just happened to be 40 when it bacame customary for women to go back to work and when more jobs became available.

Finally, there is increasing disparity between men and women as they progress along their career paths. Even if they have been pursuing careers to the same extent, in the course of time men earn higher salaries, reach higher positions, and reach them more easily.

Cohorts of women have been socialized to expect protection from society through their husbands, the traditional breadwinners. Being dependent on their husband's income resulted in an inferior economic position for women. A recent study of selected "problem groups" of old people in Chicago (Bild and Havighurst, 1976) found that the women were much more "disadvantaged" than the men, even when the data were corrected for the fact that the man's income usually supported husband and wife. More than 45 percent of single, divorced, and widowed women have incomes below poverty level compared to 33 percent of the men (Cutler and Harootyan, 1975). According to Troll and Turner (1979), "The reasons for this differential are multiple and cumulative and reflect the traditional sex roles under which the men and women who are now old were socialized and led their lives" (p. 127).

The financial abandonment of women has emerged as a new national problem; "displaced homemakers" have become an important object of legislation and general social policy. The rising tide of divorce, coupled with differential longevity, has left many older women not only without children to care for, but also without support. Even those women who remain married until the death of their husbands may find themselves in old age without any income (Schulz, 1976). Traditionally, women who are now older were not generally involved in the handling of money matters while their husbands were alive. It must come as a shock, to put it mildly, to find out at their husband's funeral, that they are now penniless.

Even those older women with an employment history outside the home are at a disadvantage. On the average, they are not as economically secure as the average older man (Atchley and Corbett, 1977). Having worked fewer total years, they have accumulated fewer retirement benefits. Their savings are apt to be less because they received lower pay than men even when they were doing approximately the same work. Having had lower-level jobs, they are less entitled to Social Security benefits or other pensions. Finally, if these women's retirement incomes have been calculated upon actuarial tables based upon average life expectancy, they are going to get less retirement money per month than men.

Troll and Turner (1979) suggest that new definitions of sex-role appropriateness might enable younger cohorts of women to take money and financial management more seriously so that they acquire more experience in sharing financial management with their husbands while they are married and are able to take care of themselves better if they are widowed or divorced. Probably many younger wives are already doing so.

### Biology: Health and Longevity

Women tend to live longer than men, with about a seven-year differential in life expectancy (U.S. Bureau of the Census, 1976). With each decade past 50 there are more older women alive than older men. Older men, furthermore, are much more likely than older women of the same age to report limitations of major work and maintenance activities due to chronic health problems. In general, women past menopause tend to be healthier than they were earlier as well as healthier than men their age (Weg, 1977).

Loss of vigor, according to Huyck (1977), can threaten men's "masculine" self-image. Further, it can lead to many women's inability to escape their nurturance role, which shifts from caring for children to caring for husband. Health differences may thus be resented by both sexes.

If vigor is central to the male role, attractiveness is central to the female role. Women's self-esteem is built on affirmations of femininity, usually defined as the ability to attract men. To the extent that physical attractiveness is dependent upon youthfulness, a woman's looks and her appeal to men succumb to age. In fact, Nowak and Troll (1974) found that middle-aged women were more concerned with youthfulness than with attractiveness per se, and Nowak (1975) later found that they even had difficulty distinguishing between youthfulness and attractiveness. If they judged a person—particularly a woman—to be attractive, they said she was years younger than if they judged her to be unattractive. Neither younger nor older women, nor men in any age group, confounded these two aspects of age identity. Signs of aging in the appearance of men were not interpreted as loss of attractiveness. In fact, young women, as compared with older women, overestimated the attractiveness of older men, just as older men overestimated the attractiveness of young women. Thus, the intersection of physical decline and sex roles—at all ages—is worth further investigation.

### Socialization

Emmerich (1973) makes the point that "adult sex roles in modern society have neither the coherence nor permanence required to serve as specific targets of early socialization" (p. 124). At least for the cohorts coming of age before 1968, early socialization encouraged the development of "masculine" personality characteristics in boys and "feminine" characteristics in girls (Kagan and Moss, 1962), so that by early adulthood inappropriate behaviors were discouraged. Longitudinal studies have shown that polarization of attributed—and, to some extent, exhibited—personality characteristics between the sexes reaches its peak during adolescence, presumably in the process of seeking a mate (Haan and Day, 1974; Livson, 1976). This is probably also the time of greatest sex-role restrictiveness. Reports of the 40 women and 40 men (born in the 1920s) who remained in the Berkeley longitudinal studies up to the time of the latest follow-up (Livson, 1976) trace patterns of similarity and divergence in personality ratings at four time periods, from early adolescence to the age of 50. When they were observed in their early teens, the girls were more assertive than the boys. By late adolescence (senior high school years) these girls had exchanged their self-assertion for flirtatious, seductive behavior, while the boys had learned to express competence, dominance, and coolness, and to suppress spontaneity and tender feelings.

The acquisition of sex-role behaviors as well as their organization have been the concern of developmental psychologists for many years. Kohlberg's (1966) cognitive-developmental theory of sex-role identity formation postulated that a child first arrives at a belief that he is a boy or she is a girl and then, largely through a process of selective modeling, adopts the behaviors he or she feels belong with that identity. While in young children the process of acquiring appropriate behaviors would be contingent upon such cognitive abilities as object constancy (when are a variety of masculine attributes all seen as masculine?) and movement from preoperational to concrete operational to formal operational ability, it is presumed that adults would at least be cognitively competent to make selections. From this theory, we would assume that even though there might be shifts in sex-role attributes in later life, they would be organized around a stable sex-role identity. A man who became more expressive or passive in later life would not necessarily view himself as other than a man. A woman who became more assertive would still feel herself to be a woman.

Some social learning theorists stress the organizing properties of social events over those of cognitive structures. According to them, each individual could have the capacity to perform a much wider array of sex-role behaviors than she or he would actually exhibit at any given time of life, since she or he would select those behaviors appropriate to time of life and situation (*competence* versus *performance*). The construct of identity would essentially be irrelevant in such a model. Other theorists (Erikson, 1959; Kohlberg, 1966, 1969; Loevinger, 1969, for example) propose sequential, stage-related "internal" mechanisms. Still others distinguish between early-formed enduring *genotypes* and later age-specific *phenotypes,* reminiscent of the competence-performance hypothesis. Four fundamental questions were posed at the beginning of this chapter. Given the background review just presented, what answers can be given to these questions?

## FUNDAMENTAL QUESTIONS

### Question 1. Are There Developmental Sex-role Changes during Adulthood?

We think that we can say that there are developmental changes, at least for some people. We know there have been marked societal shifts in sex-role norms and behaviors over the past decade. Starting with youth in the 1960s, there has been a shift toward a more balanced combination of masculine and feminine behaviors (androgyny) and away from earlier polarized and stereotyped masculinity and femininity. While this change probably began among middle-class college-educated men and women, it has become accepted by their parents' and even, to some extent, their grandparents' generations.

Changes in norms do not necessarily mean, though, that these older individuals themselves become more or less androgynous as a consequence of development, for example, in midlife transition. The popular press has been fascinated by the theories of Levinson (1978) and Gould (1972), which state that there are regular sequential shifts in sex-role behavior and feelings occurring at particular times during the adult years. Gutmann (1975) has elaborated a more sophisticated model from the same perspective, backed by data from projective tests of men (and a few women) of diverse cultures.

It may be significant that all three of these proponents of a midlife crisis or turning point have focused primarily upon men. The more recent data on women show a more complex picture. While some analyses of longitudinal data (Livson, 1976; Thurnher, 1979) reveal midlife sex-role shifts in behavior, we should note that other longitudinal data (Maas and Kuypers, 1974; Bray and Howard, 1978) seem to show more persistence than discontinuity. Which part of the elephant are we touching? Our Procrustean approach could be leading us to cut divergent data to one size.

O'Leary (1977) alerts us to the perils of concentrating on sex differences and overlooking more important sex similarities. Bem (1975) found one-third of her sample of young adults to be androgynous. High polarization was equally unrepresentative; most were low on both masculinity and femininity scales. We might conclude that midlife sex-role shifts are characteristic of only a minority, even a small minority.

One of the problems in ascertaining the presence of large-scale sex-role shifts is the global nature of the question asked. This question has several parts. Do people change their sex-role norms, their beliefs about what is appropriate behavior for men and for women, or rather, for themselves as a man or a woman? Do they change their overt sex-role behavior? Do they change their covert behavior, their self-perceptions related to their sexual identity? Do older men and women who become progressively more androgynous in their behavior see themselves any differently? Or is a shift more noticeable in self-perception and values than in behavior?

There is much more evidence for a shift in normative tolerance in other words than in actions. There is also more shift in covert than in overt behavior. At least three studies suggest that gender-linked personality characteristics are most differentiated in early adulthood and that women and men become progressively more androgynous as they move from middle to old age (Livson, 1976; Lowenthal et al., 1975; Neugarten and Gutmann, 1964). Unfortunately, most of these data are based on a relatively small number of subjects. While the data seem to show de-differentiation, we have been cautioned by Neugarten and Gutmann (1964) that this age shift is associated mostly with intrapsychic functioning (projective tests such as a Thematic Apperception Test); less often with measures of conscious material, such as self-reports; and least often with overt behavior. Age-sex norms have been seen, in a number of studies, to be much more restrictive for the events of early adulthood than for those of later life (see Troll and Nowak, 1977).

Gutmann (1964, 1974, 1975) suggests that a "normal" developmental shift occurs in middle-aged men in their 50s from an intrapsychic stance emphasizing active mastery of the environment (traditionally masculine) to a passive-receptive mode (traditionally feminine). When he asked older Americans (aged 40–70 years) to respond to a TAT-type card depicting a younger and an older couple, most of them described the old man as more passive, submissive, and easygoing than the young man. Conversely, the old woman was portrayed as a dominant authority figure and the young woman as a more passive person. If younger adult male respondents—to about their 50s—described men as wanting something, they also tended to describe them as going out and trying to get it. Men in their 50s, perhaps as a result of waning success in using an active mode, described men as turning inward, becoming more interested in feelings and ideas. They were more likely to show a *passive mastery* mode—trying to get what they wanted by appealing to greater powers. The oldest men, over 70 years old, perhaps not having found even passive mastery successful, turned to *magic mastery,* distorting reality to make themselves believe they had gotten what they wanted.

Women showed a somewhat different pattern. The younger women (under age 50) were more likely than the younger men to use *passive mastery*. After all, traditional women are trained from childhood to get what they want through others—fathers, husbands, or sons. In middle age, when men in their 50s seemed to be more passive, many of the women turned outward and became more comfortable with their assertiveness. Again, we do not know how much of what we might be seeing is developmental, and how much cohort changes or social class differences. Thus, Lowenthal and co-workers (1975) and Rubin (1975), both studying lower-middle-class and working-class older women, report more frustration with intensification or of traditional feminine behavior than a shift toward androgyny. Unhappiness with a condition does not neccessarily produce a shift away from that condition.

The Berkeley longitudinal data (Livson, 1976) as well as the seven-year follow-up of the sample of Lowenthal and colleagues (Thurnher, 1979) offer some support for a "normal" midlife-shift hypothesis. Livson found that nontraditional women—judged by personality scores—who had been following traditional sex-role behavior during their childrearing years, became more overtly assertive and thus more nontraditional during midlife. Women who had more traditional personality characteristics remained passive. They did not shift away from femininity in their middle years. Genotypic differences in passivity or assertiveness had been obscured during the restrictive childrearing years. "Naturally" assertive women behaved as passively as "naturally" passive women, producing an impression of phenotypic uniformity.

Thurnher's findings are even more interesting. The women she examined who shifted toward androgyny were those who had been living relatively good lives over the seven years of the study. Those who had troubles over that time were more likely to retain traditional feminine behavior—passivity. Similarly, those men who became more passive had had an easy time of it, while those men who remained aggressive had had a hard time.

Can we conclude, therefore, that androgyny is the condition of good mental health in middle age and that a shift toward androgyny represents a shift toward mental health? Such a conclusion would certainly be in accord with the thrust of the literature on sex-role differences and behavioral flexibility in younger adults (Bem, 1975). O'Leary's (1977) review of sex-role research arrived at two general conclusions: (1) that we tend to focus upon those characteristics which differentiate men and women to such an extent that we may be overlooking the possibility that the majority of men and women are probably androgynous—defined by Spence (1979) and Bem (1975) as a balanced combination of both sex-typed feminine and masculine characteristics; and (2) that androgynous individuals have been shown to be more flexible. They can be appropriately "feminine" or "masculine" as the situation warrants. Stereotypically "feminine" and "masculine" individuals, in contrast, are less able to adapt to situational requirements. An experiment by Bem, for example, showed androgynous women even more nurturant (toward a kitten) than feminine women. Subjects scoring high on Bem's masculinity or androgyny scales were more resistant to social pressure to conform than those who scored high on Bem's femininity scale.

A cross-sectional study of frequency of androgyny, using Bem's scale, reported sex and age differences. There were more androgynous men over 40 than under 40, and fewer androgynous women over 40 than under 40 (Hyde and Phillis, 1979). It is dangerous to extrapolate from such cross-sectional data, of course. But these findings also suggest that adult men—whose mental health is better than adult women's—make a midlife shift to androgyny more easily than do women. Srole and Fisher (1978), with more powerful longitudinal data, show that the significant improvements in mental health over the 20 years from 1954 to 1974 were primarily women. Even so, many men over 40 still do not achieve androgyny—or good mental health.

In old age, according to Neugarten and Gutmann's TAT findings (1964), both sexes turn to magic mastery. At this point of reduced power, men and women are low on both masculinity (active mastery) and femininity (passive mastery). Monge (1975) found similar age differences with a semantic-differential mastery-style instrument. Anthropological data (Gold, 1960) show a shift toward greater female dominance in later life in 14 of 26 societies. This relative shift was not, however, incorporated into the formal rules of the society, and we may wonder how much of women's increased power in such cases is attributable to the waning power of the old men.

There is evidence that the midlife transition is more problematic for women than for men. Huyck (1976) points out that jokes and social unease accompany tales of strong, dominant old women. "The old battle-axe" is deprecated; much more acceptable is the meek, kindly, "feminine" old man. The passive old man presents no generational threat to younger men, for whom he has stepped aside. Much more alarming to the younger generation—and to the husband of the older woman—is the aggressive older woman.

Social class differences can show up in the way women's greater assertiveness is expressed. Middle-class women can strive for career success or political power. The predominately lower-middle-class women studied by Lowenthal and co-workers (1975), who had fewer avenues for such expression, apparently responded by becoming more dominant in relation to their husbands, and also sometimes to their children. Their husbands, in turn, might simultaneously bask in the pampered existence their wife created for them while they decried her "bossiness." Goodchilds (1977) portrays the dilemma of the older career woman who finds herself, because of historical shifts in the 1970s, in a leadership occupational position. She is damned as a bitch if she exerts authority and damned as ineffectual if she doesn't.

As noted above, enhanced power of old wives over their husbands may be based, in part, upon the older men's physical debility. Butler and Lewis (1973) comment that society benefits from older women's enactment of the nurse role toward their husbands. Without such care, medical costs to society would spiral. The personal costs to the wives are not usually recognized. In her study of Chicago widows, Lopata (1971) found that many had nursed their husband for over a year during his final illness, rarely leaving the house or finding time for self-expression of any kind. It would seem less than accurate to label this androgynous behavior.

If we can draw any conclusions from present data, we might say that norms for appropriate sex-role behavior are more relaxed for older people than for younger, that in midlife some people shift away from rigid sex stereotyping in their feelings toward self and the world toward a more flexible androgyny—at least women seem more autonomous and men more expressive—and that some people may also change their overt sex-typed behavior, again in the direction of androgyny. We would thus expect fewer group differences—by sex—than individual differences. We can at least hypothesize a possible later change in old age toward disappearance of sex-roles by loss of both stereotypic masculine and feminine self-perceptions, norms, and even behavior. This later shift would thus remove both sex and individual differences. This is a paradox. We know that variation increases throughout life. Perhaps if we measured backward from date of death we would find a terminal drop in individual differences as well as IQ. The answer to the first question, then, is a tentative yes—for some people, at least, of present cohorts, there are developmental sex-role changes during adulthood.

**Question 2. Are Any Sex-role Behaviors Lost/Added in Later Life?**

The question here is central to personality development at any point in life. It is also central to theories of functionalism or competence versus performance and highlights the significance of age-sex norms (Neugarten, 1968) in determining behavior. Lowenthal and colleagues (1975), for example, state that different behaviors are encouraged at different ages, that the vigorous achievement-motivated men in their 40s or 50s are high in self-esteem and morale, while the same kinds of behavior reported by the men in their late 50s or 60s are associated with unhappiness.

When Kagan and Moss (1962) correlated early childhood behavior with the young adult behavior of the same individuals, they reported "sleeper effects." Characteristics displayed at one period might not be seen at the next, but would then reemerge later. Are these examples of suppression or repression of behaviors in the service of situational demands or age-appropriateness? Recent interest in functionalism brings such phenomena to the fore. If we can assume that individuals are characterized by arrays of behavioral dispositions, that behaviors can vary widely within the same time period as they are selected to fit a current situation or context, we can then ask what happens to those behaviors that are not displayed. Rather than looking at undisplayed behaviors as lost, repressed, or suppressed, we might find it more heuristic to look at them as backstage waiting for their cue. Both of Livson's (1976) reports on reappearance of adolescent sex-role attributes in middle age and Kagan and Moss' sleeper effects support hypotheses of competence versus performance and functionalism: currently inappropriate behaviors remain part of the repertoire, available for use in more appropriate contexts.

Allied to this theoretical issue of repression and recovery of behaviors from repertoires are the questions of awareness and control. Are we aware (conscious) of our unused attributes or behaviors, or are they suppressed to "below" the level of consciousness? Is our selection of behaviors controlled, or are we passive containers from which outside forces pull behaviors as necessary? It is answers to these questions that we need before we can answer the question about loss of sex-role difference or recovery of past characteristics after middle age.

**Question 3. What Causes Sex-role Transformations in Later Life?**

As noted in the introduction, various hypotheses have been advanced for explaining observed sex-role changes during the adult years. Three major causes, divided into several subcategories, are considered here: (1) biological determinants; (2) the impact of major life events and societal expectations; and (3) dialectic processes, like reciprocal socialization across generations or dyadic confrontation between men and women who may be changing in opposite directions.

*Biology.* The fact that there are significant biological changes during what could roughly be called the middle years has led many writers to connect biological changes with sex-role changes. It may even have led some theorists to look for sex-role changes as logical consequences—or perhaps analogic reasoning—of sex-related changes in fertility. If men, and particularly women, are viewed biologically and primarily as reproductive beings, they *should* show sex-role changes following menopause or decreases in sexual arousal capacity (men).

Gutmann (1975) uses the term "parental imperative" to denote the force which drives young men and women to exaggerate their differences in sex-stereotyped characteristics. Once the parenting years of a couple are over with the menopause in women, he believes that middle-aged or rather post-fertile men and women are freed to revive or reveal a wider array of behaviors. While biological events may seem logical antecedents for women, whose fertility ends more noticeably, they are less obvious for men, whose climacteric is a long, drawn-out gradual process lasting well into old age. It is curious, therefore, to use such a reason to explain male midlife crisis occurring as early as age 35.

Changes in fertility are not the only biological events, of course. The introductory section on biology in this chapter refers to loss of attractiveness in women and of muscular strength and general health in men. Biological theorists make much of such losses, as well as of confrontation with death of parents leading to recognition of mortality. The evidence here is ambiguous.

*Major Life Events.* Major events in life intrude upon daily living and often demand reappraisal of self and life situation. Whether they are events that occur only to a few people or to almost everybody, they challenge preexisting organization and could therefore lead to new attitudes and behavior. The question here is how such turning points or crises in adult life affect sex-role behavior. It might not be the emotional impact of the individual that would be instrumental in change, but placing a person in a new situation calling for different behavior. Most adults become parents and eventually also experience the end of their active childrearing years. Most adults acquire jobs, some get promoted, some get fired. Adults who survive may experience the death of their spouse, and an increasing number get divorced. The death of parents or others close to them is commonplace, and most workers eventually retire. Each of these major life events could challenge preexisting sex-role behavior or attitudes. This obvious possibility has not been overlooked in life-span research. Investigations of marriage, birth of first child, divorce, widowhood, empty nest, and retirement have all looked for significant personality changes at these times.

*Marriage.* It is in the marital arena that sex-roles are expressed most clearly. Bernard (1973) sees marriage as so different for men and women that she speaks of "his" and "her" marriages. Even present massive changes in sex-role values do not seem to have led to impressive changes in this picture (Troll and Turner, 1976). Although the age of first marriage rose significantly during the 1970s and the divorce rate leaped, most people still want to be married, and most have been married at least once.

The event of marriage itself, curiously, does not seem to be followed by marked changes in sex-role behavior. Among the younger cohorts of today, it does not even seem to be followed by marked changes in sex behavior. Since most marriages occur in the early years of adulthood, it would be more meaningful to look at data on remarriage in midlife or later—which applies more to men than to women. So far, we have no information about sex-role changes following such an event. In general, the kind of sex-role changes one might expect as a result of getting married seem to occur over the decade preceding that event, rather than following it. This is noted in the introductory section on socialization, above. While marriage might once have initiated marked personality change, it does not seem to do so among present-day cohorts, even those now in older ages.

*Parenting*. The birth of the first child, as noted by most family and developmental researchers (e.g., Aldous, 1978; Troll, 1975; Hoffman and Manis, 1978), comes closer to inducing sex-role differentiation and change than most other life events. Even in the most egalitarian couples, it seems to turn the mother toward assuming the greatest portion of responsibility for, as well as performance of, childcare and household tasks. The new father, at the same time, moves out to increase his economic contribution to the family (Hoffman, 1977; Walker, 1970). Even where women are employed, they just add on the work of the job to the work of the home. Time-motion studies like Walker's indicate no differences in household task participation between husbands of employed and of homemaker wives. This includes childcare. Husbands spend one-and-one-half hours per day in household work, on the average, compared with five hours per day for employed wives. The wives are responsible for, and actually perform, almost all janitorial services, childcare tasks, and meal preparation; husbands are responsible for, and actually perform, a very few "masculine" tasks that, in any case, require infrequent performance, such as minor repairs, shoveling snow, and mowing the grass. Emptying the garbage is an exception, requiring frequent performance (Troll and Turner, 1979).

Even though the birth of the first child tends to shift the couple's sex-role behavior toward more traditional practices, it may not alter their sex-role ideology. They may still believe in egalitarian marriage. On the other hand, cognitive dissonance theory would predict that changes in practice would lead to changes in belief.

As noted earlier, norms for child rearing, along with all other sex-role definitions, are in the process of change. For one thing, fathers expect to participate more fully in the parenting process. This attitudinal shift may not yet have affected many of the older cohorts—the grandparents—however. Bengston and Troll (1978) propose that new generational themes, which are likely to arise in particular members of the youth generation, become transmitted first to the parents of these "forerunner youth." These members of the parent generation will be more open to such ideas than others of their generation because they share basic family themes with their children.

Another significant event in the parenting process is the departure of the youngest child from the parental home ("empty nest"). While this event would once have occurred toward the end of the parents' lives, population trends of this century have moved it to middle age, sometimes early middle age. Socially oriented theorists, who are not impressed with biological causes for midlife change, often attribute it to the emptying of the nest, particularly for women.

Although the middle-aged subjects in the study by Lowenthal and co-workers (1975) looked back to the time when their children were infants as the period of greatest parental happiness, those approaching the "empty nest" did not view it as a disaster (Thurnher, 1971). Often the demands and burdens of childrearing were so immediate and overwhelming, mothers did not look ahead to their inevitable ending. In another study, both mothers and fathers reported a mixture of loss and gain in the launching of their children (Barber, 1978). Mothers tended to be more extreme than fathers in both directions, some reporting more loss than any men and some reporting more gain. The facts that middle-generation women tend to be both visiting and residential linkages to children, parents, and other extended kin, and that more and more middle-aged women complain about their children *not* leaving home may have something to do with the contradictory findings on importance of the empty nest as a significant life event.

While the birth of the first grandchild might be seen as a potential significant life event, most current research concludes that this may have less impact than other occurrences (Troll, 1980).

Divorce, being a particularly non-normative and idiosyncratic event that would not be anticipated, should provide as good a test of the life-events paradigm as we could get. Unfortunately, while the few studies that exist so far (Albrecht, 1980; Chiriboga, 1979) clearly show that divorce is accompanied by stress and loss of general societal roles, particularly at older ages, they have not looked at sex-role or allied personality variables.

Widowhood, like divorce, can occur at any time during the adult years and therefore would have different impact by age. It, like divorce, has been examined in terms of stress and identity rather than sex-role variables (Lopata, 1971, 1979). Like divorce, again, this event would have different effects on men and on women. For one thing, men are much more likely to remarry following divorce or widowhood (Troll et al., 1978). For another, women who return to the labor market face much more discontinuity than men, who have been there all along. The effect of job entry on sex-role change, though, is secondary to, and independent of, loss of spouse and will be treated in the next section, on the effect of jobs and retirement.

*Job and Retirement.* A few years ago, major life events would be separated into sex-typed categories: family events for women, and job events for men. As women would be expected to be affected by the "empty nest," men would be affected by retirement. The findings of Barber (1978) cited above show that this division is still viable though not so clear-cut as formerly.

Neugarten and Hagestad (1976), in speaking of cohort differences in the timing of role transitions, point out marked changes in the work cycle:

> The twentieth century has seen a steady decline in the proportion of men's lives spent in the labor force, with entry into work roles delayed because of prolonged education and with exit accelerated because of a drop in age of retirement. . . . For women there are often two periods in the labor force, one before and one after the early childrearing years. While in a given calendar year, work-force participation by age forms the shape of an inverted U-curve for men, it forms the shape of an M for women . . . [p. 47].

Since the entry into the job market is a major event, like the beginning of marriage or parenthood, it follows that men probably face this event only once, in early adulthood, but women twice, both in early adulthood and in middle age. Could this mean that women today are subject to more pushes for change in midlife than are men? Their second, midlife impetus could promote some of the increased assertiveness noted in research findings.

We know that there are separate career patterns for men and women, which to a large extent can be related to sex-role variables. The shaping power of the job even for an all male sample, is shown in the careers of AT&T executives (Bray and Howard, 1978). The original group of men, selected in their 20s for similarity of personality, diverged in life-styles and interests as a result of success or stalemate in their careers. Events of their first few years on the job led one-half of the group toward higher levels in the company hierarchy and the other half to slower progress. The risers showed increasing commitment to work, the non-risers a shifting of commitment and interests to non-job arenas.

Most studies report sex differences in general orientation to work. Women are more interested than men in the interpersonal and extrinsic factors of work and less interested than men in the status and achievement factors (Institute for Social Research Newsletter, 1972). Stein and Bailey (1973) concluded that although women are as motivated as men to achieve, they have a more social pattern of achievement behavior than do men.

The effects of age, marital status, and education are perhaps even more important in women's orientation to jobs than in men's. While both men's and women's employment opportunities are affected by age discrimination, women may have a doubled effect. They are the first to be laid off and they find it far more difficult to get a new job than do men in the same situation. They also average only half the number of years on a job. A more subtle kind of bias affects professional women. They are likely to be assigned to jobs on the basis of stereotyped sex-roles (Epstein, 1970; Perrucci, 1970). There is also a continuing discrepancy between men and women in top positions, partly because of differentials in reaching the highest levels of education.

Early research on retirement generally found that husbands shifted from "instrumental" to "expressive" roles, or from "masculine" (outside the home) activities to "feminine" (inside the home) activities, sharing housework with their wives. This finding has not been widely replicated, however (see Troll et al., 1978, for review). One researcher found that many retired men worked with their wives on chores that required little specialized skill and knowledge, for example, washing dishes and shopping for groceries (Lipman, 1961, 1962). However, when Ballweg (1967) compared retired husbands with employed husbands of the same age, the retirees were not more likely to be sharing household activities. Rather, they assumed responsibility for a few tasks already socially defined as "masculine." That this sex-role-defined division of labor fitted in with the values of both marital partners was attested to by Ballweg's respondents. At least among these older couples, the women had mixed feelings about the perceived intrusion of their husbands into their territory.

Another perspective on post-retirement division of labor is offered by Miller and Atchley (Troll et al., 1978), based upon longitudinal data on retired couples. In this study, there appears to be a substantial sharing of household tasks, but not along sex-stereotyped lines. It is interesting to note that in a Houston study of leisure across the life span (Gordon et al., 1976), the one activity that increased with age was cooking on the part of men. These discrepancies may themselves reveal shifting norms about shared housework. New cohorts of retired couples may reflect more androgynous, individualized values.

Golden wedding couples in New Jersey (Parron and Troll, 1978), like the respondents of Miller and Atchley's study, report sharing housework, but along more androgynous, less sex-stereotyped lines. One husband said: "We are always helping each other out. You've got to, a lot of times, to get things done." These golden wedding couples, in fact, may represent a transitional phase to the "symbiotic" arrangement of very old-age marriages described by Clark and Anderson (1967). When both husband and wife are weak, each does what he or she can (Parron, 1979).

Atchley (1976) concludes that "past assumptions about male-female differences in attitudes toward retirement have not borne the empirical test" (p. 209). Women said work was more important to them than did men. One subject that has not received much attention is the synchronization of retirement times between husband and wife. Since women usually are married to older men, who are thus more likely to reach retirement age before they do, they often find "themselves being rushed into retirement at an even earlier age than their husbands, although women may in fact be better suited to a later retirement age than men" (Ragan, 1977). Among blue-collar workers, if the wife continues to work for the same reason she has all along—money—she ends up being the sole or major breadwinner, often upsetting the traditional husband-dominant dynamics.

Although the evidence presented here for major life events serving as an impetus for sex-role change is not compelling, we may not be ready to discard this hypothesis yet. From the first study on the effects of retirement (Reichard et al., 1962), most data on life events suggest that their shadow is cast years before them. Few changes may be noted at the time of the event itself—retirement, marriage, empty nest—but years of accumulative change have often preceded that event. Neugarten (1968) used the term *anticipatory socialization* to denote the importance of these precursor effects. Widening of sex-role distinctions and restrictiveness of sex-role norms occur during adolescence, presumably leading up to mate selection and marriage. Our construct of a normal, expectable life cycle (Neugarten and Datan, 1974) could include our preparation for significant turning points.

There is a dilemma here, however. Sex-role changes during the middle years do not lead to any significant event in which greater androgyny, or cross-over of stereotyped sex-role behavior, would be advantageous. Or do they? They follow the empty nest; what do they precede? Further, why is the birth of the first child not preceded by enough anticipatory socialization to reduce its critical nature?

*Dialectic.* Riegel (1975) sees development of any kind as a dialectic process in which an existing state of equilibrium (*thesis*) faces a contradictory state or condition (*antithesis*). This confrontation leads to an integration of opposite conditions into a new *synthesis.* We could view reciprocal socialization between different generations as one such dialectic confrontation, and interaction between men and women changing in opposite directions as another. For example, reciprocal socialization, because it involves dyadic interaction or confrontation within a system like the family where harmony is desirable, presents a thesis and antithesis that results in the double-edged synthesis of new norms and values on the part of both generations.

*Reciprocal Socialization.* In the face of the major historical changes in sex-roles of recent years, present parental and grandparental generations—middle-aged and older cohorts—are confronted with new sex-role norms adopted by their children. Younger adults today tend to be less restrictive in all respects than youth of earlier times, than their parents, and than older people in general (Bengtson and Starr, 1975; Zelnick and Kanter, 1977). These older people, though, have also shifted with the times and are more permissive now than they were ten or 15 years ago (Bengtson and Troll, 1978). Although in part this is a "period effect," reflecting societal influences on all members of society, in part it also reflects "reciprocal socialization"—youth influencing their parents as parents influence them.

Some middle-aged mothers of "avant garde" youth explained to an interviewer that their attitudes had changed as a result of trying to accept the "freer" sexual behavior of their children (Angres, 1975). Hagestad (1977) similarly reports that two-thirds of her sample of mothers of college-age children said that they had been influenced by their children. The grandparents in the same sample (Hagestad, 1978) reported equivalent reciprocal influencing. That is, the young adults reported being affected by the beliefs of both parents and grandparents, just as their parents and grandparents admitted both influencing and being influenced. When she looked at sex of grandchild interaction with sex of grandparent, Hagestad found a more complex relationship. Grandfathers, but not grandmothers, tended to behave differently by sex of grandchild. The young-adult grandchildren, on the other hand, reported no sex differences in their interactions wth grandparents. Older cohorts may be more influenced by sex roles than younger, or youth may not perceive sex differences in old people. Thus, it seems that young generations see no age differences between 50-year-olds and 70-year-olds—old is old (Troll and Nowak, 1977)—and also no sex differences—again, old is old.

Another example of parent–child interactional dynamics is provided by Nydegger and Mitteness (1979). In their study of fathers, they found that fathers of young-adult children reported a more authority-related interactional style than did fathers of older adults, who described their relationship as more companionship oriented. The respondents also attributed to parents of young children sharp differences between fathering and mothering but saw these differences as diminishing over time so that parental sex-roles, in effect, converged.

Both Levinson and co-workers (1978) and Gutmann (1976) suggest that adoption or revival of cross-sex attributes by one spouse would upset the equilibrium of couple interactions and might lead, if the outcome were happy, to reciprocal cross-sex development on the part of the other spouse. Thus, increasing androgyny on the part of a wife—reviving previous autonomous and assertive characteristics—would challenge her husband's own autonomy and assertive drives and lead him to become more expressive and dependent— or vice versa. Data on husband–wife value similarity may be related to this issue. Most studies have shown higher similarity between middle aged spouses than between these individuals and their young adult child (Troll et al., 1969; Troll and Bengtson, 1979). If there is a shift in sex-role norms in midlife, then, it might be a shift on the part of both members of the couple, who, incidentally, are likely to have chosen each other initially on the basis of homogamy. Murstein (1961) made the point long ago that couples are bound to become more alike over time. The move to mutual androgyny can be viewed as a heightening of similarity behavior. So far, most of our couple data are either clinical or speculative. Until more research is based upon couples instead of men and women unconnected with each other, we can only continue to speculate on the issue.

Riegel (1975) makes the point that Americans seem to prefer the violent implications of abrupt and catastrophic transitions in contrast to Europeans, who are more prone to see a series of minute and gentle adjustments. Chiriboga (1979b), in a preliminary paper on divorce as transition, puts the concept of crisis within Van Gennep's (1960) anthropological construct of status passage. He points out that it is the "betwixt and between" position of transitions that should theoretically prove disconcerting to the individual experiencing it. Otherwise ordinary life situations become fraught with meaning, because they must now be seen in a new context and because decisions must be made about them from new perspectives.

We are apparently in the curious position of having many possible causes for an effect that may not exist. Obviously, many theorists have been so sure that sex-role changes in midlife are an inevitable part of adulthood that we went looking for explanations before they went looking for the changes themselves.

### Question 4. What Are the Consequences of Sex-role Changes in Later Life?

In the Berkeley sample (Livson, 1976) the age of 50 saw *all* of the men but only *some* of the women reviving those of their childhood characteristics traditionally assigned to the opposite sex. Independent ratings by clinical psychologists showed that those who had revived opposite-sex characteristics were more effective people than they had been before: androgyny equals good coping. All the men became more expressive; some became more nurturant and giving, others became more openly dependent. The opposite-sex characteristics added by those women who changed by the age of 50 were assertiveness and sharpness of mind; they maintained the nurturant and expressive aspects of "femininity." It may be significant that in early adolescence the women who did not add opposite-sex characteristics had been rated as particularly dependent and unassertive—poor in coping skills. At 50, this subgroup continued to be fearful and dependent, and they were more anxious than any of the other age-sex groups.

The concept of crisis implies upheaval, disorganization, or distress. If there is crossing over of sex-role attributes by men and women in middle age, seeing their former characteristics, which are no longer valued, in the other could be provoking. Men who see their wife become assertive and independent and women who see their husband become dependent and passive might not be pleased.

Even though the end result of androgyny is as beneficial to older men and women as it has been shown to be for younger men and women, the process of achieving this end state has been said to be painful and dangerous (Chiriboga, 1979a). This conclusion derives from the notion of transformation and substantive personality change. However, much of what we seem to see in the midlife changes is recovery of old characteristics in the service of greater flexibility. Are we justified in hypothesizing pain and danger?

A close look at most of our existing information leads us to feel that the notion of crisis that implies upheaval needs sharp examination. This evidence comes too frequently from clinical research, and thus nonrepresentative samples. Longitudinal date (Thurnher, 1979; Livson, 1976) that compare people who show sex-role change with those who do not indicate that such change is not associated with trauma or pathology but rather that absence of change is associated with pathology or trouble. Sinnott (1977) argues that sex-role flexibility is associated with successful aging.

It can be said that people are more at risk if they do not change in midlife than if they do. Highly feminine women, with no interests and involvement outside the family circle, are more vulnerable than more androgynous women upon widowhood, for example. Oversocialization to the feminine role can inhibit late-life development.

On the other hand, since the societal context of most people significantly older than the middle-aged samples we have been considering does not always provide opportunity for expressing all parts of their personality, the issue is one of competence versus performance. Thus, the most flexible—androgynous—older people may be paradoxically those who conform most to prevailing social requirements.

It must be emphasized that the findings of these studies do *not* document a "normal unisex of later life," as proposed by Gutmann (1975). Despite greater similarity between the sexes in personality at 50 than at 18, each sex retains same-sex characteristics as a dominant mode (Livson, 1976). In the study by Lowenthal and colleagues (1975) of four adult life transitions, sex differences were more marked than life stage differences in most realms of variables studied. Nor is it true that sex *roles* converge in old age. (See discussion of household division of labor.) In the cohorts studied, sex-role behaviors remain distinctive. To the extent that intrapsychic changes may occur, these appear to be reflected primarily in expressive interpersonal behavior: men express more tenderness, or more dependency; women express more autonomy, or more dominance. On the whole, diminished sex-role rigidity and differentiation could make late-life adaptation easier. Where resources are less, flexibility helps.

A review of available developmental data on sex-roles gives us some evidence for sex-role shifts at some point during the adult years. Some behaviors may be retrieved from the earlier repertoire, others added. An emergence of non-stereotypic behaviors can be attributed to a variety of reasons: biological changes, major life events—particularly if they are unexpected—or socialization processes. Shifts within individual development interact with shifts in cultural norms at all points. This double shift could have powerful consequences for aging.

## REFERENCES

Albrecht, S. Reactions and adjustments to divorce differences in the experiences of males and females. *Family Relations,* 1980, *29,* 59–68.

Aldous, J. *Family Careers.* New York: John Wiley & Sons, 1978.

Angres, S. Intergenerational relations and value congruence between young adults and their mothers. Unpublished Ph.D. dissertation, University of Chicago, 1975.

Atchley, R.C. Selected social and psychological differences between men and women in later life. *Journal of Gerontology,* 1976, *31* (2), 204–211.

Atchley, R., and Corbett, S. Women and work. In L. Troll, J. Israel, and K. Israel (Eds.). *Looking Ahead: A Woman's Guide to the Problems and Joys of Growing Older.* Englewood Cliffs, N.J.: Prentice-Hall, 1977.

Ballweg, J.A. Resolution of conjugal role adjustment after retirement. *Journal of Marriage and the Family,* 1967, 29 (2), 277–281.

Barber, C. Gender differences in experiencing the transition to the empty nest: Reports of middle-aged women and men. Paper presented at the 31st Annual Scientific Meetings of the Gerontological Society, 1978.

Bem, S. Sex role adaptability: one consequence of psychological androgyny. *Journal of Personality and Social Psychology,* 1975, *31,* 634–643.

Bengtson, V., and Starr, J.M. Contrasts and consensus: a generational analysis of youth in the 1970's. In R. Havighurst (Ed.), *Youth: The 74th Yearbook of the National Society for the Study of Education. Part 1.* Chicago: University of Chicago Press, 1975.

Bengtson, V., and Troll, L.E. Youth and their parents: feedback and intergenerational influence in socialization. In R. Lerner and G. Spanier (Eds.), *Child Influences on Marital and Family Interaction.* New York: Academic Press, 1978, pp. 215–240.

Bernard, J. *The Future of Marriage.* New York: World Press (Bantam Books), 1973.

Bild, B.R., and Havighurst, R.J. Senior citizens in great cities: the case of Chicago. *The Gerontologist,* 1976, *16* (1), Part II.

Bray, D., and Howard, A. Career success and life satisfactions of middle-aged managers. Paper presented at Fourth Vermont Conference on the Primary Prevention of Psychopathology, June 1978.

Butler, R., and Lewis, M.I. *Aging and Mental Health.* St. Louis: C.V. Mosby, 1973.

Chiriboga, D.A. Conceptualizing adult transitions: a new look at an old subject. *Generations,* 1979a, *4,* 4–6.

Chiriboga, D.A. Marital separation in early and later life: A comparison. Paper presented at the 32nd Annual Scientific Meetings of the Gerontological Society, Washington, D.C., 1979b.

Clark, M., and Anderson, B.G. *Culture and Aging*. Springfield, Ill.: Charles C. Thomas, 1967.

Cutler, N.E., and Harootyan, R. Demography of the aged. In D. Woodruff and J.E. Birren (Eds.), *Aging: Scientific Perspectives and Social Issues*. New York: Van Nostrand, 1975.

Emmerich, W. Socialization and sex-role development. In P.B. Baltes and K.W. Schaie (Eds.), *Life-span Developmental Psychology: Personality and Socialization*. New York: Academic Press, 1973.

Epstein, C. *Woman's Place*. Berkeley: University of California Press, 1970.

Erikson, E.H. Identity and the life cycle. *Psychological Issues,* Whole No. 1, 1959.

Gold, S. Cross-cultural comparisons of role change with aging. *Student Journal of Human Development,* Committee on Human Development, University of Chicago, No. 1, Spring, 1960.

Goodchilds, J. The older woman and power. In L. Troll, J. Israel, and K. Israel (Eds.), *Looking Ahead: A Woman's Guide to the Problems and Joys of Growing Older*. Englewood Cliffs, N.J.: Prentice-Hall, 1977.

Gordon, C., Gaitz, C.M., and Scott, J. Leisure and lives: personal expressivity across the life span. In R.H. Binstock and E. Shanas (Eds.), *Handbook of Aging and the Social Sciences*. New York: Van Nostrand Reinhold, 1976.

Gould, R. The phases of adult life: A study in developmental psychology. *American Journal of Psychiatry,* 1972, *129,* 521–531.

Gutmann, D. An exploration of ego configurations in middle and later life. In B. Neugarten (Ed.), *Personality in Middle and Later Life*. New York: Atherton, 1964.

Gutmann, D. Alternatives of disengagement. The old man of the highland Druze. In R. LeVine (Eds.), *Culture and Personality: Contemporary Readings*. Chicago: Aldine, 1974.

Gutmann, D. Parenthood: a key to the comparative study of the life cycle. In N. Datan and L. H. Ginsberg (Eds.), *Life-span Developmental Psychology: Normative Life Crises*. New York: Academic Press, 1975.

Gutmann, D. Individual adaptation in the middle years: developmental issues in the masculine mid-life crisis. *Journal of Geriatric Psychiatry,* 1976, 9, 41–59.

Haan, N., and Day, D. A longitudinal study of change and sameness in personality development, adolescence to later adulthood. *Aging and Human Development,* 1974, *5* (1), 11–39.

Hagestad, G. Patterns of communication and influence between grandparents and grandchildren in a changing society. Paper presented at the World Congress of Sociology, Uppsala, Sweden, August 1978.

Hagestad, G. O. Role change in adulthood: the transition to the empty nest. Unpublished manuscript, 1977.

Hareven, T. K. Family time and historical time. In A.S. Rossi, J. Kagan, and T. K. Hareven (Eds.), *The Family*. New York: W.W. Norton & Co., 1978.

Hoffman, L.W. Influences of the child on marital quality and parent–parent interaction. Paper presented at Conference on Human and Family Development, Penn State University, April 1977.

Hoffman, L., and Manis, J. Influences of children on marital interaction and parental satisfactions and dissatisfactions. In R. Lerner and G. Spanier

(Eds.), *Child Influences on Marital and Family Interaction.* New York: Academic Press, 1978.

Huyck, M.H. Sex, gender, and aging. Paper presented at the 29th Annual Scientific Meetings of the Gerontological Society, New York, October 1976.

Huyck, M.H. Sex and the older woman. In L. Troll, J. Israel, and K. Israel (Eds.), *Looking Ahead: A Woman's Guide to the Problems and Joys of Growing Older.* Englewood Cliffs, N.J.: Prentice-Hall, 1977.

Hyde, S., and Phyllis, D. Androgyny across the life span. *Developmental Psychology,* 1979, *15,* 334–336.

Institute for Social Research Newsletter. *Facts and Fictions about Working Women Explored: Several Stereotypes Prove False in National Study.* Ann Arbor: The University of Michigan Press, Autumn 1972.

Kagan, J., and Moss, H.A. *Birth to Maturity: A Study in Psychological Development.* New York: John Wiley & Sons, 1962.

Kohlberg, L. A cognitive-developmental analysis of children's sex-role concepts and attitudes. In E.E. Maccoby (Ed.), *The Development of Sex Differences.* Stanford: Stanford University Press, 1966.

Kohlberg, L. Stage and sequence: the cognitive-developmental approach to socialization. In D.A. Goslin (Ed.), *Handbook of Socialization Theory and Research.* Chicago: Rand-McNally, 1969.

Lamb, M.E. Influence of the child on marital quality and family interaction during the prenatal, perinatal, and infancy periods. In R.M. Lerner and G.B. Spanier (Eds.), *Child Influences on Marital and Family Interaction: A Life-span Perspective.* New York: Academic Press, 1978.

Levinson, D.J., Darrow, C.N., Klein, E.B., Levinson, M.H., and McKee, B. *Seasons of a Man's Life.* New York: Knopf, 1978.

Lipman, A. Role conceptions and morale of couples in retirement. *Journal of Gerontology,* 1961, *16,* 267–271.

Lipman, A. Role conceptions of couples in retirement. In C. Tibbits and W. Donahue (Eds.), *Social and Psychological Aspects of Aging.* New York: Columbia University Press, 1962.

Livson, F.B. Coming together in the middle years: A longitudinal study of sex role convergence. Paper presented at the 29th Annual Scientific Meetings of the Gerontological Society, New York, October 1976.

Lopata, H.Z. *Occupation: Housewife.* London: Oxford University Press, 1971.

Lopata, H.Z. *Women as Widows: Support Systems.* New York: Elsevier, 1979.

Lowenthal, M.F., Thurnher, M.T., and Chiriboga. D. *Four Stages of Life.* San Francisco: Jossey-Bass, 1975.

Lowvinger, J. Theories of ego development. In L. Breger (Ed.), *Clinical Cognitive Psychology: Models and Integrations.* Englewood Cliffs: Prentice-Hall, 1969.

Maas, H., and Kuypers, J.A. *From Thirty to Seventy: A Forty-Year Longitudinal Study of Adult Life Styles and Personality.* San Francisco: Jossey-Bass, 1974.

Monge, R.H. Structure of the self-concept from adolescence through old age. *Experimental Aging Research,* 1975, 1, 281–291.

Murstein, B.I. The complementary need hypothesis in newlyweds and middle-aged married couples. *Journal of Abnormal and Social Psychology,* 1961, 63, 194–197.

Neugarten, B.L., and Datan, N. The middle years. In S. Arieri (Ed.), *American Handbook of Psychiatry.* New York: Basic Books, 1974.

Neugarten, B.L., and Gutmann, D. Age-sex roles and personality in middle age.

A thematic apperception study. In B.L. Neugarten and associates (Eds.), *Personality in Middle and Late Life*. New York: Atherton Press, 1964, pp. 44–90.

Neugarten, B. *Middle Age and Aging*. Chicago: University of Chicago Press, 1968.

Neugarten, B., and Hagestad, G. Age and the life course. In R. Binstock and E. Shanas (Eds.), *Handbook of Aging and the Social Sciences*. New York: Van Nostrand Rheinhold Co., 1976, pp 35–57.

Nowak, C. The appearance signal in adult development. Unpublished Ph.D. dissertation, Wayne State University, 1968.

Nowak, C.A., and Troll, L.E. Age concept in women: concern with youthfulness and attractiveness relative to self-perceived age. Paper presented at the 29th Annual Meeting of the Gerontological Society, Portland, Oregon, October 1974.

Nydegger, C.N., and Mitteness, L. Transitions in fatherhood. *Generations*, 1979, *4*, 14–15.

O'Leary, V. *Toward Understanding Women*. Monterey, Calif.: Brooks/Cole, 1977.

Parron, E.M. An exploratory study of intimacy in golden wedding couples. Unpublished Master's thesis, Rutgers University, 1978.

Parron, E.M. Relationships of black and white golden wedding couples. Unpublished Ph.D. dissertation, Rutgers University, 1979.

Parron, E.M., and Troll, L.E. Golden wedding couples: Effects of retirement on intimacy in long-standing marriages. *Alternative Lifestyles*, 1978, *1* (4), 447–464.

Perrucci, C.C. Minority status and the pursuit of professional careers: women in science and engineering. *Social Forces*, 1970, *49*, 245–258.

Ragan, P. Socialization for the retirement role: "Cooling the mark out." Paper presented at the American Psychological Association, 1977.

Reichard, S., Livson, F., and Petersen, P. *Aging and Personality*. New York: Wiley, 1962.

Riegel, K.F. Adult life crises: A dialectic interpretation of development In N. Datan and L. H. Ginsberg (Eds.), *Life-span Developmental Psychology: Normative Life Crises*. New York: Academic Press, 1975.

Rubin, L. *Worlds of Pain*. New York: Basic Books, 1975.

Schulz, J. *The Economics of Aging*. Belmont, Calif.: Wadsworth, 1976.

Sinnott, J.D. Sex-role inconstancy, biology, and successful aging: a dialectical model. *The Gerontologist*, 1977, *17*, 459–463.

Spence, J. Traits, roles, and the concept of androgyny. In J. Gullahorn (Ed.), *Psychology and Women: In Transition*. Washington, D.C.: V.H. Winston and Sons, 1979.

Srole, L., and Fisher, A. The midtown Manhattan study: Longitudinal focus on aging, gender, and life transitions. Paper presented at Gerontological Society, Dallas, 1978.

Stein, A.H., and Bailey, M.M. The socialization of achievement orientation in females. *Psychological Bulletin*, 1973, *80* (5), 345–366.

Thurnher, M.I. Values and goals in later middle age. Paper presented at the 24th Annual Meeting of the Gerontological Society, Houston, Texas, 1971.

Thurnher, M. Gender experience and later life transitions. *Generations*, 1979, 9–12.

Troll, L. *Development in Early and Middle Adulthood.* Monterey, Calif.: Brooks/Cole, 1975.

Troll, L. Grandparenting. In L. Poole (Ed.), *Aging in the 1980's.* Washington, D.C.: American Psychological Association, 1980, 475–481.

Troll, L., and Bengtson, V. Generations in the family. In W. Burr, I. Reiss, R. Hill, and G. Nye (Eds.), *Contemporary Theories about the Family.* New York: The Free Press, 1979.

Troll, L., and Bengston, V. Generations in the family. In W. Burr, R. Hill, G. Nye, and I. Reiss (Eds.), *Contemporary Theories About the Family,* Vol. 1. New York: Free Press, 1979, 127–161.

Troll, L.E., Miller, S., and Atchley, R. *Families of Later Life.* Belmont, Calif.: Wadsworth, 1978.

Troll, L., and Nowak, C. How old are you? The question of age bias in the counseling of adults. In N. Schlossberg, and A. Entine (Eds.), *Counseling Adults.* Monterey, Calif.: Brooks/Cole, 1977, 98–107.

Troll, L., Neugarten, B., and Kraines, R. Similarities in values and other personality characteristics in college students and their parents. *Merrill Palmer Quarterly,* 1969, *15,* 323–337.

Troll, L.E., and Turner, B.F. Sex differences in problems of aging. In E.S. Gomberg and V. Franks (Eds.), *Gender and Disordered Behavior: Sex Differences in Psychopathology.* New York: Brunner/Mazel, 1979.

Troll, L.E., and Turner, B.F. Impact of changing sex roles on the family of later life. In C. Safilios-Rothschild (Ed.), *The Effect of Changing Sex Roles on the Family.* Detroit: Ford Foundation Conference, 1976.

U.S. Bureau of the Census. *Current Population Reports.* Series P-23, No. 59. Demographic aspects of aging and the older population in the United States. Washington, D.C.: U.S. Government Printing Office, 1976.

Walker, K. Time spent by husbands in household work. *Family Economics Review,* June, 1970, pp. 8–11.

Van Gennep, A. *The Rites of Passage.* Chicago: University of Chicago Press, 1960.

Weg, R. More than wrinkles. In L. Troll, J. Israel, and K. Israel (Eds.), *Looking Ahead: A Woman's Guide to the Problems and Joys of Growing Older.* Englewood Cliffs, N.J.: Prentice-Hall, 1977.

Women's Bureau, U.S. Department of Labor. *1969 Handbook on Women Workers.* Washington, D.C.: U.S. Government Printing Office, 1969a.

Women's Bureau, U.S. Department of Labor. *Fact Sheet on Women in Professional and Technical Positions.* Washington, D.C.: U.S. Government Printing Office, 1969b.

Zelnick, M., and Kanter, J.F. Sexual and contraceptive experience of young married women in the United States, 1976 & 1971. *Family Planning Perspectives,* 1977, *9,* 55–71.

# CHAPTER 5

# Bereavement and Grief

SUSAN K. BETTIS, PH.D. FRANCES G. SCOTT, PH.D.
CENTER FOR GERONTOLOGY
UNIVERSITY OF OREGON
EUGENE, OREGON

Bereavement in the elderly has been drawing increased attention and interest over the last 11 years. The role of loss and its impact on the lives of older people is a topic that has received a great deal of "armchair" speculation and single-case clinical observation but only limited research effort. The reasons for this void are, often, legitimate. Even in a society that seems to have become flagrantly voyeuristic, as media penetrates ever deeper into the private recesses of our lives, to request that a bereaved and elderly individual join in such a research effort is fraught with ethical issues and concerns for human kindness. A second reason for these limited investigative results lies in the problem inherent in doing research with older populations. Sampling methods, measurement, and other design problems rise up to challenge the would-be researcher before he or she ever begins.

This chapter has three purposes: (1) to review the important speculative and investigative literature concerning bereavement in the elderly, (2) to review the results of research efforts toward establishing viable and proven mental health intervention techniques in dealing with bereavement (however limited this body of information), and (3) to discuss a number of hypotheses and to evaluate the ethical and practical problems in approaching research on bereavement and to consider strategies that may be useful in overcoming these barriers.

It should be noted that this chapter will deal with the specific foci of bereavement and adjustment and not the broader range of topics involving dying and death. Other authors have adequately reviewed these subjects, and the interested reader is directed to Kalish (1976), "Death and Dying in a Social Context," as one of the best of such reviews.

## THE ROLE OF LOSS IN THE ELDERLY

Certain factors inherent in the aging process increase a person's capacity to cope with loss, while other conditions raise the level of difficulty of adjustment. As we age we encounter many stressful life experiences in which loss is the overriding factor. Having dealt with loss in any number of previous incidences, a person very often learns what is helpful to him or her in successful adjustment. Being with friends or relatives may help one individual, while quiet, solitary walks in the woods may be salutary for another.

Each person needs to have a working acquaintance with the inner process that allows him or her to make cognitive sense out of the absurdities of life. The existential uniqueness of each human life must be confronted before an individual can understand and accept the difficult times. "Being unique means being separate and alone. . . uniqueness, and therefore separateness and aloneness, are immutable conditions of human existence" (Gilmore, 1973). The development of cognitive and emotive habits that tell the individual facing loss that he or she will *eventually* be all right and that the level of pain will *eventually* diminish can be recalled from one's vast experiences. This cognitive structure often provides the individual with an explanation for the most frequently uttered question, "Why did this have to happen?" Over the span of a lifetime we develop many more or less personally satisfying answers to this question. This is not to say that the elderly do not feel pain and confusion at times, but rather that life experience probably provides some insulation.

On the negative side of this equation are those factors inherent in the aging process that heighten the untoward consequences of loss. Dealing with diminishing resources such as income, mobility, or credibility, the person must, at times, focus much of his or her physical and mental energies on sustaining himself or herself at times of crisis such as that involving significant personal loss.

While the type of loss can vary greatly in one's life, the emotional reactions to almost any dramatic deprivation are basically the same. While the focus of this chapter is on facing the death of significant others, people with whom we share an emotional investment, it must be remembered that the elderly often face multiple losses of a varying nature. The erosion of one's health and the death of one's spouse may happen concurrently, for example. The *meaning* attached to loss, as well as the intensity and duration of grief, all enter into consideration when discussing this topic.

## REVIEW OF LITERATURE

### Bereavement, Mortality, and Morbidity

Most older people are women and most outlive their husbands. This is the result of females having a longer life span than men and of women tending, at least for this age cohort, to marry men who are somewhat older. Women thus are widowed for more years than their male counterparts. Widowers tend to remarry, often a short period of time after the loss of a spouse (Cleveland and Gianturco, 1976). Widows, on the other hand, do not remarry as often or as rapidly as men; this is particularly true if the husband's death was sudden, that is, by accident (Glick et al., 1974).

In a review, Epstein and co-workers (1975) stated that individuals having recently lost a spouse face an increased risk in mortality. This was true regardless of age. In comparing the mortality rate between married and widowed populations in the United States and England, it was found that during the first six months of bereavement, the rate of death was twice that of married individuals.

Suicide, which can serve as an indicator of the level of depression and psychological adjustment of a subpopulation, is a frequent cause of death in older people. "Among the group most vulnerable to suicide, the elderly, white male, the proportion of accomplished to attempted suicide is over three times that for the entire population at the ages of sixty-three to sixty-nine, and over five times greater at the age of eighty-five. . . . Clearly, the suicidal threats and attempts in older people are almost always genuine, and involve a very great risk" (Payne, 1975).

While these statistics are for the elderly in general, that is, for people who may or may not be grieving, the data for those who are grieving reveal a disturbing picture. "The vulnerability to suicide is highest in the first year after the loss of a spouse, but remains significantly greater for over five years (Bunch, 1972; McMahon and Pugh, 1968). *For the first four years of widowhood, the number of deaths from suicide exceeds the number of deaths from all other causes*" (Bettis and Scott's italics) (Payne, 1975).

Figures published in 1967, which may at present differ slightly in one direction or another, showed that the suicide rate for individuals living alone was three times higher than for those who shared a residence. In considering the newly widowed, 80 percent of the suicides were committed by those living alone (Payne, 1975). While the statistics for the late 1970s may be somewhat different, the devastating effects of bereavement, particularly in situations that present few positive life-style alternatives, are clearly seen.

Morbidity rates, including mental and physical health problems, have also been investigated. An increase in the number of visits to physicians and somatic complaints have been found (Parks, 1964; Clayton et al., 1971; Madison, 1972; Skelskie, 1975). Somatic disruption seems to be more severe and long-lasting for the bereaved over the age of 65. The interpretation of these results must be mediated by a realization of problems inherent in this type of research. The role of "masked" depression (Kielholz, 1973), pre-existing health problems, and attention needs all skew accurate results.

The fact that bereavement has a major deteriorative effect on mental health (in addition to depression and suicide, as discussed above) is established and common information (Clayton et al., 1971; Harvey and Bahr, 1974). The impact can often surface in unexpected symptoms. Studying agoraphobics, Roth (1959) states that the initial breakdown and symptom onset was often associated with bereavement:

> The association with calamitous circumstances was striking. The illness had frequently followed on a bereavement or a suddenly developing illness in a close relative or friend [p. 591].

## Psychological Reactions in Grief and Bereavement

The most immediate problem in discussing bereavement in the elderly concerns these questions: (1) What do we know about bereavement generally? (2) What do we know specifically about the role it plays in the lives of the elderly? Many investigators have spoken to the first question without monitoring age factors within their research. Lindemann's work (1944) is a good example of such. Studying the survivors who lost loved ones in the Coconut Grove fire in the early 1940s where 491 persons lost their lives, survivors consistently reported somatic distresses including tightness in the throat, shortness of breath and sighing, lack of muscular power, an empty feeling in the abdomen, and tension and mental pain.

Schor (1974) spoke to behavioral changes in grief as being a result of the nonfunctional cognitive-perceptual structuring. Schor sees the interaction with others, particularly those as significant as a spouse, as being a major organizing factor in one's life. The loss of a spouse serves to disorganize the mental and behavioral habits in life. The fact that marriages have often existed for anywhere from 30 to 50 or more years underlines the criticalness of this loss. Bettis (1978) has also spoken to these cognitive-perceptual habits. If an elderly person is already suffering some mental confusion, this loss can only exacerbate the problem.

In reviewing the writings on psychological reactions in bereavement it was found that the effort toward developing an epigenetic, emotional response model of dying, death, and bereavement is monumental. It should be pointed out that this approach has resulted not from good scientific research but, rather, from unsystematic observation. The review of this topic will be brief.

**Emotional Adjustment to Loss**

The concept of working through bereavement has often been perceived as a series of epigenetic emotional stages that are common to most individuals in grief. Several theorists have posited models of grief which consist of critical emotional encounters that one must struggle through prior to gaining acceptance of loss. While the models have differed from one author to another in both the order and content of emotions, the theorists do share some basic beliefs. Most generally agree on the emotions to be faced by the grieving person. The individual differences found in the grieving process allow the models to *explain* a complex human reaction but not to prescribe how one *should* face death. The observation that adjustment comes in stages is useful in helping individuals who are in mourning understand their own complex and even irrational emotions. Professionals in a wide variety of disciplines can understand and perhaps then refrain from making negative evaluations of behavior based on preconceived values of how one *should* grieve. As Ramsay states (1979):

> . . . it is useful to have a general idea of what a grief process consists of, even though individual differences are great. For example, there is almost invariably a stage of desolation, with uncontrollable crying outbursts. If this has not occurred, we can be fairly sure that the whole process has been delayed or distorted. If there has been no experience of protest and aggression that lends weight to our hypothesis of pathology [p. 220].

The person who can be credited with popularizing an emotional-stage approach in bereavement is Kübler-Ross (1969). While her work was originally intended to describe the stages one goes through in facing one's own death, it was soon generalized to losses of any nature.

Kavanaugh (1972), a Catholic priest, has dealt with the bereaved as a part of his vocation. He has observed seven stages of grief: (1) shock, (2) disorganization, (3) volatile emotions, (4) guilt, (5) loss and loneliness, (6) relief, and (7) reestablishment.

Lindemann (1944) also saw common stages in emotional adjustment. He identified only three, however: (1) denial, (2) depression, and (3) readjustment.

Ramsay and Happee (1977) speak of seven components rather than stages, including: (1) shock, (2) denial, (3) depression, (4) guilt, (5) anxiety, (6) aggression, and (7) reintergration.

While it would be possible to list other models, they would only replicate the approach, in one form or another, of these four. It should be noted that these models are the result of unsystematic observation, and that while they share many components, there is a lack of agreement on these observations. These issues will be considered later in this chapter when implications for research are discussed.

Lately, it seems to have become almost fashionable to criticize an epigenetic emotional-stage response to loss. The lack of research and inter-model disagreement are used as reasons to approach each individual case as unique, without prior expectations concerning stages and order. As Bugen (1979) states, "the existence of *a variety of emotional states* is the essential point and *not* the need to order them" (p. 34). It is the strong recommendation of these authors that the "baby not be thrown out with the bath," and that these models be experimentally analyzed before such an abandonment. The practitioner or the bereaved herself or himself may find this approach to be both pragmatic and explanatory of a mysterious and elusive process.

## Predictors of Psychological Adjustment in Bereavement

In order to give a full representation of psychological adjustment to loss one needs to begin by standing back from the bereavement literature and consider some facts concerning the general mental health status of our elderly. Given that loss (not limited to the death of a spouse) is a predominant event in the lives of the elderly, it is not at all surprising that the depression rates for this group are so high. It has been estimated that 30 percent of all those over the age of 60 show symptoms of depression (Dovenmuehle and McGough, 1970). Other researchers have estimated a higher prevalence, including one study that found such symptoms in 65 percent of a population over age 60 (Pfeiffer and Busse, 1973).

Depression in the elderly, as compared to the young, is not a time-limited occurrence but rather worsens and becomes very resistant to change after approximately two years (Jarvik, 1978). A poor prognosis is seen in individuals where the onset of depression comes after the age of 70 (Gerner et al., 1979). It should be underlined that Busse (1970) found that 85 percent of the depressions in the elderly he studied were the result of specific events and losses.

While a more extensive discussion of the topic of depression and the elderly is not within the scope of this chapter, it is critical that the interested professional realize that bereavement, particularly pathological grief and depression in the elderly, are intertwined. A complete study of one necessitates a full exposure to the other.

A second major area that has been considered, as it relates to adjustment, concerns anticipatory grief. The main question being, does an individual who has time to prepare for the death of a loved one have a better post-death adjustment than one who is faced with the sudden, unexpected loss? Fulton (1970), arguing for the concept that anticipatory grief aids in this adjustment, differentiates between *high grief* responses to sudden loss and/or the death of a young person and *low grief,* which results from an anticipatory period before the death and/or the death of an old person. Fulton's beliefs are challenged by Glick and colleagues (1974), who argued that the responses prior to the actual death cannot be considered grieving. Research results shed little light on these opposing views.

Clayton and co-workers (1973) found that survivors who had been depressed as a part of the anticipatory period did not show significantly more or less depression than those who didn't experience the pre-loss depression. Schwab and colleagues (1975) reported a different outcome. In a population where 65 percent of the subjects were over age 65, the more intense grief reactions were seen in the survivors of deaths that came after at least a one-year or longer anticipatory period.

Gerber and co-workers (1975), using medical adjustment as a criterion, found that longer periods of anticipatory grief were associated with *higher* medical risk, with widowers showing more problems than widows.

While the role of anticipation remains unclear, Gerber's effort does introduce the topic of sex differences in emotional and behavioral adjustment. Men and women make different adjustments to the loss of a spouse (Berardo, 1970). Men tend to be overwhelmed by problems of daily maintenance; cooking, cleaning, and other household tasks. Strong societal values concerning the division of labor by a husband and wife prevent many men from developing such skills.

Women's problems more often involve finances, legal concerns, and the grieving process itself. Women have an easier time than men in dealing with the death of a spouse resulting from a long illness (Gerber et al., 1975). Widows run a greater risk of developing psychological adjustment problems than men (Volkart and Michael, 1957).

Men who face the death of a spouse after 65 years of age tend to have more problems adjusting to the single life than do women in that age group (Berardo, 1970). Atchley, on the other hand, observing older people of both sexes, concluded that no generalization could be made about the adjustment of men to the loss of a spouse. For women, it was found that among working-class widows concerns about financial difficulties and threatened mobility may cause lower social participation and increased loneliness and anxiety (Atchley, 1975).

Lopata, conducting several research projects on urban widows in the Chicago area, has concluded that women's adjustment to widowhood depends on factors such as personality, attitudes, and ethnic status. Investigating the phenomenon of husband sanctification, Lopata found several correlates between the grieving process and demographic status such as race, educational level, age, and income level prior to the husband's death. It was observed by Lopata during a series of projects (1973, 1974, and 1979) that women tend to sanctify their deceased husbands. Using a semantic differential evaluation, Lopata's theory was supported by the data. Within this study, other findings showed that women who thought their former husbands to be superior failed, however, to rate them as friendly, warm, or "useful." It could be suggested that men who behave in ways that are stereotypically male, that is, cool, controlled, masterful, are seen as fulfilling the expectations involved in being a good husband.

Women who were in the least-educated strata differed from the rest of the widows in their memories of their husbands. They did not rate their former husbands as superior or their former marriages as being above average, nor did they remember shared activities. Women with 16 or more years of education rated their marriages and former husbands positively.

"The disruptive consequences of the death of a member of a marital dyad, seen as a social unit, upon the survivor depends on several factors" (Lopata, 1975). This disruptiveness seems to depend on the number of roles the marital unit shared, that is, friend, advisor, sports partner; and the psychological and environmental resources of the widow. Where the partners shared major roles and where the contributions of the deceased to the marriage were intense, bereavement may be more difficult to contend with and the restructuring of the survivor's life is correspondingly difficult. Widowhood disrupts survivors by altering their membership within social groups. Doors may close at times when the person needs most to have them remain open. Having access to new social groups or the changing of the definition of one's role within a community can serve to dilute the pain involved in losing one's spouse and then losing some of one's friends who are threatened by the widow's new status.

Positive adjustment to widowhood is correlative with access to social groups and good interpersonal relationships. This desertion of the new widow by old friends is not a myth, but was found often in Lopata's work (1973).

Clayton (1975), failing to show significant differences in adjustment between persons living alone versus those living with families three months after conjugal loss, did find that after *one year* depression was significantly greater in those living solitarily.

Rosen (1973) found higher morale in widows who had access to group participation and a confidante. This research showed interaction with family and neighbors to be basically innocuous. Arling's (1976) investigation supported these results.

The criticalness of social participation and group validation as a necessary condition for adjustment to conjugal loss will become even more apparent in the discussion of mental health intervention.

## MENTAL HEALTH INTERVENTIONS

The bottom line for many professionals is to answer the question: "What do the bereaved elderly need and what proven methods are available as mental health interventions?" The greatest percentage of literature written to answer this question is speculative. So scant is this information that sections of a chapter can exist on this without even one reference to any research results (see Bugen 1979, pp. 43–44, for example). In a very recent major review, *Grief, Death, and Dying* (Spikes, 1980), no reference to specific mental health intervention research was made. While some single case examples were used to illustrate helpful techniques, the void of a solid research base in the field was readily apparent.

Ramsay (1979) has taken existing behavioral treatments and applied them to aspects of pathological grief. The use of *flooding* to help an individual work through unresolved grief is an example of this application. Ramsay saw this approach as being helpful to only certain individuals who are arrested at specific points in their bereavement. Using single case observations of 23 subjects, Ramsay stated that "my subjective ratings of improvement, for what they are worth, were 9 highly improved, 9 moderately improved, 4 slightly improved, 1 unchanged, and none worse" (p. 245). The limitations of this approach are obvious and result not from poor work, but from the unavailability of good research models.

The use of peer counselors and widow-to-widow groups have found a great deal of support. This type of intervention can aid in the emotional validation in the initial period after the loss and provide important group affiliation (Pressey 1973; Silverman and Cooperband, 1975). It should be noted that no statistical results exist to support this contention.

In two doctoral dissertation research studies conducted at the University of Oregon, it was found that widowed women in the older age bracket did not gain from training for the modification of specific behaviors. Page (1977), using a formative design, attempted to develop methods for teaching self-modification and self-reinforcement skills to older women. Knowing that older people typically do not seek counseling from professionals, Page stated that "since the great majority of old people rely on 'self-treatment' for psychological problems, it makes sense to help these individuals maximize their potential for *effective* self-treatment" (p. 48).

Page's finding showed that this training did not significantly increase behavioral skills for self-reward and self-modification. She did find, however, that the social interaction among the group members was reported by the subjects as being a valued benefit of the educational sessions. The one participant who seemed to implement the training was the only married subject in Page's sample.

In a study conducted by Bettis (1978), two methods of assertiveness training with widowed women over the age of 40 were investigated. The training methods included coaching and covert rehearsal. While some movement toward assertiveness and *aggressiveness* was noted, it was not significant in either training method. As with Page's sample, Bettis reported finding that the social contacts with group members and resulting friendships were mentioned by the subjects as an important outcome of the workshop, though no emphasis was placed on this during training. The widows also reported a general sense of urgency about the absence of a clear direction in their lives.

These studies used behavior-modification procedures and failed to show significant changes from the interventions. Both researchers felt strongly that these findings resulted from a misdiagnosis of the needs of the widowed women, that is, because the subjects had undergone a major structure loss (death of a spouse), life planning and long-term restructuring would have been the treatment of choice, rather than behavior modification.

Further experimental evidence that supports this can be found in Lindbloom's (1974) work with mature momen. In his study of factors that influenced the implementation of life planning with mature women, he found that loss of structure through the death or divorce of a spouse was a major contributor to change. "A woman was more likely to change her work pattern if she had lost a spouse during the period of time covered by the study than if she had continued in a stable marriage" (p. 143).

To state that rich opportunities exist for meaningful research in mental health needs and interventions for the bereaved is a dramatic understatement. The fact that abundant problems also exist should come as no surprise. The next section will address these issues in relation to research in bereavement.

## RESEARCH ON GRIEF AND BEREAVEMENT

The purpose of this final section is to identify the critical questions that need to be subjected to research, the practical problem (including ethical considerations) in such investigations, and some strategies that may be most effective in approaching this research while minimizing the concomitant obstacles.

It is admittedly difficult to conduct even minimal research study using as subjects newly—or even recently—bereaved prsons. It seems especially unfeeling to contemplate using bereaved *older* persons as research subjects. But researchers must confront such distasteful issues and proceed to design and implement research studies in this important content area. The primary issue must become not whether to do our research on loss and bereavement as opposed to some other, more easily approached problem area but whether to focus on applied questions which may produce immediate results usable by practitioners who desperately need this knowledge or to give prior attention to questions of broader theoretical significance in the field of loss and bereavement. We can only exhort researchers to attempt both types of studies simultaneously, an age-old exhortation which, unfortunately, is usually impossible in application.

Investigators should begin, then, by asking what it is that we most critically need to know. What information would make the most significant positive impact in the lives of the bereaved? A rational answer to this can go a long way toward illuminating one major ethical problem but avoiding voyeuristic inquiry.

If the identification of mental health needs and valid interventions is the most important question, as the authors of this chapter think they are, it is possible to begin there and, in effect, work backwards. Delineation of each piece of missing information becomes possible. Examples of this are as follows:

1. What constitutes a "good" adjustment to the loss of a significant other? Is depression, morale, and/or medical services utilization the best indicator(s) of this adjustment?
2. What do the bereaved, at various points in the grieving process, see as their most critical need? What does the mental health professional and paraprofessional have to add to this assessment?
3. Should the development of intervention strategies be aimed exclusively at those experiencing pathological grief, or should the normal grieving processes be considered? How may these two types of bereavement differ? To whom do most of the bereaved turn for help?

4. Is there a critical path in treatment? For example, during the initial phases is one best aided by group or individual treatment? Must emotional resolve precede long-term restructuring? Are specific behavioral interventions more effective at certain times and cases than others? Does the path differ for men versus women, the older and infirm elderly?
5. How *much* loss constitutes a critical mass, and does this vary with age and sex? For example, if a person loses three close friends, is this equivalent to losing a spouse? Or can losses other than deaths ultimately "add up" to a level as significant as the loss of a person (e.g., loss of health, loss of one's home because of institutionalization, etc.)?
6. The question that has received the most speculation is in critical need of investigation. Are there epigenetic emotional stages common in the grieving process? This information should not be sought for the purpose of developing a prescription for normal grief, but as a general indicator of adjustment and the grieving trajectory. As an aid to the bereaved in understanding their responses and having some element of predictive control over life, the value of this effort cannot be overstated.

It almost goes without saying that the controversy over stages has generated innumerable researchable hypotheses. Regardless of one's theoretical preferences, however, the gerontologist cannot be sanguine about the ability of mental health practitioners—or of anyone else in modern society—significantly to aid the older American in bereavement until our nation's researchers provide something more than "armchair philosophies" as the basis of knowledge.

Once these questions have been addressed and an informational foundation established, it becomes more possible to track down answers to more general inquiries. If we know what constitutes a good adjustment in bereavement then the question concerning the *impact* of anticipatory grief can be more adequately ferreted out.

At this initial stage of generating critical research areas, the ethical questions involved with studying this vulnerable population can never be overlooked. Perhaps the most important queries are the ones the investigator must constantly ask concerning: (1) What is my purpose in conducting this study? (2) Why is it important that this specific question be answered? (3) How can I conduct the effort with an absolute minimal risk to my sample?

## Research Problems

Beyond the ethical and conceptual concerns in approaching bereavement, there are many problems inherent in doing research with older populations. True experimental designs are simply impossible unless populations are limited by definition. Using volunteer samples will always have some impact on the generalizability of results, but when one considers the limitations in trying to find volunteer samples among the depressed, an obvious pitfall exists: when individuals are depressed there is a reduction in behavior, affect, and risk taking. It is frustrating to realize that the very individual who may be best helped by the results of our investigations will probably never be included in large studies. There are single case study methods where this severely depressed individual may become involved, but again only limited amounts of information can be gleaned from these methods.

While the barriers exist there are also many viable methods and designs that can be used. Many of them are not well known in gerontological science. The authors of this chapter do not wish to represent themselves as knowing all of those procedures. A full discourse on such topics would take volumes. However, several approaches that are particularly effective and are being used with increased frequency will next be discussed.

## Research Strategies

In trying to locate the effects of individual differences on a process such as grieving, the use of multivariate techniques is a recommended procedure.

> *Multiple regression analysis* is a method for studying the effects and the magnitudes of the effects of more than one independent variable or one dependent variable using principles of correlation and regression [Kerlinger, 1973, p. 603].

When one looks at the contradictory results of research in bereavement, the impact of anticipatory grief, for example, subjecting the data to multiple regression techniques would ferret out the role of the independent variable, which could go a long way toward clarifying the results.

Another, often overlooked method appropriate for testing treatment techniques is formative-design evaluation. The tendency to develop an intervention method, test it on a summative basis, and accept the results as representing the total picture is seen time and again in psychological research. Page's (1977) use of a formative design in measuring the impact of training in self-modification techniques for older women is one good example of how experimental questions can be answered through evaluative procedures. The nonstatic nature of this approach is ideal.

A third strategy, often considered less vigorous than more standard approaches, is the in-depth interview. While descriptive data exists and individual interviews have been conducted with a scattering of individuals, there is no example of using a systematic, *controlled* in-depth reconstruction of the grieving process with many and varied individuals. While limitations exist the amount of information that could be gleaned is considerable. Questions concerning epigenetic emotional stages in grief could well be addressed with this method in the initial stages. More specific hypothesis testing could result from there.

Finally, while single case experimental design may offer limited information, it is, at times, the only method available to the investigator. Methods involved in this type of research are becoming quite refined. The reader is directed to Hersen and Barlow's (1976) volume for a full discussion of these methods.

As stated earlier, empirical research in the area of grief and bereavement is a requisite. Many methods, including those listed above, can add useful information. The field is wide open, the speculations useful, but as a science it is time for bereavement research to come of age.

## REFERENCES


Arling, G. The elderly widow and her family, neighbors and friends. *Journal of Marriage and the Family*, 1976, *38*, 757–768.

Atchley, R. C. Dimensions of widowhood in later life. *Gerontologist*, 1975, *15* (2) 176–178.

Berardo, F. M. Survivorship and social isolation: a case of the aged widower. *Family Coordinator*, 1970, *19*, 11–25.

Bettis, S. K. R. Assertiveness training with widowed women. Doctoral dissertation, University of Oregon, Eugene, Ore., 1978.

Bugen, L. A. *Death and Dying: Theory/Research/Practice*. Dubuque, Iowa: Wm. C. Brown, 1979.

Bunch, J. Recent bereavement and suicide. *Journal of Psychosomatic Research*, 1972, *163*, 361.

Busse, E. W. Psychoneurotic reactions and defense mechanisms in the aged. In E. Palmore (Ed.), *Normal Aging*. Durham, N.C.: Duke University Press, 1970.

Clayton, P. The effects of living alone on bereavement symptoms. *American Journal of Psychiatry*, 1975, *132*, 133–137.

Clayton, P. J., Halikas, J. A., and Maurice, W. L. The bereavement of widows. *Diseases of the Nervous System*, 1971, *32*, 597–604.

Clayton, P. J., Halikas, J. A., Maurice, W. L., and Robins, E. Anticipatory grief and widowhood. *British Journal of Psychiatry*, 1973, *122*, 47–51.

Cleveland, W. P., and Gianturco, D. T. Remarriage probability after widowhood: a retrospective method. *Journal of Gerontology,* 1976, *31,* 99–103.

Dovenmuehle, R. H., and McGough, W. E. Aging, culture and affect: predisposing factors. In E. Palmore (Ed.), *Normal Aging.* Durham, N. C.: Duke University Press, 1970.

Epstein, G., Weitz, L., Roback, H., and McKee. Research on bereavement: a selective and critical review. *Comprehensive Psychiatry,* 1975, *16,* 537–546.

Fulton, R. Death, grief, and social recuperation. *Omega: Journal of Death and Dying,* 1970, *1,* 23–28.

Gerber, I., Rusalm, R., Hannon, N., Battin, D., and Arkin, A. Anticipatory grief in aged widows and widowers. *Journal of Gerontology,* 1975, *30,* 225–229.

Gerner, R. H., Post, R. M., and Bunney, W. E. Biological and behavioral effects of one night's sleep deprivation in depressed patients and normals. *Journal of Psychiatric Research,* 1979, *15,* 21–40.

Gilmore, S. K. *The Counselor in Training.* New York: Appleton-Century-Crofts, 1973.

Glick, I. O., Weiss, R. S., Parks, M. C. *The First Year of Bereavement.* New York: Columbia University Press, 1974.

Harvey, C. D., and Bahr, H. M. Widowhood, morale and affiliation. *Journal of Marriage and the Family,* 1974, *36,* 97–106.

Hersen, M., and Barlow, D. H. *Single Case Experimental Designs: Strategies for Studying Behavioral Change.* New York: Pergamon Press, 1976.

Jarvik, L. Personal communication, January 1978. Department of Psychiatry, University of California at Los Angeles. In R. H. Gerner, *Depression in the Elderly* and in O. J. Kaplan, *Psychopathology of Aging.* New York: Academic Press, 1979.

Kavanaugh, R. E. *Facing Death.* Baltimore: Penguin Books, 1972.

Keilholz, P., (Ed.). *Masked Depression.* Vienna: Hans Huber, 1973.

Kerlinger, F. N. *Foundations of Behavioral Research,* 2nd ed. New York: Holt, Rinehart and Winston, 1973.

Kübler-Ross, E. *On Death and Dying.* New York: Bantam Books, 1969.

Lindbloom, C. G. Factors influencing activity changes following career change with mature women. Doctoral dissertation, University of Oregon, Eugene, Ore., 1974.

Lindemann, E. Symptomatology and management of acute grief. *American Journal of Psychiatry,* 1944, *101,* 141–148.

Lopata, H. J. *Widowhood in an American City.* Cambridge, Mass.: Schenkman Publishing Company, Inc. 1973.

Lopata, H. J. On widowhood: grief work and identity reconstruction. *Journal of Geriatric Psychiatry,* 1974, *8,* 41–55.

Lopata, H. J. Widowhood: societal factors in life-span disruptions and alternatives. In N. Datan and L. Ginsberg (Eds.), *Life-Span Developmental Psychology: Normative Life Crises.* New York: Academic Press, 1975.

Lopata, H. J. Widowhood and husband sanctification. In L. A. Bugen, (Ed.), *Death and Dying: Theory/Research/Practice.* Dubuque, Iowa: Wm. C. Brown, 1979.

Maddison, D. Bereavement. *Mental Health in Australia,* 1972, *5,* 30–32.

McMahon, B., and Pugh, T. Suicide in the widowed. *American Journal of Epidemiology,* 1968, *81,* 23.

Page, F. I. The development and evaluation of a self-management training program for older adults. Doctoral dissertation, University of Oregon, Eugene, Ore., 1977.

Parks, C. M. Effects of bereavement on physical and mental health: a study of the medical records of widows. *British Medical Journal*, 1964, *2*, 274–279.

Payne, E. C. Depression and suicide. In J. G. Howells (Ed.), *Modern Perspectives in Psychiatry of Old Age*. New York: Brunner/Mazel, 1975.

Pfeiffer, E., and Busse, E. W. Mental disorders in later life—affective disorders, paranoia, neurotic, and situational reactions. In E. W. Busse and E. Pfeiffer (Eds.), *Mental Illness in Later Life*. Washington, D. C.: American Psychiatric Association, 1973.

Pressey, S. Age counseling crisis, services, potentials. *Journal of Counseling Psychology*, 1973, *20*, 356–360.

Ramsay, R. W. Bereavement: a behavioral treatment of pathological grief. In P. Sjoden, S. Bates, and W. Dockens III (Eds.), *Trends in Behavior Therapy*. New York: Academic Press, 1979.

Ramsay, R. W., and Happee, J. A. The stress of bereavement: components and treatments. In C. Spielberger and I. Sarason (Eds.), *Stress and Anxiety*, Vol. 4. London: John Wiley, 1977.

Rosen, D. H. Social relationships and aging among the widows. *Dissertation Abstracts International*, 1973, *34*, 2029A.

Roth, M. The phobia anxiety-depersonalization syndrome. *Proceedings of the Royal Society of Medicine*, 1959, *52*, 587–595.

Schor, A. G. Acute grief in adulthood: toward a cognitive model of normal pathological mourning. *Dissertation Abstracts International*, 1974, *35*, 2447B.

Schwab, J. J., Chalmers, J. M., Conroy, S. J., Farris, P. B., and Markush, R. E. Studies in grief: a preliminary report. In B. Schoenberg, I. Gerber, A. Wiener, A. H. Kutscher, D. Peretz, and A. Carr (Eds.), *Psychosocial Aspects of Bereavement*. New York: Columbia University Press, 1975.

Silverman, P.R., and Cooperband, A. On widowhood: mutal help in the elderly widow. *Journal of Geriatric Psychiatry*, 1975, *8*, 9–27.

Skelskie, B. E. An exploratory study of grief in old age. *Studies in Social Work*, 1975, *45*, 159–182.

Spikes, J. Grief, death, and dying. In G. Busse and D. Blazer (Eds.), *Handbook of Geriatric Psychiatry*. New York: Van Nostrand Reinhold, 1980.

Volkart, E. H., and Michael, S. T. Bereavement and mental health. In A. H. Leighton, J. A. Clausen, and R. N. Wilson (Eds.), *Explorations in Social Psychiatry*. New York: Basic Books, 1957.

# CHAPTER 6

# Behavior Therapies

ROBERT G. RIEDEL, PH.D.[1]
DEPARTMENT OF PSYCHOLOGY
SOUTHWEST STATE UNIVERSITY
MARSHALL, MINNESOTA

The focus of this chapter is on papers published from 1975 on. On occasion an older paper is included where it represents an earlier effort of an ongoing project or program and it is essential to understanding the program as a whole. Some earlier papers are included because of historical significance (e.g., Lindsley, 1964) or when they appear to have been passed over in earlier reviews. The conception of behavioral approaches taken here is very broad so as to include more than just contingency management but include also such approaches as biofeedback which are essentially behavioral in their approach. At the same time studies that take on a strictly environmental or ecological approach are not included because they are covered in a chapter by Howell (1980) which appeared in the prior volume of this series.

One of the difficulties in finding relevant articles in the behavioral area is that age is frequently not mentioned. For example, Keefe and Surwit (1978) list a most significant article under the keywords "biofeedback," "electromyograph," and "neuromuscular disorders," yet the disorders they review contain many syndromes common in the elderly. Since research reviewed therein indicates that most persons benefit from behavioral therapies, they claim research is needed on patient characteristics that relate to successful and unsuccessful outcome. Surprisingly, they do not mention age as one of the characteristics that might relate to outcome.

Since an earlier review (Riedel, 1974) there has been a great increase in the relevant literature concerning behavioral approaches to geriatric problems. Two points made in that review are still correct:

[1]I wish to thank Valerie Helling and Lynn Annis for their assistance in the literature search, reprint acquisition, correspondence, and filing involved in preparing this chapter.

1. The behavioral approach to the elderly was a positive one, an alternative to the decline or disease model.
2. Many of the early works in the area of token economies and other institutional applications were done in chronic populations which were, in large part, geriatric.

Richards and Thorpe (1978) also add that behavior therapy is directed at *problems*, not *populations*. Very little has been done on the theme of *population-specific* procedures. The work of Keefe and Surwit (1978) represents one of the few attempts to point out that patient characteristics are very important and that virtually no work exists which attempts to relate patient characteristics to outcome. There is also little work on the differences between contexts such as a nursing home, a large or small hospital, a mental hospital or any other type of setting. What works for old may not work for young, and what works for old in a hospital setting may not work in a nursing home. Many studies include subjects whose ages are as much as 60 years apart, yet not one mentions that inter-subject differences associated with age do or do not occur. The conceptualization of *population-specific* and *context-specific* differences remains an imperative for the research of the 1980s in the field of applied analysis of behavior as a whole.

The concentration on problems rather than on populations and on individuals rather than on groups confounds the reviewer in this area. One must look at virtually all research in behavior therapy since any given report might include the entire range of ages from very young to very old. Articles with significant geriatric populations often occur in places where one does not usually search for geriatric literature, and no cross-listing under "geriatric" is mentioned for the purposes of a computer-based search.

For example, I found 19 reports of token economies that had subject populations whose median ages were 40 years or older in the earlier review (Riedel, 1974). None of these studies were performed in a nursing home or in a facility that would be considered geriatric in the usual sense. Two of the studies did not report ages of the subjects. One of these articles was included because a personal correspondence with the author verified the ages of the population to be appropriate for inclusion, and the other was included because the very nature of the problems (chronic schizophrenics with multiple years in the hospital) indicated that a significant portion of subjects must have been elderly. Table 6.1 shows a sample of some of these studies that one finds frequently mentioned in the operant literature but which are usually not identified as being geriatric in populations. While many of the problems targeted in these studies are appropriate and common to the geriatric *population*, most of these arti-

Table 6–1.
Summary of Token Economies as Applied to Older Subjects

| *Investigator, Date* | *Age Years* | *Subject characteristics* | *Setting* | *Size of sample* | *Target behaviors* | *Results* |
|---|---|---|---|---|---|---|
| Atthowe and Krasner, 1968 | Mdn. = 57 ⅓ over | Chronic mental patients | V.A. Hospital closed ward | 60 | Personal care, activity attendance, help on ward, increased responsibility | Significant increase in performance of reinforced behavior. Improvement in patient initiative, responsibility, and social interaction. |
| Ayllon and Azrin, 1968 | Mdn. = 50 | Female chronic | Mental hospital | Not Given | Self-care and work activity | Increased self-care and work activity. |
| Beal, Sletten, Ognjanov, and Hughes, 1969 | 15–58 | Withdrawn patients | Mental hospital | Not Given | Desired behaviors (things patients wanted to do but failed to do) | Found nondeprivation more humane, easier to administer, and brought about as much desired behavior. |

| | | | | | | |
|---|---|---|---|---|---|---|
| Bok, 1971 | 55–75 | Ambulatory continent chronic (8–35 years) mental patients | Mental hospital | 84 | Participation in activities | Participation in activities in creased from 14.8 to 22.5 hours per week. |
| Dubey, 1968 | All but two over 60 | Over 60, ambulatory nonpsychotic | Geriatric ward | 50 | Self-care | Increased discharge rate of 1.250%. |
| Mueller and Atlas, 1972 | 50, 60, 67, 81, and 82 | Ambulatory regressed patients | County hospital | 5 | Social interaction | Subjects social interaction increased for each subject from 1 to 6.82, 1 to 5.17, 1.5 to 6.17, 0 to 7.0 and .75 to 4.22 interactions with reinforcement given contingent upon social interactions. |
| Shean and Zeidberg, 1971 | Exp. = 43.9 Cont. = 44.15 | Mental patients | Mental hospital | 26 in each group | Resocialization, instrumental role performance, and bizarre behavior | Improvement greater for token group. |

Source: Riedel, 1974.

cles are not part of what is generally considered to be the geriatric literature. It is imperative in the future that articles delineate the differential effectiveness of their interventions in relation to patient characteristics such as age, or indicate that none exists, or at least that there are not significant numbers in the appropriate categories to test differences. Only one report was found in the present search that indicated a *planned* attempt to look at the interaction between age and the type of reinforcement; this study did not include anyone above school age. There is some evidence from outside the area of therapy that at least some behavioral techniques operate with effectiveness across the entire life span. One such study by Denney, Jones, and Krigel (1979) found that both young children and elderly adults improved their performance under two different types of strategy-modeling techniques on the 20-questions game.

The major changes that have occurred in the last few years are:

1. A greater number of relevant articles.
2. Fewer disguised populations (i.e., increased rigor on the part of investigators and demands by editors have led to more accurate and complete delineation of sample characteristics in published reports). Also more studies were found to be included in commonly known geriatric sources such as the bimonthly Shock bibliographies in the *Journal of Gerontology*.
3. More work is being done with older populations in situations where the populations are generally older, such as nursing homes.

## THEORETICAL ISSUES AND REVIEWS

### Beyond the Behavioral Model

There is a growing trend in the gerontological literature to take a broader view of intervention with the elderly than simply to look at the environment, or at the history, or at any other one factor. Whitbourne (Glenwick and Whitbourne, 1977–78; Whitbourne and Weinstock, 1979) has presented a transactional theory of personality development in later life that is particularly relevant to the present discussion. In her view, any person reacts to a combination of events that include internal ones such as physiologic, sensory, and behavioral changes; and external ones such as the immediate environmental setting, social situations, and the general cultural milieu. All of these variables interact simultaneously to bring about any given response. Rebok and Hoyer (1977) indicate that persons inclined toward a behavioral position tend to eschew the developmental and historical elements that are readily available. They state:

> . . . behavior analysts have ignored descriptive developmental data. That is, the extant knowledge base with regard to age changes and differences in intellectual, memory, perceptual, and sensory capacities, is generally not taken into account in design of behavioral treatment programs. *Individualization* is a reasonable response to intersubject variance [e.g., see Hoyer, 1974]. However, a more informed selection of kinds and intensities of treatments, for example, is possible when developmental descriptions are considered [Rebok and Hoyer, 1977, p. 28–29].

Not only are treatments that include the "whole person" more likely to be effective but they are more likely to lead to longer-lasting results. This result may be on the very simple level of awareness of competing contingencies or a more complex level of interaction between the several concurrent parameters that Lazarus (1971) describes. Lazarus (1971) states that he was concerned about the high rate of recidivism in his phobic patients; when he analyzed their case records he found that those who had remained symptom free were patients with whom he had made case notes about "wasting" a lot of time discussing philosophies, self-concept, and the like. He began to program these "wasting time" variables into his therapeutic approach and his general recidivism rate declined significantly.

Baltes and Barton (1979) review many of the available data relative to the operant model. They argue that there is too much emphasis in the aging literature on a one-sided approach. They found five models to predominate in the literature: (1) the decrement model; (2) the life-span developmental model; (3) the socio-environmental model; (4) the biobehavioral model; and (5) the operant-learning model.

The operant model terms a behavior an operant if it changes when environmental conditions change. The behavioral decline noticed with aging could be a function of behavior–environment relationships such as (1) the absence of positive consequences; (2) the presence of negative consequences; (3) lack of discriminative stimuli or the ability to detect those that are present; and (4) the presence of discriminative stimuli which inhibit behavior. Baltes and Barton (1979) give several examples of each of the four which are common in the elderly, and how they can be identified and modified, and thereby bring about a behavioral improvement. After a review of much of the literature, they argue that working with the operant model promises to enhance the effectiveness of long-range intervention programs with the elderly.

### Reinforcement and Expectations

As Rebok and Hoyer (1977) point out, an internal set of values may act as a set of contingencies in the same way as external variables. The values more correctly determine *which* contingencies will be effective for the individual. Since our range of possible reinforcers is limited (by both practical and ethical considerations, (see Harris et al., 1977), we must be aware of people's value systems if we are to program for them effectively. This means going beyond the functional analysis of behavior and seeing what purpose the behavior serves in the total context of the person's history, present, and future. Without this total analysis unintended consequences such as undesired changes in behavior in other situations might occur. Rebok and Hoyer (1977) cite as an example of how a narrow perspective can lead to unforeseen negative consequences the study by Proshansky, Ittelson, and Rivlin (1970) in which environmental remodeling reduced standing behavior in the ward, but increased it in other areas of the hospital.

Rebok and Hoyer (1977) also make the same point that Lindsley (1964) made in the first attempt to marry behavioral ecology with behavioral therapy: behavioral approaches are of high benefit when working with the elderly because they deal with *present* behavior and they utilize the contingencies *presently* available. If a therapy requires considerable additional expenditure of staff time or financial resources, it is unlikely that it will be implemented even if it improves behavior.

Similar points are made by Eisdorfer, Cohen, and Preston (1978) when they state that reliance on a single approach, be it behavioral or whatever, is artificial. In the applied context we must always deal with the biological, psychological, and social as inseparable entities. Time after time we read in literature that staff attitudes and expectations are some of the most important determinants of outcome in any therapy. The assumptions of the behavioral approach, that behavior is related to present contingencies and that alteration of the contingencies will bring about change, is a heuristic approach that encourages the therapist to begin with positive expectations. Too many therapists of all persuasions have negative ideas about the elderly that not only influence the outcome of therapy but even determine the willingness of therapists to start therapy in the first place. As Eisdorfer, Cohen, and Preston (1978) put it:

> Outcome is also related to the therapeutic model which is chosen in a given clinical instance. For example, the presumption that there is a paucity of available psychic energy, or that the aged are too rigid in their traits to undergo major character changes, doubtless was a factor in the reluctance of psychodynamically oriented psychotherapists to accept older patients until only a short time ago. The belief that older persons cannot learn could thus lead to exclusive reliance on medications and failure to institute behavioral therapies [p. 8].

Eisdorfer and colleagues (1978) see too much dependence on the use of edibles in behavior therapy with older persons and too little use of the

*Premack Principle* (Premack, 1959) where a high-probability behavior is made contingent upon the performance of a low-probability target behavior. Another problem with some therapies, such as reality orientation, is that they do not generalize to behaviors in other contexts very well (Citrin and Dixon, 1977). Reality orientation, in particular, has not resulted in documented improvement using objective behavior-rating devices (Barnes, 1974; Harris and Ivory, 1976). What is needed is an approach that will allow for the maximum generalization of newly developed behaviors to all life situations. While Eisdorfer and colleagues (1978) have restricted their review to the patient with cognition impairment, their statements hold equally well for all geriatric patients. They state:

> There are several components of effective cognitive enhancement strategies and each aspect requires an empirical data base: 1) appropriate techniques for identifying and monitoring cognitive skills; 2) appropriate reinforcers for the older male and female patients; 3) individual differences; 4) the integration of cognitive enhancement strategies into a system of comprehensive care; 5) environmental contingencies, especially those factors that sustain the individual's attention to and interest in the environment. We would also speculate that cognition would be enhanced by encouraging appropriate play activity (Vandenberg, 1978), and it is not unreasonable to suspect that play and games could be used to develop and exercise sensory-motor, cognitive and social skills in the impaired elderly [Eisdorfer et al., 1978, p. 24].

In their review of therapies with the elderly, Woods and Britton (1977) conclude that existing data point to the fact that behavioral therapies are very beneficial with geriatric subjects. Shedletsky (1977) makes the same point and reinforces the idea that the lack of behavioral applications to older persons may be due to the attitude that older persons are incapable of learning. Ingebretsen (1977), writing with a psychodynamic bias, does not mention behavior modification in her review of psychotherapy with the elderly but makes much the same points when discussing Freud's views that the elderly lacked flexibility and motivation and were thus not good candidates for psychotherapy. It is interesting that some of Freud's early followers such as Abraham (1919) and Fenichel (1946) and current psychodynamically oriented therapists such as Rosenthal (1959) disagree with Freud and point to positive results using dynamically oriented therapy with older persons. In their comprehensive review of therapy with the elderly, Eisdorfer and Stotsky (1977) come to the same conclusion concerning negative attitudes on the part of therapists and the generally good results resulting from behavioral and psychodynamically oriented approaches. A more complete discussion of psychodynamically oriented therapy may be found in Blum and Tross (1980).

Shedletsky (1977) cites a paper by Atthowe (1975) that found staff attitudes to be *the* critical factor in outcome. A second source of agreement found in most reviews is that maximum benefit occurs when behavior therapy is used in conjunction with other interventions. Shedletsky cites the successful example of psychoactive medication in conjunction with behavioral therapies. Neither acts as a substitute for the other in the vast majority of cases.

### Self-control

Research such as that of Carp (1976) showed that elderly subjects who selected their own parameters of desirable change agreed with the staff's perceptions of what were problem behaviors. If an older patient is not seriously mentally deranged and can be shown that a program will improve behavior or feelings of well-being, he will often opt for the implementation of the program. Even though self-control procedures have been found to be highly effective with most groups, little has been attempted with the elderly. Since these procedures are highly effective with other populations (see, e.g., Mahoney and Thoresen, 1974) we need to determine whether they will also be useful with the elderly. There is absolutely no reason to suppose *a priori* that they will not. (See the summary of Bellucci, 1976; Melamed and Siegel, 1975; Weiner, 1977; on page 182 of this chapter).

### Age Differences, Context, and Reinforcement

Because of the apparent lack of interest in differential age response to various types of behavioral procedures, there is a paucity of information relative to age differences. Johnson (1977) tried three different types of bar-press response-elimination procedures with the elderly and found differences between their responses and those reported for younger subjects. All three response-elimination procedures were found to be equally effective. He concluded that older subjects tend to misinterpret certain types of feedback as positive even though they were negative, which caused some types of negative feedback to be less effective. Jones (1977) found no difference after training in asking sex- or age-efficient questions for the 20-questions game. Henthorn (1975) found that there was a high correlation between the level of disengagement and the anticipated level of reinforcement of nursing home subjects; they were higher in disengagement and thus lower in level of expected reinforcement.

### Operant Models

The Living Environments group at the University of Kansas has made several contributions to the literature. Risley and Edwards (1978) summarized a behavioral systems approach to nursing homes which treated various components as subsystems, for example, activity subsystem, dietary subsystem, nursing care subsystem, and training and supervision. Each of these subsystems has unique sets of problems and unique methods must be developed to cope with them. In addition, some way must be developed in the overall system to coordinate and integrate the programs and elements of each subsystem. Edwards (1979), in reviewing problems relating to the dietary subsystem, identified eight problem areas that could be approached and ameliorated with behavioral methods. The eight areas he identified were wandering, problems with eating, entering and leaving the dining room, fine motor movements, placement or seating, unusual food preferences, dressing for meals, and compulsive behavior. He does not claim that this is an exhaustive list, but a list of the most common problems mentioned by staff. Edwards (1978) also reviewed the behavioral approach to the problems of "senile behavior" in the elderly. His final paragraph summarizes the major differences between the pure medical model approach and the behavioral approach, pointing out the benefits of the latter as an addition to the medical approach. He concludes:

> Medical treatments for the various disorders commonly collected under the heading of "senility" have been less than successful over the range of people and disorders. Behavioral treatments may not "cure" all of the "senile" all of the time, but working toward restoration seems to be a necessary step prior to medical treatment. We know that the general sequence toward death follows this pattern: 1) those behaviors controlled by the social environment disappear, then 2) those controlled by nonsocial events (i.e. psychological supports) fall out, and finally, 3) those controlled by biological functions no longer continue (Health Resources Administration, 1974). It is within the range of the expertise of the behavioral scientist, utilizing the behavioral model, to deal with the first two. By concentrating on appropriate models, we may be far more successful in the treatment of the elderly, and those successes would make the elderly a far more pleasurable population to work with. Professionals from relevant fields should then be more likely to work more effectively with this group which has been so sadly ignored in the past [Edwards, 1978, p. 23–24].

### Observational Studies

Baltes and her colleagues have conducted a number of operant observational studies. Studies of this type are performed to demonstrate the functional relationship of behavior to environmental events. They have demonstrated such behaviors as dependency (Barton et al., in press) and behaviors that indicated engagement in activity of some sort (Baltes et al., n.d.) to show a functional relationship to present, naturally existing antecedents and consequences in the nursing home environment.

One of the more important elements is staff behavior, which acts as a strong reinforcer. Many nursing homes operate under a "medical model" appropriate for acute care, which fosters dependency and other behaviors that are maladaptive in a long-term-care setting. Moreover, staff are most commonly trained in acute medical settings and bring a whole set of medical-model behaviors with them into long-term care. Observational studies are the first line of research that can be used to convince staff of the importance of behavior on their part that supports appropriate patient behaviors.

Page (1978) summarized some of the necessary elements of a good behavioral approach and some of the difficulties in applying the approach to an elderly population, especially where the elderly are allowed to select their own problems and monitor their own evaluations. She lists the following emphases:

Defining problems in behavioral terms
Systematic self-observations
Setting realistic goals
Self-contracting
Preparation for maintenance and generalization

She concluded:

1. Most participants had great difficulty identifying a target behavior to change.
2. Most of the participants were able to understand the self-management techniques, but implemented them only sporadically.
3. Almost all participants objected to and resisted the use of self-reward methods. The most frequently expressed reason for this resistance was the notion that "virtue should be its own reward."
4. Most participants showed progress on their target behavior during the group.
5. At the one-month follow-up most had maintained at least some of the improvement on their target behavior. Only one participant had applied the self-management methods to other problems.
6. Participants appeared to be motivated more by an interest in socialization and concern about the larger issues of finding satisfying new life goals rather than working toward specific behavior changes [Page, 1978, p. 393].

## TOKEN ECONOMIES AND OTHER GROUP APPROACHES

Group approaches have the advantage of being less expensive than individual approaches and additionally, where social interaction is a problem, of facilitating social interaction while dealing with other difficulties. Much of the popularity of methods like reality orientation (Folsom, 1967; Stephens, 1969; Taulbee and Folsom, 1966) and remotivation therapy (Robinson, n.d.) lies in their simplicity and the fact that they are implemented by lower-paid staff rather than highly trained and highly paid professional therapists. Training manuals are available from the American Psychiatric Association for reality orientation (Stephens, 1969) and for remotivation, a kit containing several articles, an audiovisual list, a bibliography, and a manual (Beckenstein, 1966; Garber, 1965; Long, 1962; and Robinson, n.d.) is available from the same source.

As stated earlier, Eisdorfer, Cohen, and Preston (1978) conclude that the evidence available in regard to reality orientation paints a mixed picture. Gains were not substantiated with geriatric rating scales. There was a lack of generalizability and some gains were shown to have been short-lived. Other group techniques used frequently in nursing homes are summarized by Barns, Sack, and Shore (1973). The most comprehensive treatment of group work with the elderly to date occurs in Burnside (1978). Burnside makes three references to behavior modification in her index, but all of these refer simply to changes in behavior rather than the formalized use of behavior-therapeutic techniques.

Behavior therapists themselves have not devoted much time to the development of group methods. Rather, the major impetus in group work has come from the field of social work, where behavioral approaches were brought into social-work groups rather than groups having been developed from a behavioral viewpoint. Recent compendiums of the behavioral approach (e.g., O'Leary and Wilson, 1975; and Redd et al., 1978) do not mention group work within this perspective at all. In his second edition of *The Practice of Behavior Therapy*, Wolpe (1973) describes two processes done in groups, but these are really nothing more than individual processes applied at the same time to a group of individuals such as the systematic relaxation of a group of people rather than just one person at a time. There is no opportunity for interaction in the group approaches he describes.

### Remotivation and Reality Orientation Compared to Operant Approaches

Toepfer, Bicknell, and Shaw (1974) compared remotivation therapy to behavior therapy and concluded that the gains in remotivation therapy would be increased if there were more operationally defined behaviors; if direct quantitative measures of patients' responses were obtained; and if differential reinforcement was focused on the goal behaviors of each patient, as is done in behavior therapy. Reality orientation has also been compared with other forms of therapy such as sheltered workshop (MacDonald and Settin, 1978) and been found to be inferior to the more specific approaches. Bernstein and Dvorkin (1978) reported difficulty in the implementation of reality orientation, which led them to develop a "behavioral-analytic" approach that addressed specific problem situations developed for individual patients rather than the general goals of a typical reality-orientation program. They found that the revised approach was superior in enhancing the "ongoing functioning" of a sample of impaired elderly.

## Behaviorally Oriented Social Work Groups

Typical of the behaviorally oriented group work methods developed by social workers is one reported by Linsk, Howe, and Pinkston (1975). (This article also contains a good review of the behaviorally oriented social work literature for those who are interested.) Groups of nursing home residents were led by a variety of staff. Using a behavior coding measure reminiscent of those developed by Bales (1950), leader and group member behaviors were studied in a baseline period of three sessions. After this, leaders and experimenters viewed a videotape and signed a contract concerning the development of more appropriate verbal behavior in residents through the use of questions and reinforcement. After a 12-session reinforcement period, a reversal procedure was implemented. After ten reversal sessions a return to the reinforcement–questioning approach was reinstated. A record of leader behaviors showed that they were following the reinforcement and reversal procedures in that the number of questions during treatment periods was several times that during baseline periods. Data plots of appropriate verbalization per minute by resident as well as percentage of residents who verbalized appropriately in each session closely paralleled the reinforcement and reversal. Verbal behavior and appropriate attention of individual residents also followed the reinforcement reversal but not as closely. Thus, even a simple implementation such as the directing of appropriate questions by the group leader significantly affects group member behavior. The advantage of this approach over more general group methods should be obvious since it is directed at specific behaviors of specific residents through the manipulation of leader behaviors.

Toseland (1978) used three group methods: a behavioral role-play method, a problem-solving method, and a discussion social-group work method. He assessed outcome using a role-play test that consisted of four situations that were included in the training and four situations in which generalization could be expected. Immediately after training, the behavioral role-play and the problem-solving methods were superior to the social-group work method; however, at a three-month follow-up measurement while the behavioral role-play and the problem-solving groups simply maintained their gains, the social-group work method members improved to the point where there was no significant difference between any group.

Mishara (1977, 1978) compared a token economy program with a general milieu program. After randomly assigning chronic geriatric hospital patients to wards which were virtually identical, staff was given training appropriate to the program on their ward. Each staff received equal amounts of training. Significant behavioral improvements were noted on both wards. Incontinence decreased immediately after transfer and bizarre and unusual behaviors decreased significantly within months. While there was improvement on both wards, certain patient characteristics were found to be strongly related to one approach using multiple discriminant analyses. Patients who improved under the token economy program were less "institutionalized," which Mishara defines as exhibiting active psychotic behaviors and sloppy dressing habits, needing less staff care, being in better physical condition, having been recently admitted, and being actively discontented. Those who responded under the general milieu condition were best discriminated by the fact that they responded less to an interviewer. It is not surprising that different patients responded to the very different demands made by the programs, but this is the first controlled comparison of the two approaches in the literature.

An interesting sidelight to the differential changes which occurred in patients was the responses of the staff. Staff in the token economy ward often reported they were doing well in their efforts, while staff in the general milieu ward reported they were getting nowhere. These differences were most likely due to the fact that there is more structure for the staff behaviors on the token economy ward, as well as detailed records being available of patient behavior. Under the general milieu condition, staff often had to rely on their "intuition" about how to behave and also to evaluate patient progress.

The major conclusion from this study is that different patients respond to different programs. Although not analyzed in this study, it is also likely that different staff characteristics would be associated with comfort and effectiveness under one condition rather than the other. Future research should be directed at finding the patient and staff characteristics associated with various treatment approaches so that they may be brought together to provide the most effective treatment program designed for any given combination of staff and patients.

### Assertion Training

Another set of behavioral procedures that has recently been used with older samples is assertion training. Assertion training is not necessarily done in groups, although it frequently is. Originally developed as an adjunct to individual therapy, the more recent assertion techniques tend to be implemented with groups (e.g., Lange and Jakubowski, 1976). Five studies were found applying assertion training and/or assertion measures to elderly populations (Corby, 1975; Edinberg, 1976; Edinberg et al., 1977; Kazdin, 1976; Toseland, 1978). Corby's article explores the use of assertion procedures with the elderly and concludes that they are appropriate for a wide range of complaints and problem behaviors of the elderly. Further, while elderly persons might not participate in "therapy," the use of the word *training* does not seem to carry the same negative connotations. Corby (1975) also found that the elderly are less fearful of assertion training when it is labeled "effectiveness training," since they tend to equate assertiveness with aggressiveness.

Edinberg (1976) developed an assertiveness assessment technique consisting of four assertion-relevant situations. Two situations were listened to on an audiotape and two were role-played by the subjects. He used this device to assess the difference between post-treatment scores for a group that had undergone assertion training, another group that had participated for an equal length of time in discussion, and a no-training group. He found no difference between the groups. In a later study Edinberg, Karoly, and Gleser (1977) developed an assertiveness assessment procedure following the behavioral-analytic model utilizing eight situations for which they found good concurrent validity. They found that assertiveness is highly situation-specific and this might explain the lack of difference between the three groups on the first study. This lack of difference following general assertiveness training between groups with and without treatment is a problem of generalizability of training and is consistent with the caveat given by the behaviorally oriented group workers just reviewed. Group methods have to be based on objective observation and differential reinforcement of individual target behaviors. The generalized assertiveness training methods thus suffer from the same lack of generalizability as do the reality orientation methods and probably also have short-lived effectiveness since once the formal period of intervention is concluded, the skills are often not practiced. Likewise Kazdin (1976) used assertiveness training in a group of subjects 15–59 years old and found no age differences worthy of mention. In a study comparing three group methods, behavioral role play, problem solving, and a discussion social work group method, Toseland (1978) found that only the first two methods demonstrated any change in social skills in older clients at both an immediate post task analysis and at a three months delayed follow-up.

## Token Economies

The Living Environments group in Lawrence, Kansas (e.g., McClannahan, 1973a, 1973b; McClannahan and Risley, 1973, 1974, 1974–75, 1975) found great improvement using relatively simple interventions with a group of seriously demented patients. Manipulanda such as strings and beads were simply made available and convenient. Patients' behavioral improvement was shown both in the data and in a set of before-and-after slides (available from the center) illustrative of the essentials of their program. Another member of the Living Environments group, Pierce (1975), after leaving the center, demonstrated in Canada that operant techniques similar to those used by Risley and McClannahan would work in increasing attendance and participation in a senior citizen center.

Tamburela[2] (1972, 1976) has developed a token economy system for a ward of twenty chronic schizophrenics who have been long-term hospital residents. Their median age was 61 years and their median length of hospitalization 35 years. What makes his program unique in this day and age is the total absence of psychopharmocologic intervention in his sample. Even though all had been on a phenothiazine before the study, he was able to remove all patients from medication in order to conduct his second study. Reinforcement consisted not only of tangible back-up rewards, but implementation of the Premack Principle (Premack, 1959) where high-probability behaviors were made contingent upon lower-probability behavior. Examples given in the paper included ice cream cones and the privilege of napping on a couch. An extensive Activities of Daily Living (ADL) checklist was used for each patient and before and after measurements of status were assessed using the Lorr Psychiatric Inpatient Profile (PIP) (Lorr and Vestre, 1969). Baseline measurements were followed by reinforcements made contingent upon target behaviors selected for each patient, with a final period in which reinforcement was withdrawn. Differences on virtually all of the PIP dimen-

[2]I wish to thank Professor Joseph Amato for his help in translating portions of the Tamburela articles from Italian.

sions were significant in the expected direction; only one value did not significantly improve, although it was in the expected direction. ADL also showed improvement.

In a pair of much-cited studies, Rodin and Langer (Langer and Rodin, 1976; Rodin and Langer, 1977) found that a simple autonomy-inducing intervention such as having responsibility for the personal care of a plant was associated with improvement in several measured parameters among nursing home residents. The follow-up study in 1977 found that the intervention had sustained its beneficial effects, as indicated by the nurses' ratings, health, and mortality rate. They ascribed this beneficial effect largely to greater feelings of control and consequently improved self-concept. Table 6-1 summarizes the results of some token economy studies.

### Continuity and Gaps in Treatment

McClannahan (1974) has criticized the current system of treating the elderly as having too many discontinuities, such as the concentration on either chronic-care facilities or totally independent living, with virtually no alternatives in between such as group homes or foster homes. These discontinuities force unnecessary institutionalization, loss of independence, and increased cost. Her treatment model provides a continuum of behavioral services at different levels, which attempt to: (1) make an early determination of which persons are in need of assistance, (2) provide services to these persons as soon as possible, (3) deliver services only at the level at which they are needed, and (4) provide different levels of service designed to allow independent living for as long a time as possible and also permit people to return to more independent forms of living after institutionalization. In her model, an entry-prevention unit has the job of identifying a service need and plugging the individual into the system at an appropriate level. A premise of her approach is that all of these different levels of service would be available *and* that as many persons as possible would be able either to be maintained outside of a chronic care facility or return to the community from such a facility. This type of model has worked with other groups such as the mentally retarded and problem adolescents and has been shown to reduce costs overall. Most elderly would undoubtedly prefer virtually any alternative to permanent placement in a chronic-care facility. Shedletsky and Voineskos (1976) concluded that the beneficial effects of an institutional token economy system were useless unless this system was merged with the community mental health system so as to maintain treatment effects after removal from the token economy.

## INDIVIDUAL APPROACHES AND CASE HISTORIES

In some of the articles summarized in this section, the procedures were applied to more than one patient, and in some they were actually done as a group, but they are included here rather than in the group section because they were essentially individual procedures applied to more than one person and no advantage was taken of the group interaction processes.

### Socializing and Skill Training

One of the commonly mentioned problems with nursing home residents is the lack of social behavior caused either by a lack of desire or a lack of social skills. Skills such as talking or even, in the case of severely demented or retarded patients, vocalization, may be lacking. Other skills such as problem solving atrophy for lack of practice or stimulation and this will affect other day-to-day behaviors in a nursing home. Several of the studies to be reviewed here attacked one or more of these types of problems.

The earlier work of McClannahan and Risley (e.g., 1975) demonstrated that very simple arrangements of activities and contingencies increased attendance at activity programs. Blackman, Howe, and Pinkston (1976) found that providing coffee and orange juice in a pleasant area at a time when very little social gathering and interaction occurred (before breakfast) improved residents' social interaction. Peterson and coworkers (1977) found that rearrangement of the furniture in a nursing home had little effect on any behavioral parameter other than amount of talking. Using structured learning therapy (Goldstein, 1973), which involved modeling, role-playing, social reinforcement, and transfer training, Lopez (1978) found that social interaction increased for all groups except the one group in which the skill was practiced to overlearning. She hypothesized that this effect was probably due to the hostility engendered by the enforced repetition in the overlearning group. Sachs (1975) also found behavioral intervention with a single resident beneficial in increasing desired social interaction.

Clark and colleagues (1978) compared operant procedures with sensory-integrative procedures, and a combination of the two, as a means of increasing and improving vocalization in 27 ambulatory mentally retarded people. They found that all treatment groups showed improvement and there was no significant difference between the approaches. In the cognitive area, Labouvie-Vief and Gonda (1976) showed that not only did training in covert self-monitoring strategies in reasoning problems raise performance on the training task, but the gain was also evident on a transfer task. They also demonstrated that both the task and the transfer improvements were maintained for a period of two weeks. On the other hand, Berger and Rose (1977) found improvement to have occurred only on the trained task with no generalization occurring. The difference between the two studies is that in the prior study, laboratory tasks were used to test generalization while in the second study, generalization to real living situations was tested.

### Self-Care and the Activities of Daily Living

Older persons may lose the ability to maintain themselves adequately for many reasons. When losses are due to irreversible physical disabilities, appropriate environmental or personal assistance in performing the tasks is required. On the other hand, when the loss is due to a lack of appropriate reinforcement, or the reinforcement of antagonistic behaviors such as dependency, then the behavioral approach should prove quite useful in reversing the loss.

Self-care skills as diverse as oral hygiene (Sachs, 1975), bathing (Rinke et al., 1978), adherence to a medical regime (Dapich-Miura and Hovell, 1979), eating (Blackman et al., 1979), and walking (Sachs, 1975) have all been successfully attacked utilizing operant procedures.

Sachs (1975) worked with three nursing home residents who exhibited very poor oral hygiene and was able to reinstate the performance to acceptable levels in two of the patients. By definition, the procedures followed were not reinforcing for the one patient since they did not bring about a sufficient increase in the target behavior. Since compliments about appearance were not reinforcing to this patient, perhaps utilization of the Premack Principle or other tangible reinforcers would have been appropriate.

Rinke and colleagues (1978) used prompting and reinforcement with four nursing home residents and found that either procedure separately increased self-bathing, while the combined procedure was not significantly better than either procedure used singly. The most convenient and economical single procedure to use would be the one effective with a particular patient. Two studies dealt with problem eating behaviors. Baltes and Zerbe (1976) reestablished self-feeding behaviors in two residents with a relatively simple behavioral intervention. Blackman and coworkers (1979) were able to develop appropriate use of utensils during eating in three severely demented nursing home residents of ages 85, 87, and 95. Inappropriate eating behavior, defined as eating with the hands, varied from 25 to 100 percent during most of the baseline period. During the training and maintenance periods, it remained virtually at zero percent with only one occasion going above 20 percent. When appropriate eating behavior was analyzed during lunch, the baseline figures were 25, 30, and 42 percent. With training, appropriate behavior increased to 96, 97, and 98 percent. Edwards (1979), in an excellent review, summarizes the major variables that are related to appropriate eating and socialization behavior in an institutional setting based on his experience in the Living Environments context in Lawrence, Kansas.

Dapich-Miura and Hovell (1979) worked with an 82-year-old subject after a myocardial infarction. They utilized a token-economy approach where the patient received poker chips for adhering to various parts of his medical regime, which was monitored at home by his daughter, who was a registered nurse. The initial back-up reinforcer for the poker chips was the privilege of selecting the menu for the evening meal. More involved contingencies earned more poker chips and eventually poker chips were able to earn the privilege of selecting a restaurant for the evening meal. The value of the poker chips was diminished and the activities required to earn them were increased as the patient's progress warranted. Under baseline conditions, the subject did not take any of the walks directed by his physician, he drank only one glass of orange juice every other day, and took from three to six pills of the nine prescribed. Under the token economy system, he took between two and three walks per day, drank three glasses of orange juice, and missed taking the nine pills only once. A removal of the token system resulted in a rapid return to the baseline levels. When the tokens were restored, the three behaviors returned to acceptable levels.

### Problem Behaviors and Rehabilitation Programs

Undesirable behaviors that are the result of the aging process, disease processes, or simply behaviors that are troublesome to the person involved or other residents and staff, are included in this section.

*Incontinence* is a problem for many older persons in nursing homes. Decreased sensory acuity coupled with a decreased ability to postpone onset of urination leads to accidents that are embarrassing and unpleasant to the individual. Howe (1975) developed a strategy for decreasing accidents, which was expanded upon by Blackman (1977) with six incontinent nursing home residents at the Drexel Home in Chicago. After the intervention, four residents' incontinence was at a level 50 percent or less of their baseline level; one was unchanged, and one was at a higher level than at baseline.

Haynes, Price, and Simons (1975) treated four subjects, ages 22, 25, 46, and 71, who were suffering from *insomnia.* They used the simple intervention of changing where the subjects slept, since the researchers considered the insomnia to be under stimulus control. They accomplished improvement in all subjects, which was maintained at a nine-month follow-up measurement.

Two associated problems were successfully dealt with in a pair of studies. *Wandering* is a problem for many residents and *dawdling* for others. Wandering may involve simple pacing if the person is restrained within a relatively restricted area, while with no restrictions the person may wander all over the facility, perhaps tiring himself or herself unnecessarily or causing or worsening foot problems. The wanderer may also annoy or interfere with other residents or staff. The wandering serves no useful immediate purpose, but rather seems related to confusion and anxiety. When anxiety, confusion, and disorientation are lessened, the wandering lessens. Snyder and colleagues (1978) used behavioral mapping to compare the difference between wanderers and nonwanderers. They developed a typology of wanderers as follows:

1. Those who were constantly searching for something lost, such as their husband.
2. Those who seemed to have a need to be busy all the time.
3. Those who wander aimlessly, diverted by one stimulus and then another with no desirable purpose.

Not only did they differentiate between types of wanderers, but they differentiated the wanderers' motivations. The three major forms of motivation were:

1. Life-long patterns of coping with stress.
2. Previous work roles.
3. Search for security.

While the discussion by Snyder and co-workers (1978) does not provide definitive strategies for dealing with the wandering problem, it does highlight the issues of which one must be aware in designing a behavioral program to modify this type of behavior.

*Dawdling* is the tendency of institutionalized persons to return from an activity so slowly that they either have to be supervised or their participation in the activity has to be curtailed. Cuvo (1976) worked with a 66-year-old mentally retarded person with a reversal design, where candy bars were the tangible reward. During baseline she took between ten and 25 minutes to return. Four days of reinforcement produced times of four, ten, nine, and 12 minutes. When reinforcement was again not given, she took over a half hour to return for each of four days. When reinforcement was reinstated, she reached a fairly stable rate of close to ten minutes.

*Choreal movements* associated with Sydenham's chorea and tardive dyskenesia are physiologically based movements that are unpleasant and unbecoming. While medication is sometimes helpful, two studies attempted purely behavioral approaches to counteract the undesirable movements. Taylor, Zlutnick, and Hoehle (1979) trained two subjects who exhibited tardive dyskenesia using overcorrection and both positive and negative feedback. Both subjects showed a significant decrease in symptoms within the training situation, and one generalized outside the treatment situation to the point where there was a complete absence of any symptoms. Longin, Kohn, and Macurik (1974) worked with a 63-year-old male suffering from chronic Sydenham's chorea. He was trained toward incompatible responses on a lever-pull button-press apparatus. There was a decrease in inappropriate spasmodic movements during training that generalized toward behavior and was maintained at a follow-up measurement 20 weeks later.

Another problem that occurs more often in elderly persons than in the young is the need for operations and other medical procedures. Cohort differences in experience and familiarity with such procedures are very great. Fifty years ago one thought of going to the hospital only to avoid dying, while today it is quite common to go for a great variety of non-life threatening problems. Two studies have dealt with the reduction of *fear in connection with medical procedures,* one with an elderly population, and the other for a problem common among the elderly. Kendall and colleagues (1979) worked with 44 male subjects preparing to undergo cardiac catheterization. Their age range was 39–77 years with a mean age of 56.5 years. There were two treatment and two control conditions. The two treatments were a cognitive-behavioral approach and a patient-education approach. The first control group was treated by the standing policy and conditions in the hospital, and the second was given additional attention equal to the time involved in the intervention groups. Ratings of patient anxiety were made by the persons performing the procedure as well as the patients themselves. Both treatment groups showed lowered anxiety by both staff and self-ratings; the cognitive-behavioral intervention was superior to the patient-education treatment.

Similarly, Shipley and co-workers (1978) studied 60 subjects aged 22–80 years (mean = 53 years) who were preparing to undergo an endoscopy examination. Subjects viewed a tape of the procedure either zero, one, two, or three times. Three exposures to the tape of the procedure was more effective than two, which in turn was more effective than one, which was more effective than no exposure. In a follow-up experiment with the same group of subjects (Shipley et al., 1979) re-exposure to the taped procedure showed an anxiety decrease in those subjects who were classified as sensitizers on the Repression-Sensitization Scale (Byrne, 1961). An increase in anxiety was experienced by those who were classified as repressors. This is one of the few studies in which attempts were made to differentiate on the basis of personality variables in response to behavioral interventions.

Another problem that many elderly persons suffer from is *pressure sores* resulting from being confined to a wheelchair or bed without relieving pressure through appropriate changing of position. Malament, Dunn, and Davis (1975) taught a group of five subjects in wheelchairs how to do wheelchair pushups to relieve pressure. They were then given a 30-second alarm pulse if they did not do a pushup within a ten-minute period. In order for the alarm to be shut off, a four-second-long pushup was required. The method proved to be highly effective in relieving pressure sores, but for various reasons, including transfer to another floor, only two subjects completed the program. The authors conclude that this is a simple, effective, and highly useful approach that deserves more trial.

*Obsessive-compulsive behavior* is common among older persons. Foa and Goldstein (1978) worked with 21 obsessive compulsive patients of ages 18–58 years. One-third were compulsive checkers and two-thirds were compulsive cleaners and washers. They used in vivo flooding procedures, for example, a washer was required to hold a "contaminated" object such as a dirty piece of cloth for increasing lengths of time. Twelve clients were totally asymptomatic after treatment, one had mild symptoms remaining, three were moderate, and three remained very symptomatic. No mention of age or sex differences are made in the article, although several other variables are listed to account for the differences in treatment effectiveness. Melamed and Siegel (1975) worked with a 63-year-old compulsive checker and used self-directed in vivo procedures which were found to be highly effective in reducing symptoms.

Self-direction or self-reinforcement during behavior therapy is a major advantage where it is possible, since expensive and often limited therapist and staff time is minimized. Weiner (1977) found self-reinforcement to be an effective procedure with older patients, just as Melamed and Siegel (1975) did. Bellucci (1976) found that younger subjects reinforced themselves more and evaluated themselves more positively than did older subjects under a self-reinforcement procedure. Treatment raised self-reinforcement levels as well as self-evaluation; the increase was greater for the older subjects but they remained below the young in the treatment condition.

Cicirelli (1976) reinforced the presence of early-loss themes during interviews with a group of 64 subjects aged 65–88 years, of whom half were living in the community and half in nursing homes; half were female and half male. Reinforcement was given to the experimental group for producing early-loss themes but was not given to a control group. When there was no reinforcement for early-loss themes, there was no difference in their frequency of production between community-living and nursing-home elderly. The reinforced community group, however, showed higher production of such themes than did the reinforced nursing home group. This demonstrates that even apparently simple procedures like intake interviews can be affected by interviewer behaviors, which could lead to distorted perception of patients. The verbalization of problems is also an operant.

Bardin-Ayers, Potter, and McDearmon (1975) worked with 78 *aphasics,* many of whom were older, who had become aphasic as the result of a cardiovascular accident. They concluded that the method could be used effectively with paraprofessional therapists because of its relative simplicity. It also provided a clarification of lesson objectives and a means of continuous and long-term recordkeeping of client response and therapy activity.

Whitman and Lukes (1975) have even proposed that *undesirable behaviors associated with terminal illness* could be modified using an operant approach. Such patients were trained to become more able to deal realistically with their condition and improve communication with staff and family. In addition, they were found to be grateful for the intervention.

Finally, Flannery (1974) worked with a 77-year-old man who was referred by his physician for "*agitated depression and grief* because of the death of one sister six months prior, right-sided headaches, sexual arousal with concomitant guilt and insomnia" (Flannery, 1974, p. 199). The client and the therapist contracted for:

1. Not going to other agencies or physicians for medicine.
2. To throw away all medications in the house.
3. To use only the medications prescribed by the clinic, and to use only one pharmacy (specified).
4. In case of physical or psychiatric emergency, he was to go only to his family physician or Cambridge Hospital (back-up unit for this agency).
5. To attend daily the Elderly Drop-in Center (Flannery, 1974, p. 199).

The patient showed marked improvement in all parameters, which was interpreted not only as testimony favoring the efficacy of the treatment but also for a method of behavioral contracting and assessment.

## Biofeedback and the Elderly

Biofeedback consists of measuring the electrical changes that accompany the body's physiologic processes, amplifying them, and feeding them back to the individual in either a visual or auditory signal. Biofeedback is a behavioral approach since it involves control and alteration of response and stimulus by arranging contingencies. In the case of biofeedback, the reinforcement is the signal indicating success in attaining the physiologic state desired. Since learning theory states that we need feedback in order to learn, making people aware of changes in physiologic processes as they occur provides the mechanism for establishing control of them. Measures that are typically used are muscle tension, sweat gland activity, temperature, heart rate, and brain wave activity. Using these and other measures, symptoms of many medical problems such as asthma, hypertension, Raynaud's syndrome, and various other forms of psychosomatic distress have been successfully attacked (Brown, 1974). Since many of these medical problems are common in the elderly, and it has been demonstrated that the elderly do have learning ability, it is not surprising that biofeedback is finding its way into geriatrics. In a literature search there is the same problem as mentioned earlier in this chapter; that is, problems rather than patients are highlighted and therefore one must examine virtually all biofeedback literature to determine which studies are pertinent to the elderly. The articles reviewed in this section are limited to those that involve older persons except where the problem dealt with among younger people is also a common one for older persons.

Woodruff (1971) was apparently the first to point to the possibilities of biofeedback as a tool for remediating the problems of the elderly and for doing research on the psychophysiology of aging. Not only are many disorders in the elderly amenable to treatment by biofeedback techniques, but the tantalizing possibility exists of using biofeedback to study and perhaps reverse some of the changes in brain and other physiologic activity that seem to be related to decline in the elderly. Marsh and Thompson (1977) agree that biofeedback research with the elderly is a priority, especially as a means of determing whether the brain wave changes observed under stress are tied to cardiac responses to stress or directly to the stress task itself.

Woodruff (1975) found that there was a significant relationship between EEG speed and reaction time. She hypothesized further that learning to increase EEG speed might increase reaction time in older persons and thereby have a beneficial effect on many problematic behaviors associated with slowed reaction time, such as decision making, problem solving, and even low scores on IQ tests.

Noda's (1979) study of electromyogram and temperature feedback among rheumatoid arthritis patients was inconclusive, because of a small number of subjects, a short total training time, and difficulty in establishing adequate response to the biofeedback. The occurrence of marginally positive results in a disease entity that has been so refractory to even symptomatic relief indicates that more extensive work is justified.

Nadler (1979) studied 46 volunteers from two senior centers between the ages of 61 and 85 years. Thirty-one subjects received temperature feedback training combined with relaxation training and the remaining 15 subjects served as a no-treatment control group. Physical symptoms and sense of well-being significantly improved in experimental as compared to control groups; depression scores declined but not significantly. The entire study lasted only five weeks with two sessions per week.

Brannon (1977) divided his elderly subjects into two experimental groups of eleven each and a third group of 14. The first group received auditory feedback contingent upon production of EEG waves in the alpha band without any instructions concerning brain waves but, rather, instructions to simply increase the sound. The second group received recorded auditory feedback not contingent on the production of alpha waves. The third group received contingent feedback, but was also given detailed instructions concerning alpha waves. Only the last group showed significant improvement on depression scores, and the author concluded that an understanding of the task and the development of cognitive strategies are necessary for improvement to occur.

Melzack and Perry (1975) used alpha feedback training and hypnosis for pain in subjects who ranged in age from 28 to 70 years with a mean age of 48. Both the feedback and hypnosis were effective in the reduction of pain. However, concerning alpha feedback training they concluded:

> the contribution of the alpha training procedure to pain relief is not due to increased EEG alpha as such but, rather, to the distraction of attention, suggestion, relaxation, and sense of control over pain which are an integral part of the procedure [Melzack and Perry, 1975, p. 452].

One is led to wonder whether other forms of distraction and relaxation may not be less expensive and easier to use in most settings than biofeedback.

Surwit and his colleagues have been somewhat critical of the biofeedback approach. In a study of the efficiency of a portable blood pressure feedback device as compared to meditation plus relaxation, Hager and Surwit (1978) found that both methods were able to decrease blood pressure but, while the difference for both methods was *statistically* significant for the diastolic pressure, the amount of reduction was not *clinically* significant. There was no significant difference between the biofeedback and the meditation conditions. Another study (Surwit et al., 1978) compared cardiovascular feedback, neuromuscular feedback, and meditation. It also found no superiority for the biofeedback conditions, nor were the decreases clinically significant. In this latter study a one-year follow-up measure showed that the initial decreases observed were not maintained. Finally, Surwit and Keefe (1978) compared the amount of relaxation obtained with frontalis EMG (muscle feedback to the frontalis muscle in the forehead) training and concluded that biofeedback was not superior to relaxation training, which is far less costly and much simpler to use.

Another study that contrasted biofeedback measures with relaxation treatment utilized subjects with a history of migraine headaches (Blanchard et al., 1978). These researchers found that both methods significantly decreased the frequency, duration, and peak estimates of pain, while no such improvement was noted in a control group. Relaxation training proved initially superior to biofeedback, but there was no significant difference between the two methods at one-, two-, and three-month follow-up times. West (1978) studied the differential effects of relaxation and biofeedback on stress indicators in a group of 41 elderly residents of a nursing home. She concluded that there was no significant difference for biofeedback used with relaxation as opposed to relaxation alone. She also concluded that both methods appear equally effective in improving psychologic measures of tension and fatigue and physiologic measures of sleep disturbances, aches and pains, and systolic blood pressure.

Manuso (1977) used temperature feedback training with a 60-year-old woman who had suffered from chronic eczematous dermatitis of the hands for six years. She had attempted several medical interventions such as creams and medication with no success. After a baseline period of measurement, she was given temperature feedback training for 13 weekly sessions of 15 minutes each. She was also given training in relaxation and how to identify when the temperature of her hands was low. Whenever her hand temperature was likely to be low, she was to spend five minutes using the relaxation procedure and trying to raise her hand temperature using the mental imagery that was successful during the feedback training sessions. The subject was able to raise her skin temperature from the low 70s to the low 90s. After a six-month period, she was still able to increase her skin temperature to the same level. At the end of treatment, her dermatitis had completely remitted and she ceased all dermatologic treatment. Her dermatitis had not returned at a six-month follow-up examination.

In general the results of the application of biofeedback with the elderly has generated mixed results. Part of the problem is in the scope and duration of the studies. It may be that persons with these disorders have to utilize biofeedback continuously (or relaxation or a combination) in order to maintain the beneficial effects observed in a short-term experiment. What seems to be needed is a series of studies on the optimal utilization of these procedures in a clinical situation.

## CONCLUSION

In the last five years, the number and variety of applications of behavioral interventions with older subjects has increased dramatically. With few exceptions, the techniques have proven useful and effective with this population and with a wide variety of problems. In the behavioral literature, there is a strong tendency to deal with problems rather than with patient variables. While this is useful in showing the wide applicability of the methods for a great variety of problems, the reader has to infer that there are no age differences rather than being explicitly told so. In most cases, no mention is made of any attempt to assess the differential effects of any method or problem on specific patient subpopulations. In the next decade, care should be taken to include an assessment and reporting of any differential effects associated with particular patient characteristics. For the geriatric practitioner, it is satisfying and encouraging to see a study with an age range of 15–78 years, but when some subjects show little or no treatment effects, it is essential that the author indicate whether there was any relationship of age, sex, or other characteristics to the effectiveness of the experimental conditions. Such a post hoc analysis does not involve repeating any experiment or program, but rather requires only a more thorough analysis of the available data.

Where the techniques have been demonstrated to be useful with older persons, or with problems that are common in older people, their usefulness may be enhanced if they can be cast in the framework of self-monitored or paraprofessional-monitored interventions. Behavioral techniques are also useful because it is usually not necessary to deprive anyone of anything or add expensive reinforcers to those already in existence. The task is simply the rational *and* humane *and* contingent use of already available reinforcers.

In addition to the fact that behavioral approaches work, they can sometimes be self-applied and they are not expensive. Behavioral interventions also make positive assumptions about the client and put the burden of failure on the therapist. If the technique is not successful with a given person at a given time, behavioral psychologists assume it is because the technique is not adequate, not that the patient is "showing resistance" or that "this particular problem is irreversible." Seemingly impossible problems, such as tardive dyskinesia and choreal movements, have been successfully dealt with in some patients. The question is not why this particular patient did not benefit, but what *other method* we can *try* with this patient.

Cautela and Mansfield (1977) have concluded:

> While it is known that organic deficits do influence behavior, it does not follow that treatment has to be focused mainly on changing related behaviors by electric shock, drugs, or some other direct method such as surgery. It can be of practical and heuristic value to assume that many behaviors can at least be modified somewhat by applying specific behavior therapy procedures regardless of past history or organic involvement [Cautela and Mansfield, 1977, p. 23].

Let us move into the 1980s with a concentrated attack on those problems that interfere with the dignity and independence of our older citizens. For as Fischer (1978) stated:

> Gerontophobia is a highly destructive attitude, destructive most of all to those who adopt it—for in the end it is always directed inward upon the mind it occupies. Gerontophobia begins as a loathing of something in others; it ends as a loathing of something in oneself. In the end, the discovery that one is old is inescapable [Fischer, 1978, p. 134].

Let us prepare for our future rewards by supporting the notion that favorable outcomes are reinforcing for the elderly.

## REFERENCES


Abraham, K. *The Applicability of Psychoanalytic Treatment to Patients at an Advanced Age.* (1919). New York: Basic Books, 1953.

Atthowe, J. M. Controlling nocturnal enuresis in severely disabled and chronic patients. In R. C. Katz and S. Zlutnick (Eds.), *Behavior Therapy and Health Care: Principles and Application.* New York: Pergamon, 1975.

Atthowe, J. M., and Krasner, L. Preliminary report on the application of contingent reinforcement procedures (token economy) on a "chronic" psychiatric ward. *Journal of Abnormal Psychology,* 1968, *73,* 37–43.

Ayllon, T., and Azrin, N. H. Reinforcer sampling: a technique for increasing the behavior of mental patients. *Journal of Applied Behavior Analysis,* 1968, *1,* 13–20.

Bales, R. F. *Interaction Process Analysis.* Reading, Mass.: Addison-Wesley, 1950.

Baltes, M. M., and Barton, E. M. Behavioral analysis of aging: a review of the operant model and research. *International Journal of Behavioral Development,* 1979, *2,* 297–320.

Baltes, M. M., Honn, S., Barton, E. B., and Lago, D. Interaction between engagement behavior of nursing home residents and their social environment: an operant-observation study. Mimeo. No date.

Baltes, M. M., and Zerbe, M. B. Re-establishing self-feeding in a nursing home resident. *Nursing Research,* 1976, *25,* 24–26.

Bardin-Ayers, S. K., Potter, R. E., and McDearmon, J. R. Using reinforcement therapy and precision techniques with adult aphasics. *Journal of Behavior Therapy and Experimental Psychiatry,* 1975, *6,* 301–305.

Barnes, J. A. Effects of reality orientation classroom on memory loss, confusion, and disorientation in geriatric patients. *Gerontologist,* 1974, *14,* 138–142.

Barns, E. K., Sack, A., and Shore, H. Guidelines to treatment approaches. *Gerontologist,* 1973, *13,* 513–527.

Beal, E., Sletten, I. W., Ognjanov, V., and Hughes, D. Nursing care approaches for operant reinforcement with psychiatric patients. *Journal of Psychiatric Nursing and Mental Health Services,* 1969, *7,* 157–159.

Barton, E. M., Baltes, M. M., and Orzech, M. J. On the etiology of dependence in older nursing home residents during morning care: the role of staff behavior. *Journal of Personality and Social Psychology,* in press.

Beckenstein, N. Remotivation: a first step to restoration. *Hospital and Community Psychiatry,* 1966, *17,* 115–118.

Bellucci, G. Effects of feedback on self-reinforcement in elderly and young adults. *Dissertation Abstracts International,* 1976, *36,* 5246.

Berger, R. M., and Rose, S. D. Interpersonal skill training with institutionalized elderly patients. *Journal of Gerontology,* 1977, *32,* 346–353.

Bernstein, R., and Dvorkin, L. An alternative to reality orientation: a "behavioral-analytic" approach. Paper presented at the 31st Annual Scientific Meeting of the Gerontological Society, Dallas, Texas, Nov. 16–20, 1978.

Blackman, D. K. Control of urinary incontinence among the institutionalized elderly. Paper presented at the 11th annual convention of the Association for the Advancement of Behavior Therapy, Atlanta, Georgia, December 1977.

Blackman, D. K., Gehle, C., and Pinkston, E. M. Modifying eating habits of the institutionalized elderly. *Social Work Research and Abstracts,* 1979, *14,* 18–24.

Blackman, D. K., Howe, M., and Pinkston, E. M. Increasing participation in social interaction of the institutionalized elderly. *Gerontologist,* 1976, *16,* 69–76.

Blanchard, B., Theobald, D. E., Williamson, D. A., Silver, B. V., and Brown, D. A. Temperature biofeedback in the treatment of migraine headaches: a controlled evaluation. *Archives of General Psychiatry,* 1978, *35,* 581–588.

Blum, J. E., and Tross, S. Psychodynamic treatment of the elderly. In C. Eisdorfer (Ed.), *Annual Review of Gerontology and Geriatrics,* vol. 1. New York: Springer, 1980.

Bok, M. Some problems in milieu treatment of the chronic older mental patient. *Gerontologist,* 1971, *11,* 141–147.

Brannon, L. J. The effects of biofeedback training of EEG alpha activity on the psychological functioning of the elderly. *Dissertation Abstracts International,* 1977, *37 (11B),* 5875.

Brown, B. B. *New Mind, New Body.* New York: Harper and Row, 1974.

Burnside, I. M. (Ed.). *Working with the Elderly: Group Processes and Techniques.* North Scituate, Mass.: Duxbury Press, 1978.

Byrne, D. The repression-sensitization scale: rationale, reliability, and validity. *Journal of Personality,* 1961, *29,* 334–349.

Carp, F. M. User evaluation of the housing of the elderly. *Gerontologist,* 1976, *16,* 102–111.

Cautela, J. R., and Mansfield, L. A behavioral approach to geriatrics. In W. D. Gentry (Ed.), *Geropsychology: A Model of Training and Clinical Service.* Cambridge, Mass.: Ballinger Publishing Co., 1977.

Cicirelli, V. G. The relationship of task reinforcement to personal loss themes revealed in earliest memories of elderly subjects. *Journal of Experimental Aging Research,* 1976, *2,* 435–447.

Citrin, R. S., and Dixon, D. N. Reality orientation: a milieu therapy used in an institution for the aged. *Gerontologist,* 1977, *17,* 39–43.

Clark, A., Miller, L. R., Thomas, J. A., Kucherawy, D. A., and Azen, S. P. A comparison of operant and sensory integrative methods on developmental parameters in profoundly retarded adults. *American Journal of Occupational Therapy,* 1978, *32,* 86–92.

Corby, N. Assertion training with aged populations. *Counseling Psychologist,* 1975, *5,* 69–74.

Cuvo, A. J. Decreasing repetitive behavior in an institutionalized mentally retarded resident. *Mental Retardation,* 1976, *15,* 22–25.

Dapich-Miura, E., and Hovell, M. F. Contingency management of adherence to a complex medical regimen in an elderly heart patient. *Behavior Therapy,* 1979, *10,* 193–201.

Denney, N. W., Jones, F. W., and Krigel, S. H. Modifying the questioning strategies of young children and elderly adults with strategy-modeling techniques. *Human Development,* 1979, *22,* 23–36.

Dubey, E. Intensive treatment of the institutionalized ambulatory geriatric patient. *Geriatrics,* 1968, *23,* 170–177.

Edinberg, M. A. Behavioral assessment and assertion training of the elderly. *Dissertation Abstracts International,* 1976, *36,* 4865–4866.

Edinberg, M. A., Karoly, P., and Gleser, G. G. Assessing assertion in the elderly: an application of the behavioral-analytic model of competence. *Journal of Clinical Psychology,* 1977, *33,* 869–874.

Edwards, K. A. Restoring functional behavior of "senile" elderly. In V. Ferguson and C. B. Taylor (Eds.), *Comprehensive Handbook of Behavioral Medicine.* New York: Spectrum Press, 1978.

Edwards, K. A. Dining experiences in the institutionalized setting. *Nursing Homes,* 1979, *28,* 6–17.

Eisdorfer, L., Cohen, D., and Preston, C. Behavioral and psychological therapies for the older patient with cognitive impairment. Paper delivered at the NIH Conference on Behavioral Aspects of Senile Dementia, Washington, D.C., December, 1978.

Eisdorfer, C., and Stotsky, B. A. Intervention, treatment and rehabilitation of psychiatric disorders. In J. E. Birren and K. W. Schaie (Eds.), *Handbook of the Psychology of Aging.* New York: Van Nostrand, 1977.

Fenichel, O. *The Psychoanalytic Theory of Neurosis.* London: Routledge and Kegan, Paul, 1946.

Fischer, D. H. *Growing Old in America.* New York: Oxford University Press, 1978.

Flannery, B. Behavior modification of geriatric grief: a transactional perspective. *International Journal of Aging and Human Development,* 1974, *5,* 197–203.

Foa, E. B., and Goldstein, A. Continuous exposure and complete response prevention in the treatment of obsessive-compulsive neurosis. *Behavior Therapy,* 1978, *9,* 821–829.

Folsom, J. C. Intensive hospital therapy of geriatric patients. In J. H. Masserman (Ed.), *Current Psychiatric Therapies,* vol. 7. New York: Grune and Stratton, 1967.

Garber, R. S. A psychiatrist's view of remotivation. *Mental Hospitals,* 1965, *16,* 219–221.

Glenwick, D. S., and Whitbourne, S. K. Beyond despair and disengagement: a transactional model of personality development in later life. *International Journal of Aging and Human Development,* 1977–78, *8,* 261–267.

Goldstein, A. P. *Structured Learning Therapy: Toward a Psychotherapy for the Poor.* New York: Academic Press, 1973.

Hager, J. L., and Surwit, R. S. Hypertension self-control with a portable feedback unit or meditation-relaxation. *Biofeedback and Self-regulation,* 1978, *3,* 269–276.

Harris, C. S., and Ivory, P. B. C. B. An outcome evaluation of reality orientation therapy with geriatric patients in a state mental hospital. *Gerontologist,* 1976, *16,* 496–503.

Harris, S. L., Snyder, B. D., Snyder, R. L., and MacGraw, B. Behavior modification therapy with elderly demented patients: implementation and ethical considerations. *Journal of Chronic Disease,* 1977, *30,* 129–134.

Haynes, S. N., Price, M. G., and Simons, J. B. Stimulus control treatment of insomnia. *Journal of Behavior Therapy and Experimental Psychiatry,* 1975, *6,* 279–282.

Health Resources Administration. *Working with Older People: A Guide to Practice. Volume II. Biological, Psychological and Sociological Aspects of Aging.* DHEW Publication No. HRA 74-3117. Rockville, Md.: Department of Health, Education and Welfare, 1974.

Henthorn, B. S. Disengagement and reinforcement in the elderly: an exploratory survey. Unpublished doctoral dissertation, University of Oklahoma, 1975.

Howe, M. W. Behavior management of urinary incontinence in the elderly. Unpublished doctoral dissertation, University of Chicago, 1975.

Howell, S. Environments and aging. In C. Eisdorfer (Ed.), *Annual Review of Gerontology and Geriatrics,* vol. 1. New York: Springer Publishing Co., 1980.

Hoyer, W. J. Aging as intraindividual change. *Developmental Psychology,* 1974, *10,* 821–826.

Ingebretsen, R. Psychotherapy with the elderly. *Psychotherapy: Theory, Research and Practice,* 1977, *14,* 319–332.

Johnson, T. A. A comparison of three response-elimination techniques among gerontological subjects. *Dissertation Abstracts International,* 1977, *38,* 1440–1441.

Jones, F. W. Modifying the questioning strategies of young children and elderly adults by strategy modeling training instructions. *Dissertation Abstracts International,* 1977, *38,* 904.

Kazdin, A. E. Assessment of imagery during covert-modeling of assertive behavior. *Journal of Behavior Therapy and Experimental Psychiatry,* 1976, *7,* 213–219.

Keefe, F. J., and Surwit, R. S. Electromyographic biofeedback: behavioral treatment of neuromuscular disorders. *Journal of Behavioral Medicine*, 1978, *1*, 13–24.

Kendall, C., Williams, L., Pechacek, T. F., Graham, L. E., Shisslak, C., and Herzoff, N. Cognitive-behavioral and patient education interventions in cardiac catheterization procedures: The Palo Alto Medical Psychological Project. *Journal of Consulting and Clinical Psychology*, 1979, *47*, 49–58.

Labouvie-Vief, G., and Gonda, J. N. Cognitive strategy training and intellectual performance in the elderly. *Journal of Gerontology*, 1976, *31*, 327–332.

Lange, A. J., and Jakubowski, P. *Responsible Assertive Behavior: Cognitive/Behavioral Procedures for Trainers*. Champaign, Ill.: Research Press, 1976.

Langer, E. J., and Rodin, J. The effects of choice and enhanced personal responsibility for the aged: a field experiment in an institutional setting. *Journal of Personality and Social Psychology*, 1976, *34*, 191–198.

Lazarus, A. A. *Behavior Therapy and Beyond*. New York: McGraw-Hill, 1971.

Lindsley, D. R. Geriatric behavior prosthetics. In R. Kastenbaum (Ed.), *New Thoughts on Old Age*. New York: Springer Publishing Co., 1964.

Linsk, N., Howe, M. W., and Pinkston, E. M. Behavioral group work in a home for the aged. *Social Work*, 1975, *20*, 454–463.

Long, R. S., Jr. Remotivation—fact or artifact. *Mental Hospital Service*, 1962, No. 151, 1–8.

Longin, H. E., Kohn, J. P., and Macurik, K. M. The modification of choreal movements. *Journal of Behavior Therapy and Experimental Psychiatry*, 1974, *5*, 263–265.

Lopez, M. A. Establishing and maintaining a social skill among elderly psychiatric patients. *Dissertation Abstracts International*, 1978, *39*, 987–988.

Lorr, M., and Vestre, M. P. The psychotic inpatient profile: a nurse's observation scale. *Journal of Clinical Psychology*, 1969, *25*, 137–140.

MacDonald, M. L., and Settin, J. M. Reality orientation versus sheltered workshops as treatment for the institutionalized aging. *Journal of Gerontology*, 1978, *33*, 416–421.

Mahoney, M. J., and Thoresen, C. E. *Self-control: Power to the Person*. Monterey, Calif.: Brooks/Cole, 1974.

Malament, I. B., Dunn, M. E., and Davis, R. Pressure sores: an operant conditioning approach to prevention. *Archives of Physical Medicine and Rehabilitation*, 1975, *56*, 161–164.

Manuso, S. The use of biofeedback—assisted handwarming training in the treatment of chronic eczematous dermatitis of the hands: a case study. *Journal of Behavioral Therapy and Experimental Psychiatry*, 1977, *8*, 445–446.

Marsh, G. R., and Thompson, L. W. Psychophysiology of aging. In J. E. Birren and K. W. Schaie (Eds.), *Handbook of the Psychology of Aging*. New York: Van Nostrand Reinhold, 1977.

McClannahan, L. E. Recreation programs for nursing home residents: the importance of patient characteristics and environmental arrangements. *Therapeutic Recreation Journal*, 1973a, *7*, 26–31.

McClannahan, L. E. Therapeutic and prosthetic lining environment for nursing home residents. *Gerontologist*, 1973b, *13*, 424–429.

McClannahan, L. E. A proposal for a continuum of behavioral treatment services for the aged. Paper presented at the Annual Convention of the American Psychological Association, New Orleans, 1974.

McClannahan, L. E., and Risley, T. R. A store for nursing home residents. *Nursing Homes*, 1973, *22*, 10–11, 29.

McClannahan, L. E., and Risley, T. R. Design of living environments for nursing home residents: recruiting attendance at activities. *Gerontologist*, 1974, *14*, 236–240.

McClannahan, L. E., and Risley, T. R. Design of living environment for nursing home residents: increasing participation in recreation activity. *Journal of Applied Behavior Analysis*, 1975, *8*, 261–268.

McClannahan, L. E., and Risley, T. R. Activities and materials for severely disabled geriatric patients. *Nursing Homes*, 1974–1975, *24*, 10–13.

Melamed, B.G., and Siegel, L. J. Self-directed *in vivo* treatment of an obsessive compulsive checking ritual. *Journal of Behavior Therapy and Experimental Psychiatry*, 1975, *6*, 31–35.

Melzack, R., and Perry, C. Self-regulation of pain. The use of alpha-feedback and hypnotic training for the control of chronic pain. *Experimental Neurology*, 1975, *46*, 452–469.

Mishara, B. L. Geriatric patients who improve in token economy and general milieu programs: a multivariate analysis. Paper presented at the meeting of American Psychological Association, San Francisco, September 1977.

Mishara, B. L. Geriatrics patients who improve in token economy and general milieu treatment programs: a multivariate analysis. *Journal of Consulting and Clinical Psychology*, 1978, *46*, 1340–1348.

Mueller, D. J., and Atlas, L. Resocialization of regressed elderly residents: a behavioral approach. *Journal of Gerontology*, 1972, *27*, 390–392.

Nadler, D. B. Temperature biofeedback and relaxation training for older adults. *Dissertation Abstracts International*, 1979, *39*, 3532.

Noda, H. H. An exploratory study of the effects of EMG and temperature biofeedback on rheumatoid arthritis. *Dissertation Abstracts International*, 1979, *39*, 3532–3533.

O'Leary, K. D., and Wilson, G. T. *Behavior Therapy: Application and Outcome.* Englewood Cliffs, N.J.: Prentice-Hall, 1975.

Page, F. I. The development and evaluation of a self-management training program for older adults. *Dissertation Abstracts International*, 1978, *39*, 393.

Peterson, R. F., Knapp, T. J., Rasen, J. C., and Pither, B. F. The effects of furniture arrangement on the behavior of geriatric patients. *Behavior Therapy*, 1977, *8*, 464–467.

Pierce, C. H. Recreation for the elderly: activity participation at a senior citizen center. *Gerontologist*, 1975, *15*, 202–205.

Premack, D. Toward empirical behavior laws: positive reinforcement. *Psychological Review*, 1959, *66*, 219–233.

Proshansky, H. M., Ittleson, W. H., and Rivlin, L. G. (Eds.). *Environmental Psychology*. New York: Holt, Rinehart and Winston, 1970.

Rebok, G. W., and Hoyer, W. J. The functional context of elderly behavior. *Gerontologist*, 1977, *17*, 27–34.

Redd, W. H., Porterfield, A. L., and Anderson, B. L. *Behavior Modification: Behavioral Approaches to Human Problems*. New York: Plenum Press, 1978.

Richards, W. S., and Thorpe, G. L. Behavioral approaches to the problems of later life. In M. Storandt, I. C. Siegler, and M. E. Elias (Eds.), *The Clinical Psychology of Aging*. New York: Plenum Press, 1978.

Riedel, R. G. Experimental analysis as applied to adulthood and old age: a review. Paper presented at the Annual Convention of the American Psychological Association, New Orleans, August 1974.

Rinke, C. L., Williams, J. J., Lloyd, K. E., and Smith-Scott, W. The effects of prompting and reinforcement on self-bathing by elderly residents of a nursing home. *Behavior Therapy,* 1978, *9,* 873–881.

Risley, T. R., and Edwards, K. A. Behavioral technology for nursing home care: toward a system of nursing home organization and management. Paper presented at the Nova University Behavioral Conference on Aging, Port St. Lucie, Florida, May 1978.

Robinson, A. M. *Remotivation Technique: A Manual for Use in Nursing Homes.* Washington, D.C.: American Psychiatric Association, no date.

Rodin, J., and Langer, E. J. Long-term effects of a control-relevant intervention with the institutionalized aged. *Journal of Personality and Social Psychology,* 1977, *12,* 897–902.

Rosenthal, H. R. Psychotherapy of the aging. *American Journal of Psychotherapy,* 1959, *13,* 55–65.

Sachs, D. A. Behavioral techniques in a residential nursing home facility. *Journal of Behavior Therapy and Experimental Psychiatry,* 1975, *6,* 123–127.

Shean, G. D., and Zeidberg, Z. Token-reinforcement therapy: a comparison of matched groups. *Journal of Behavior Therapy and Experimental Psychiatry,* 1971, *2,* 95–105.

Shedletsky, R. Behavior modification and the hospitalized elderly. *Essence,* 1977, *2,* 25–31.

Shedletsky, R., and Voineskos, G. The rehabilitation of the chronic psychiatric patient: beyond the hospital-based token economy system. *Social Psychiatry,* 1976, *11,* 145–150.

Shipley, R. H., Butt, J. H., Horwitz, B., and Farby, J. E. Preparation for a stressful medical procedure: effect of amount of stimulus preexposure and coping style. *Journal of Consulting and Clinical Psychology,* 1978, *46,* 499–507.

Shipley, R. H., Butt, J. H., and Horwitz, E. A. Preparation to reexperience a stressful medical examination: effect of repetitions, videotape exposure and coping style. *Journal of Consulting and Clinical Psychology,* 1979, *47,* 485–492.

Snyder, L. H., Rupprecht, P., Pyrek, J., Brekhus, S., and Moss, T. Wandering. *Gerontologist,* 1978, *18,* 272–280.

Stephens, L. P. *Reality Orientation.* Washington, D.C.: American Psychiatric Association, 1969.

Surwit, R. S., and Keefe, F. J. Frontalis EMG feedback training: an electronic panacea? *Behavior Therapy,* 1978, *9,* 779–792.

Surwit, R. S., Shapiro, D., and Good, M. I. Comparison of cardiovascular biofeedback, neuromuscular biofeedback, and meditation in the treatment of borderline essential hypertension. *Journal of Consulting and Clinical Psychology,* 1978, *46,* 252–263.

Tamburello, A. Un programma di "Token Economy" in un ambiente ospedaliero italiano. *Rivista di Psichiatria,* 1972, *2* (no pages given).

Tamburela, A. Institutional setting based on learning theory principles of behavior in chronic schizophrenics of long standing: results of an experimental study (original in Italian). *Archivio di Psicologia, Neurologia e Psichiatria,* 1976, *37,* 272–298.

Taulbee, L. R., and Folsom, J. C. Reality orientation for geriatric patients. *Hospital and Community Psychiatry*, 1966, *17*, 22–25.
Taylor, C. B., Zlutnick, S. I., and Hoehle, W. The effects of behavioral procedures on tardive dyskinesias. *Behavior Therapy*, 1979, *10*, 37–45.
Toepfer, C. T., Bicknell, A. T., and Shaw, D. O. Remotivation as behavior therapy. *Gerontologist*, 1974, *14*, 451–453.
Toseland, R. W. A comparison of three group methods to train social skills in older persons. *Dissertation Abstracts International*, 1978, *38*, 6324–6325.
Vandenberg, B. Play and development from an ethological perspective. *American Psychologist*, 1978, *33*, 724–737.
Weiner, H. R. Self-reinforcement in the elderly as a function of feedback and modeling. *Dissertation Abstracts International*, 1977, *37*, 4230.
West, H. L. The differential effects of biofeedback/relaxation training on elderly people. *Dissertation Abstracts International*, 1978, *39*, 1523–1524.
Whitbourne, S. K., and Weinstock, C. S. *Adult Development: The Differentiation of Experience*. New York: Holt, Rinehart and Winston, 1979.
Whitman, H. H., and Lukes, S. Behavior modification for terminally ill patients. *The American Journal of Nursing*, 1975, *75*, 98–101.
Wolpe, J. *The Practice of Behavior Therapy*. New York: Pergamon, 1973.
Woodruff, D. Biofeedback—implications for gerontology. Paper presented at the annual meeting of the Gerontological Society, Houston, Texas, October 1971.
Woodruff, D. S. Relationships among EEG alpha frequency, reaction time, and age: a biofeedback study. *Psycho-physiology*, 1975, *12*, 673–681.
Woods, R. T., and Britton, P. G. Psychological approaches to the treatment of the elderly. *Age and Ageing*, 1977, *6*, 104–112.

SECTION III

# Health and Clinical Practices

# CHAPTER 7

# Drug Treatment of Cognitive Impairment in the Elderly

JEROME A. YESAVAGE, M.D.
PSYCHIATRIC INTENSIVE CARE UNIT
VETERANS ADMINISTRATION MEDICAL CENTER
PALO ALTO, CALIFORNIA
DEPARTMENT OF PSYCHIATRY AND BEHAVIORAL SCIENCE
STANFORD UNIVERSITY MEDICAL SCHOOL
STANFORD, CALIFORNIA

ROY KING, M.D., PH.D.
DEPARTMENT OF PSYCHIATRY AND BEHAVIORAL SCIENCE
STANFORD UNIVERSITY MEDICAL SCHOOL
STANFORD, CALIFORNIA

In addition to work on the pharmacologic treatment of senile psychoses, involutional depression and neurotic disorders, considerable searching in geriatric psychopharmacology has been done for drugs to improve cognitive function in the elderly (Hollister, 1975; Reisberg et al., 1979). Both normal and pathologic cognitive decline have been well documented in the psychological and public health literature (Birren and Schaie, 1976; Butler, 1978; Eisdorfer, 1978). Despite these efforts, pharmacologic treatments for dementias remain controversial. This chapter defines the classes of medications involved and the rationales for their usage; lists specific agents available in this country and abroad, citing recent research on such agents; and finally discusses their clinical applications.

## BIOCHEMICAL RATIONALE

Current concepts of cognitive impairment in the elderly do not include the historical view that "senility" is due to the death of neurons secondary to cerebral atherosclerosis. Although the effects of atherosclerosis

This research has been aided in part by the Veteran's Administration Medical Research Service and by the Geriatric Research Educational and Clinical Center, VA Medical Center, Palo Alto.

cannot be denied in certain cases, the vasculature is quite intact in many others; hence specific biochemical causes of dementias have been sought (Ingvar and Lassen, 1975; Meier-Ruge et al., 1975; Simard et al. 1971). This search is important, since if the basis of certain dementias is biochemical, the process is potentially reversible by pharmacologic intervention. This area has been the subject of detailed review (Yesavage, 1979a), but the major possibilities for reversible biochemical defects are summarized for reference. These possibilities are impaired glycolytic metabolism, changes in neuroregulatory systems, and neurotransmitter changes.

### Glycolytic Metabolism

Neuronal stability, maintenance of ionic balance, and synthesis and reuptake of some neurotransmitters is adenosine triphosphate (ATP)-dependent (Ingvar and Lassen, 1975) and requires large quantities of energy-rich compounds. There appears to be abnormal DNA–RNA transcription and abnormal enzymatic activity in the aged brain (Jarvik, 1974; Terry and Gershon, 1976). Rational pharmacologic manipulation of some basic metabolic functions of the neuron may eventually lead to improved overall neuronal function and less neuronal dropout in the aged.

### Regulatory Mechanism

There are several levels at which alteration in neuroregulatory mechanisms may affect the aged brain. First, at the level of neuropeptides, several investigators have examined the enkephalins (de Weid, 1977). These peptides appear to play a role in regulating a number of psychological functions, including aspects of cognition, perception of pain, hormonal levels, and sleep. At a second level, hormonal factors may be involved with cognitive changes in aging (Fedor-Freybergh, 1977). Finally, the regulation of cyclic nucleotide levels, predominantly through changes in activities of phosphodiesterase in the aged, may produce several age-related physiologic changes (Meier-Ruge et al., 1975; Weiss and Hait, 1977).

### Neurotransmission

Changes in functional levels of neurotransmitters at the synapse may be the final common pathway for behavioral expression of many neurochemical changes. This area has been reviewed in detail elsewhere (Samorajski, 1975; Yesavage, 1979a); however, it is important to underline certain changes (Yesavage, 1979a). Several studies using histologic and spinal fluid data have indicated reduced functional levels of biogenic amines in elderly with cognitive deficits (Samorajski, 1975), sometimes associated with increased levels of monoamine oxidase (MAO) activity (Robinson, 1975). Furthermore, numerous studies have linked acetylcholine levels with major cognitive effects (Davis and Berger, 1979). As is the case with biogenic amines, lower functional levels of acetylcholine at the synapse are associated with cognitive impairment.

## SPECIFIC CLASSES OF MEDICATIONS

The classes of compounds tried in the treatment of senile dementias are listed in Table 7–1.

Table 7–1
Agents Available to Treat Cognitive Dysfunction in Elderly

| | |
|---|---|
| *Vasodilators* | *Neuropeptides* |
| Cyclandelate | ACTH 4-10 |
| Papaverine | Vasopressin |
| Nylidrin | Enkephalins |
| *Metabolically active drugs* | *Hormones* |
| Ergot Alkaloids | Estrogens |
| Piracetam | *Neurotransmitters* |
| Naftidrofuryl | Choline |
| Vinca Alkaloids | Physiostigmine |
| *Phosphodiesterase Inhibitors* | L-dopa |
| Flavonoids | *Nonspecific Agents* |
| Pthalazinol | CNS Stimulants |
| Pentifylline | Antidepressants |
| | Antipsychotics |
| | Anxiolytics |

### Vasodilators

A recent review of 102 studies of vasodilators in senile dementias found less evidence for clinical effect of these drugs in the dementias than for drugs which appear to act primarily on cerebral metabolism (Yesavage et al., 1979b). In fact, there have been five direct comparisons between the vasodilator papaverine and ergot alkaloids; and ergot alkaloids were found to be superior in each case. But another vasodilator, cyclandelate, may have a prophylactic effect in dementias which appear to have a vascular origin (Rao et al., 1977). And a recent multicentered study has shown efficacy of nylidrin in dementias (Gaitz et al., 1979). Most current data suggest that drugs which appear to act upon neuronal glycolytic metabolism are superior to drugs acting upon vasculature.

## Stimulants of Cerebral Metabolism

These medications are not direct vasodilators despite the possibility that they may secondarily increase cerebral blood flow by increasing cerebral oxidative metabolism. They include the ergot and vinca alkaloids, and two purely synthetic compounds, piracetam and naftidrofuryl.

*Ergot Alkaloids.* Dihydroergotoxine mesylate (DEM, Hydergine®) is probably the most commonly used medication worldwide in the attempt to improve cognitive function in the elderly. Recent reviews of the literature have concluded that the drug does have a small but statistically significant effect on improving some of the cognitive loss associated with senile dementias; but others argue that the mild drug effect is rarely clinically useful (Hughes et al., 1976; Yesavage et al., 1979b). A new approach used in the United States to augment the efficacy of the medication has been to increase the daily dosage from 3 to 6 mg per day, consistent with European dosage. A preliminary report suggested that this higher dose might be of benefit to select patients, and these findings are now being replicated in a large-scale study (Yesavage et al., 1979a).

Other investigators have suggested a prophylactic effect of DEM, slowing the decline associated with progressive dementias (Kugler et al., 1978). Unfortunately, such studies are rare and tedious and may yield contradictory results. One such study found reduced rating-scale evidence for clinical efficacy in a nine-month follow-up, but also found that patients on active medication may have needed less hospital care (Soni and Soni, 1975). Further study of the public health issues of the long-term and prophylactic use of this drug is indicated.

The actual biochemical effect of ergot alkaloids remains unclear and probably involves multiple factors. The drug is known to have mixed agonist and antagonist effects on dopaminergic receptors, to inhibit and stimulate phosphodiesterase activity, and to increase the activity of certain enzymes in glucose metabolism (Berde and Schild, 1978). These multiple effects will complicate further research with the medication.

*Vinca Alkaloids.* These compounds are used widely in Europe for the same indications as the ergot alkaloids. They seem to have a similarly wide range of neurochemical effects, but there have been fewer double-blind studies of clinical effect compared with the ergot alkaloids (Theil,

1975). At present, the manufacturers of this compound have no plans for clinical testing or marketing in the United States.

*Piracetam.* This European medication is a new synthetic compound originally produced in the search for a gamma-aminobutyric agonist. Despite its hypothesized effects on neurotransmission and studies which have shown the effect on ATP/ADP ratio in animal brain, this drug has been labeled "nootropic" to describe its stimulant action on neuronal metabolism (Giurgea, 1972).

A recent review of the piracetam literature documented its efficacy (Reisberg et al., 1979), but there has been at least one negative study (Gustafson et al., 1978). A particularly relevant study of aged memory impairment involved a primate model (Bartus, 1979). In this elegant series of experiments, piracetam was better than two other stimulants of cerebral metabolism (ergot and vinca alkaloids), while in the same model, general CNS stimulants (magnesium pemoline, methylphenidate, Metrazol®, and caffeine) showed little positive and some negative effects.

*Naftidrofuryl.* This synthetic compound has been used in Europe for over ten years in the treatment of peripheral vascular diseases and dementias. It appears to increase the activities of certain Krebs cycle enzymes, as shown by histologic studies in animals. In clinical trials in demented elderly in Europe, eight double-blind studies have shown positive effects (Yesavage et al., 1979b). These results have been replicated in at least one preliminary study in the United States (Branconnier and Cole, 1977). A second study recently completed in the United States has confirmed some of the biochemical effects of the medication, in particular reducing spinal fluid lactic acid levels in demented elderly (Yesavage et al., 1979c). Further studies of clinical efficacy are underway in the United States.

### Medications Affecting Neuroregulation

The distinction between neuroregulator and neurotransmitter is at times arbitrary, and certain entities may clearly act as both; but organizationally, we will now consider drugs which primarily affect neuroregulation, including phosphodiesterase inhibitors, neuropeptides and hormones.

*Phosphodiesterase Inhibitors.* Increased levels of intracellular cyclic adenosine 3′,5′-monophosphate (cAMP) produced by inhibition of phosphodiesterase may have widespread physiologic effects. Although some stimulants of cerebral metabolism discussed above may inhibit phosphodiesterase, several primarily phosphodiesterase inhibitors potentially useful in the dementias (Weiss and Hait, 1977) include the flavonoids, phthalazinol and pentifylline.

1. *Flavonoids.* The flavonoids are a large group of polyphenolic com-

pounds synthesized by plants. Comprising as much as 5 percent of the dry weight of some herbal teas, they are an important constituent of some preparations used in folk medicine (Geissman, 1962). These compounds are now under scientific investigation.

Pharmacologic studies have noted that flavonoids may dilate coronary arteries, are spasmolytic, block reserpine-induced hyperactivity, and enhance amphetamine-induced hyperactivity (Bhattacharya et al., 1972; Jongebreur, 1952; Willaman, 1955). At a cellular level, flavonoids inhibit catechol-O-methyl transferase and Na/K-dependent ATPases and elevate intracellular levels of cAMP (Ferrel et al., 1979; Graziani et al., 1977). Recent evidence indicates that flavonoids are extremely potent inhibitors of cAMP phosphodiesterases. This inhibition is competitive with cAMP, and structure/activity studies and quantum chemical calculations indicate that flavonoids stereochemically and in charge distribution mimic the adenine nucleus of cAMP (Ferrel et al., 1979).

Aside from their traditional use in teas as "tonics," human clinical studies of flavonoids are sparse, several suggesting that they reduce capillary fragility (Grubich, et al., 1979; Willaman, 1955). One could speculate that flavonoid-induced inhibition of phosphodiesterase may affect cognitive function.

2. *Phthalazinol.* This powerful phosphodiesterase inhibitor developed in Japan is reputed, in uncontrolled trials, to help patients having various degenerative central nervous system diseases (Shimamoto et al., 1976). The manufacturers have not disclosed their plans, if any, for testing the medication in the United States.

3. *Pentifylline.* This compound, similar to theophylline, has been used for its stimulant properties in European elderly and has been studied extensively in animals (Stefanovich and Joh, 1974). There is one positive controlled study of the substance in dementia (Kirchberger et al., 1969).

*Neuropeptides.* There have been recent detailed reviews of the role of neuropeptides in the central nervous system and in cognitive function (Reisberg et al., 1979; de Weid, 1977). Two general categories of peptides have attracted most attention: those secreted by the pituitary, namely ACTH, MSH, and vasopressin; and the enkephalins. Currently most attention has centered on the ACTH 4-10 fragment which has been tested with mixed results in geriatric populations (Branconnier et al., 1978; Will et al., 1978). Neuropeptides will continue to be studied as agents for potentially reversing cognitive deficits in the elderly.

*Hormones.* The major work with classically defined hormones in geriatrics has been with estrogens in postmenopausal women. Studies have indicated that estrogens may have a beneficial effect on both cognition and affect in selected patients (Fedor-Freybergh, 1977); but concern for carcinogenesis has limited their use.

It should be noted that antidepressants may improve cognition in depressed patients, and the effect of estrogens may be primarily on mood with secondary improvement in cognition (Sternberg and Jarvik, 1976).

### Neurotransmitters

Despite one report of the use of the gamma-aminobutyric acid (GABA) agonist muscimol in the treatment of dementia, the major work using neurotransmitters in dementias has been with the cholinergic and, to a lesser extent, adrenergic systems.

*Cholinergics.* A recent volume contains extensive reviews of the complex relationships of the cholinergic system to memory and cognition (Davis and Berger, 1979). The basic theoretical argument is that a relative cholinergic deficiency exists, primarily in the temporal cortex, which leads to impaired learning in the elderly. Elegant animal work, showing the effect of cholinergic agonists and antagonists on memory, has been replicated by even more elegant work in normal human volunteers (Davis et al., 1978; Deutsch, 1971). However, documenting a positive response in the elderly has proved more difficult, probably because of the lack of efficient cholinomimetic agents and a wide variety of cerebral pathologies in the demented elderly, only some of which respond to cholinomimetics (Mohs et al., 1979). Dosage effects are also important since overdosage of cholinomimetics can result in as much impairment as anticholinergics. Nevertheless, clinical research will continue in this area because of its strong theoretical basis.

*Adrenergic Agents.* Most of the work using adrenergic agonists in dementias, aside from the use of stimulants such as amphetamine or antidepressants, has centered on the use of L-dopa in Parkinsonism (Caine et al., 1975). Cognitive function may improve in some Parkinsonism patients treated with L-dopa, suggesting possible efficacy beyond motor disorders, especially in view of the clinical similarities between Parkinsonism and of primarily degenerative dementias, such as Alzheimer's type dementias, who may show considerable motor difficulties (Walton, 1977). L-dopa treatment of demented patients without motor disorders has had mixed results (Barbeau, 1972).

### Nonspecific Agents and Factors

General reviews of psychopharmacology in the elderly have argued that antipsychotics, anxioloytics, and antidepressants are more useful than any of the medications previously mentioned (Hollister, 1975; Jarvik et al.,

1972; Jarvik and Milne, 1975; Yesavage, 1979b). Their emphasis on using generally lower doses in the elderly need not be elaborated here. Some reviews have also argued that general CNS stimulants or analeptics such as amphetamines, magnesium pemoline, Metrazol, and caffeine are of little use and may in fact be detrimental. This argument has recently received support from careful learning experiments in primates (Bartus, 1979) and from the Food and Drug Administration (Crook, 1979). The successful use of general psychotropic medication in the elderly depends upon careful evaluation to rule out reversible causes of organic mental disorders and depression.

The differential diagnosis of reversible causes of organic mental disorders is extensive, and one of the authors has developed a mnemonic device (Yesavage, 1979b) using the word *dementia* as an acronym, representing the following classes of reversible factors: Drug intoxications; Emotional illness; Metabolic imbalances; Endocrine disorders; Normal pressure hydrocephaus and Nutritional deficiences; Tumor and Trauma; Infections; and Atherosclerotic disease. Excluding these reversible factors and occult depression are essential in successful psychopharmacologic treatment in the elderly.

The differentiation of dementia from depression in the elderly has been discussed in detail by Wells, who has listed a series of useful points which allow the distinction to be made often on clinical grounds alone (Gaitz, et al., 1977; Wells, 1979). Normal electroencepholograms and computerized axial tomography (CAT scans) suggest the possibility of depression or other reversible causes. Despite these clues, a pharmacologic trial of antidepressants may be indicated in unclear cases (Hollister, 1975).

If the diagnosis seems to be an Alzheimer's type dementia, ergot alkaloids should be tried. Miracles should not be expected, but some improvement has been seen in numerous studies by competent investigators. These effects seem to be distinct from those of antidepressants (Gaitz et al., 1977; Yesavage, 1979c).

Successful treatment of cognitive disorders in the elderly is also dependent upon nonpharmacologic factors. For example, careful record keeping, including use of rating scales, monitoring of dosages, and serum levels, should be used with antidepressants and antipsychotics. Support is necessary and placebo value should be enhanced. Furthermore, the clinician should be aware that there are specific psychotherapies recommended for cognitive deficits which may be of benefit alone or in combination with medications (Labouvie-Vief, 1976; Zarit et al., 1979). These purely psychological treatments, modeled after those used in brain-damaged patients, may rival the effectiveness of medication in dementias (Luria et al., 1969; Yesavage et al., 1979d).

## References

Barbeau, A. Dopamine and mental function. In S. Malitz (Ed.), *L-DOPA and Behavior*. New York: Raven Press, 1972, pp. 9–34.

Bartus, R. Four stimulants of the central nervous system: effects on short-term memory in young versus aged monkeys. *Journal of the American Geriatrics Society*, 1979, *27*, 289–297.

Berde, B., and Schild, H.O. (Eds.). *Ergot Alkaloid and Related Compounds*. Berlin: Springer-Verlag, 1978.

Bhattacharya, S., Sanyal, A., and Ghosal, S. Monoamine oxidase inhibiting activity of mangiferin isolated from canscora decussata. *Naturwissenschaften*, 1972, *59*, 651–652.

Birren, J.E., and Schaie, K.W., (Eds.). *Handbook of the Psychology of Aging*. New York: Van Nostrand Reinhold, 1976.

Branconnier, R.J., and Cole, J.O. A memory assessment technique for use in geriatric psycho-pharmacology: drug efficacy trial with naftidrofuryl. *Journal of the American Geriatrics Society*, 1977, *25*, 186–188.

Branconnier, R., Cole, J.O., and Gardos, G. ACTH 4-10 in the amelioration of neuropsychological symptomatology associated with senile organic brain syndrome. *Psychopharmacology Bulletin*, 1978, *14*, 27–30.

Butler, R.N. Overview on aging, In G. Usdin and C.K. Hofling (Eds.), *Aging: The Process and the People*. New York: Brunner/Mazel, 1978, pp.1–19.

Caine, D., Chase, T., and Barbeau, A. (Eds.). *Dopaminergic Mechanisms*. New York: Raven Press, 1975.

Crook, T. Central-nervous-system stimulants: appraisal of use in geropsychiatric patients. *Journal of the American Geriatrics Society*, 1979, *27*, 476–477.

Davis, K.L., and Berger, P.A. (Ed.). *Brain Acetylcholine and Neuropsychiatric Disease*. New York: Plenum Press, 1979.

Davis, K.L., Hollster, L.E., and Berger, P.A. Improvement of long-term memory processes in normal humans. *Science*, 1978, *201*, 272–274.

Deutsch, J.A. The cholinergic synapse and the site of memory. *Science*, 1971, *174*, 788–794.

Eisdorfer, C. Psychophysiologic and cognitive studies in the aged. In G. Usdin and C.K. Hofling (Eds.), *Aging: the Process and the People*. New York: Brunner/Mazel, 1978, pp. 96–128.

Fedor-Freybergh, P. The influence of oestrogens on the well-being and mental performance of climacteric and postmenopausal women. *Acta Obstetrica et Gynecologica Scandinavica*, 1977, 1–91.

Ferrell, J.E., Chang-Sing, P., Loew, G., King, R., Mansour, M., and Mansour, T. Structure activity studies of flavonoids as inhibitors of cyclic AMP phosphodiesterase and relationship to quantum chemical indices. *Molecular Pharmacology*, 1979, *16*, 141–153.

Gaitz, C.M., Varner, R.V., and Overall, J.E. Pharmacotherapy for organic brain syndrome in late life. *Archives of General Psychiatry*, 1977, *34*, 839–845.

Gaitz, C.M., Garetz, F.K., Goldstein, S.E., Greenblatt, R., Hollinsworth, S.W., Mattheis, D.B., Rao, D.B., and Soong, B. Nylindrin in Dementia. Presented at the Scientific Exhibit, American Gerontological Society, Washington, D.C., November 1979.

Geissman, T.A. The occurrence of flavonoid compounds in nature. In T.A. Geissman, *Chemistry of Flavonoid Compounds*. New York: Macmillan, 1962, pp. 1–5.

Giurgea, G. Vers une pharmacologie de l'activité integrative du cerveau: tentative du concept nootrope en psychopharmacologie. *Actualités Pharmacologiques,* 1972, *25,* 115–156.

Graziani, Y., Winikoff, J., and Chayoth, R. Regulation of cAMP level and lactic acid production in ehrilick ascites tumor cells. *Biochemical and Biophysical Acta,* 1977, *497,* 499–506.

Grubich, V., Fever, L., Turma, Z., and Unyi, G. Cardiovascular properties of 7-isopropoxy-isoflavone. *Lancet,* 1979, *1,* 211–212.

Gustafson, L., et al. Effects of piracetam on regional cerebral blood flow and mental functions in patients with organic dementia. *Psychopharmacology,* 1978, *56,* 115, 7.

Hollister, L.E., Risberg, J., Johanson, M., Fransson, M., and Maximilian, A. Drugs for mental disorders of old age. *Journal of the American Medical Association,* 1975, *234,* 195–198.

Hughes, J.R., Williams, J.G., and Currier, R.D. An ergot alkaloid preparation in the treatment of dementia: a critical review of the literature. *Journal of the American Geriatrics Society,* 1977, *24,* 490–497.

Ingvar, D.H., and Lassen, N.A. *Brain Work: The Coupling of Function, Metabolism and Blood Flow in the Brain.* Copenhagen: Munksgaard, 1975.

Jarvik, L.F. Chromosomes and mental status. *Archives of General Psychiatry,* 1974, *30,* 186–190.

Jarvik, L.F., and Milne, J.F., Gerovital-$H_3$: A review of the literature. In S. Gershon and A. Raskin (Eds.), *Aging,* vol. 2. New York: Raven Press, 1975.

Jarvik, M., Gritz, E., and Schneider, N. Drugs and memory disorders in human aging. *Behavioral Biology,* 1972, *7,* 643–668.

Jongebreur, G. Relation between the chemical constitution and the pharmacologic action, especially on the coronary vessels of the heart, of some synthesized pyrones and khellin. *Archives Internationales de Pharmacodynamie et de Therapie,* 1952, *90,* 384–411.

Kirchberger, F., Kehl, R., and Gutmann, W. Zur behandlung zerebraler Ernahrungestorungen. *Medizinische Welt,* 1969, *27,* 1542–1546.

Kugler, J., Oswald, W.D., Herzfeld, U., Scus, R., Pingel, J., and Welzel, D. Langzeitherapie Altersbedingter Insuffizienzerscheinungen des Gehirns. *Deutsch Medizinische Wochenschrift,* 1978, *103,* 456–462.

Labouvie-Vief, G. Towards optimizing cognitive competence in later life. *Educational Geriatrics,* 1976, *1,* 75–92.

Luria, A.R., Naydin, V.L., Tsvetkova, L.S., and Vinarskays, E.N. Restoration of higher cortical function following local brain damage. In P.J. Vinken and G.W. Broyn (Eds.), *Handbook of Clinical Neurology.* Amsterdam: North Holland, 1969, pp.368–433.

Meier-Ruge, W., Enz, A., Gygax, P., Hunziker, O., Iwangoff, P. and Reichlmeier, K. Experimental pathology in basic research of the aging brain. In S. Gershon and A. Raskin (Eds.), *Aging,* vol. 2. New York: Raven Press, 1975, pp. 55–126.

Mohs, R.C., Davis K.L., Tinklenberg, J.R., Hollister, L.E., Yesavage, J.A., and Kopell, B.S. Choline chloride treatment of memory deficits in elderly. *American Journal of Psychiatry* 1979, *136,* 1275–1277.

Rao, D.B., Georgiev, E.L., Paul, P.D., and Guzman, A.B. Cyclandelate in the treatment of senile mental changes: a double blind evaluation. *Journal of the American Geriatrics Society,* 1977. *25,* 548–551.

Reisberg, B., Ferris, S., and Gershon, S. Psychopharmacologic aspects of cognitive research in elderly: some current perspectives. *Interdisciplinary Topics in Gerontology*, 1979, *15*, 132–152.

Robinson, D.S. Changes in MAO and monoamines with human development and aging. *Federation Proceedings*, 1975, *34*, 103–107.

Samorajski, T. Age related changes in brain biogenic amines. In H. Brady and D. Harman (Eds.), *Aging*, vol. 1. New York: Raven Press, 1975, pp. 119–214.

Shimamoto, T., Murase, H., and Numano, F. Treatment of senile dementia and cerebeller disorders with phthalazinol. *Mechanisms of Aging and Development*, 1976, *5*, 241–250.

Shock, N.W. Biological theories of aging. In J.E. Birren and K.W. Schaie, (Eds.), *Handbook of the Psychology of Aging*. New York: Van Nostrand Reinhold, 1976, pp. 103–116.

Simard, D., Oleson, J., and Paulson, O.B. Regional cerebral blood flow and its regulation in dementia. *Brain*, 1971, *94*, 273–288.

Soni, D., and Soni, S. Dihydrogenated alkaloids of ergotoxine in nonhospitalized elderly patients. *Current Medical Research and Opinion*, 1975, *3*, 464–468.

Sternberg, D.E., and Jarvik, M.E. Memory function in depression. *Archives of General Psychiatry*, 1976, *33*, 219–223.

Stefanovich, V., and Joh, P. Concerning the effect of theophylline and pentifylline on the energy metabolism of rat brain. *Experimental Gerontology*, 1974, *24*, 1974.

Terry, R.D., and Gershon, S. (Eds.). *Aging*, vol. 3, *Aging and the Human Brain*. New York: Raven Press, 1976.

Theil, P. *La Perivincamine Dans le Mond La Medicine Practicienne*. Paris: Laboratoires Dausse, Jan., 1975, No. 571.

Walton, J.N. (Ed.). *Brain's Diseases of the Nervous System*. New York: Oxford University Press, 1977, pp. 587 ff.

de Weid, D. Peptides and behavior. *Life Sciences*, 1977, *20*, 195–204.

Weiss, B., and Hait, W.N. Selective cyclic nucleotide phosphodiesterase inhibitors as potential therapeutic agents. *Annual Review of Pharmacology and Toxicology*, 1977, *17*, 441–477.

Wells, C.E. Geriatric organic psychoses. *Psychiatric Annals*, 1979, *8*, 57–73.

Will, J.C., Abuzzehab, F.S., and Zimmerman, R.L. The effects of ACTH 4–10 versus placebo in the memory of symptomatic geriatic volunteers. *Psychopharmacology Bulletin*, 1978, *14*, 25–27.

Willaman, J.J. Some biological effects of flavonoids. *Journal of the American Pharmaceutical Association*, 1955, *44*, 404–407.

Yesavage, J. Pharmacotheraphy of the aged central nervous system. In H.L. Klawans (Ed.), *Clinical Neuropharmacology*, vol. IV. New York: Raven Press, 1979a, pp. 199–220.

Yesavage, J.A. Drugs to alter cognitive function in the elderly. *Geriatrics*, 1979b, *9*, 51–59.

Yesavage, J. Practical points in the use of dihydroergotoxine mesylate. *Psychiatric Annals*, 1979c, *8*, 74–83.

Yesavage, J., Burian, E., and Hollister, L. Hydergine in senile dementias, 6 mg versus 3 mg dosage: a preliminary report. *Journal of the American Geriatrics Society*, 1979a. *27*, 80–84.

Yesavage, J., Tinklenberg, J., Berger, P., and Hollister, L. Vasodilators in senile dementias: a review of the literature. *Archives of General Psychiatry*, 1979b, *36*, 220–223.

Yesavage, J., Tinklenberg, J., Berger, P., and Hollister, L. Submitted for publication, 1979c.

Yesavage, J., Westphal, J., and Rush, L. Combined pharmacological and psychological treatment for dementias. Presented at the Annual Scientific Meeting, American Gerontological Society, Washington, D.C., November 1979d.

Zarit, S.H., Gallagher, D., and Krauer, N. Memory training in the community aging. *Educational Gerontology*, 1979, in press.

# CHAPTER 8

# Aging and Drug Therapy

Joy B. Plein, Ph.D. Elmer M. Plein, Ph.D.
Department of Pharmacy Practice
University of Washington
Seattle, Washington

While it is still true that the elderly are "therapeutic orphans" (Butler, 1978), since approximately 1974 there has been very noticeably increased interest in the effects of aging on drug therapy. This interest by pharmaceutical and medical scientists and by practitioners is manifested by increased numbers of reviews of drug therapy for the elderly and publications relating to pharmacokinetics and aging, drug misuse and abuse by the elderly, education of older patients about their medications, improved professional pharmacy services for older persons, and use of specific drugs or groups of drugs in the treatment of elderly patients. The reports of effects of aging on drug therapy have not only increased in number but also are scattered throughout basic science and clinical literature, reflecting wide interest (and, incidentally, increasing the complexity of monitoring the literature).

We will review clinically relevant research concerning the effects of aging on pharmacokinetics and on susceptibility to drug action. Our review will be limited to data in humans and will exclude developments in pharmacotherapeutics of cognitive disorders, which are reviewed in this volume by Dr. Yesavage in Chapter 7. Also excluded are studies of drug regimen compliance or drug misuse and abuse by the elderly.

Although both the quantity and the sophistication of research concerned with aging's effect on drug therapy have increased in the past six or seven years, there are still relatively few drugs that have been carefully

The authors acknowledge with appreciation the review of the manuscript and valuable suggestions of Milo Gibaldi, Ph.D., and Jeffrey R. Koup, Pharm. D., both at the School of Pharmacy, University of Washington. They also thank Jean Pasche, M.Lbr., Research Librarian, Institute of Aging, University of Washington, for her continued assistance in monitoring the pertinent literature.

studied in the elderly, and there are few generalizations that can be made about the effects of aging on drug disposition and response. The literature must be reviewed carefully since some investigators have failed to recognize a few rather characteristic pitfalls in interpretation or in study design. For example, some studies have compared drug effects in geriatric patients with effects in healthy young adults, and then attributed differences to age alone rather than either age or disease, or both variables. Second, limitations of the specific methodology used have gone unrecognized in some investigator's interpretations of their pharmacokinetic studies; and third, a number of comparisons of drug metabolism in young and old subjects have failed to include consideration of the effects of cigarette smoking. In addition, current comparisons of drug effects are of course subject to the limitation of being cross-sectional comparisons rather than measures of longitudinal changes in the way drugs affect humans and the way humans handle drugs.

In spite of these limitations much progress has recently been made in describing the effects of aging on human response to specific drugs. This knowledge can, and should, be applied in treating patients.

## PHARMACOKINETICS AND AGING

Much recent human pharmacologic research in aging has been pharmacokinetic. The interrelationships of drug absorption, distribution in the body, binding to proteins, metabolism, and excretion are illustrated diagrammatically in Figure 8–1. Each of the processes shown may be influenced by the quantitative changes in body composition and physiologic function that occur normally as the body ages. Such pharmacokinetic changes obviously may alter the concentration and persistence of drugs at receptor sites. With the exception, however, that aging can be expected to decrease the elimination rate of drugs that are excreted intact (unchanged) by the kidney, few generalities can be used to predict the effects of aging on the pharmacokinetics of specific drugs. Those drugs that have been studied pharmacokinetically in the elderly represent a few pieces of a large jigsaw puzzle; and additional pieces of the puzzle can be obtained only by additional research.

Symbols used in both text and tables of this review are identified in Table 8–1. Throughout this review the probability level for statistical significance is $p < 0.05$.

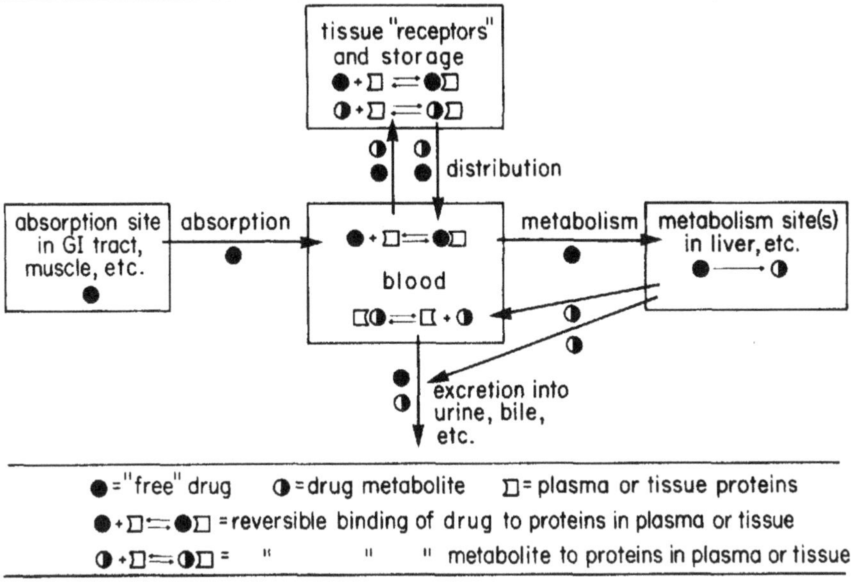


**Figure 8–1.** Schematic representation of the processes of drug absorption, distribution, metabolism, and excretion, all of which may be affected by aging.

## Absorption

For drugs that are administered by mouth, it is reasonable to expect that age-related changes in gastrointestinal physiology would alter the rate or extent of drug absorption. In aged persons the volume of salivary secretion and the secretion of gastric acid, intrinsic factors, and pepsin decrease. Few data are available on age-related changes in the morphology or secretory activity of the small intestine. There is also little information on the effect of aging on gastric emptying time and gastrointestinal motility, despite the widespread assumption that constipation in the elderly is due in part to a reduction in colonic peristalsis (Bhanthumnavin and Schuster, 1977; Goldman, 1979).

With advanced age, there appears to be impaired absorption, and also decreased renal excretion, of D-xylose (Bhanthumnavin and Schuster, 1977). Stevenson and co-workers (1979) concluded, however, that the apparent reduction in xylose absorption is probably due to its decreased rate of urinary excretion. Calcium absorption, which occurs via an active transport mechanism in the proximal small intestine, is impaired in the elderly (Bhanthumnavin and Schuster, 1977; Goldman, 1979). One study in animals showed decreased uptake of iron with aging (Goldman, 1979), and diminished absorption of iron and vitamin $B_{12}$ may result from the

Table 8–1
Symbols Used

| *Symbol* | *Term* |
|---|---|
| AUC | area under the curve (area under the plasma concentration vs. time curve) |
| β | apparent first-order elimination rate constant |
| Css | plasma concentration at steady state |
| Cmax | maximum plasma concentration |
| Cl | clearance (plasma clearance) |
| Clcr | creatinine clearance |
| Kabs | absorption rate constant |
| NSD | not significantly different ($p > 0.05$) |
| po | by mouth (oral administration) |
| iv | intravaneous administration |
| Scr | serum creatinine |
| $t_{1/2}$ | half-life |
| $t_{1/2}$ abs. | absorption half-life |
| $t_{1/2}\beta$ | elimination half-life |
| $t_{Cmax}$ | time from drug administration to maximum concentration in plasma |
| Vd | apparent volume of distribution |
| Vdβ | volume of distribution during the elimination phase |
| Vdss | volume of distribution at steady state |

decrease in gastric secretions noted above (Bhanthumnavin and Schuster, 1977; Goldman, 1979). Thiamine may also be absorbed less well in old age (Goldman, 1979). The dietary substances cited above are absorbed, at least in part, by active transport mechanisms; most drugs, however, are absorbed by passive diffusion (Crooks et al., 1976; O'Malley et al., 1980; Vestal, 1978).

Several reviewers have pointed out that data concerning age-related changes in drug absorption are limited (Crooks et al., 1976; Stevenson et al., 1979; Vestal, 1978). Some recent studies, however, add to the older information suggesting that in general aging probably does not appreciably affect absorption of most drugs.

Data from age-related absorption studies of 11 different drugs are summarized in Table 8–2. The extent of drug absorption following oral administration can be quantified by comparing plasma concentration versus time curves (AUC) following intravenous and oral administrations of the drug (Gibaldi, 1977). Cusack and colleagues (1979) used this method to compare absorption of digoxin by six "young" (mean age 47 years) and seven "elderly" (mean age 81 years) patients. As shown in Table 8–2, mean extent of absorption of orally administered digoxin, approximately 76 percent of the dose in the older group and 84 percent in the younger, was not significantly different in the two groups. Fulton and co-workers

(1979) compared the pharmacokinetics of acetaminophen in 11 young (mean age 24 years) and 12 elderly (mean age 76 years) individuals. The authors report bioavailability of 0.98 in the younger individuals and 0.95 in the elderly group. (The method of calculating bioavailability was not included in their brief report). Somogyi and co-workers (1980) used the AUC method to determine the extent of absorption of cimetidine by 12 patients who ranged in age from 28 to 64 years. There appeared to be a trend toward greater oral absorption by the younger individuals, but this age-dependence was not statistically significant in this small population. Kampmann and colleagues (1979) used the AUC method to determine the bioavailability of propylthiouracil in nine elderly patients aged 74–86 years. The extent of bioavailability was not significantly different from that previously determined for a younger group (see Table 8–2).

Comparisons of extent of absorption can also be made from determinations of the amounts of unchanged drug excreted in the urine following oral administration. Gibaldi (1977) points out that the usefulness of this method depends upon the extent of urinary excretion of the drug, the sensitivity of the assay method, and the variability in urinary output. Triggs and co-workers (1975) administered single, oral doses of sulfamethizole, a drug excreted primarily intact in the urine, to six young men (mean age 24 years) and seven elderly men (mean age 81 years). The percentages of the dose excreted as unchanged drug and as metabolite were not significantly different between the two age groups. Triggs and co-workers (1975) also administered oral acetaminophen to the same two groups of subjects and found that the total percentage of the dose excreted in the urine, mostly as metabolites, was similar for the two age groups. However, the percent of the dose that was excreted as metabolites was more variable in the older group. Simon and colleagues (1972) determined urinary excretion of propicillin following administration of a single oral dose of propicillin K to ten healthy subjects aged 20–30 years and to 16 patients aged 60–80 years who did not have renal or cardiac pathology. In the nine-hour period after administration, similar total mean percentages of the dose (53.4 percent for the younger and 51.8 percent for the older group) were recovered in the urines of the two groups.

Aging also seems to have little effect on rate of absorption. As shown in Table 8–2, the absorption rate constants of aspirin and practolol were similar in young and old subjects, while the absorption rate constant of propylthiouracil was found to be less in a group of nine elderly patients than in a group of six young subjects studied previously. The absorption rate constant of chlordiazepoxide was less in the elderly than in the young group; however, the difference was not statistically significant because of the large standard error in the younger individuals (Shader et al., 1977).

Table 8–2
Drug Absorption in "Young" and "Old" Following Oral Administration of Single Doses

| Drug | Age group in yrs range (n) [mean] | | Extent of absorption | | Rate of absorption | | Reference |
|---|---|---|---|---|---|---|---|
| | "YOUNG" | "OLD" | $AUC_{po}/AUC_{iv}$ | MEAN % OF DOSE EXCRETED IN URINE | Kabs/hr | $t_{Cmax}$ (hr) | |
| Acetaminophen | 22–30 (6) [24] | 73–91 (7) [81] | — | NSD young vs. old (see text) | — | 0.67 young 0.74 old | Triggs et al., 1975 |
| Acetaminophen | — (11) [24] | — (12) [76] | NSD (see text) | — | — | — | Fulton et al., 1979 |
| Antipyrine (in combination with aspirin and *d*-propoxyphene) | 24–37 (8) [—] | 74–75 (6) [—] | — | — | — | 1.2 young 1.0 old | Melander et al., 1978 |
| Aspirin | — (6) [29] | — (11) [84] | — | — | 4.3 young 3.4 old | 0.7 young 0.7 old | Castleden et al., 1977b |
| Aspirin | — (7) [21] | — (15) [77] | — | — | NSD young vs. old[a] | — | Cuny et al., 1979 |
| Aspirin | 20–40 (—) [—] | > 65 (5) [—] | — | — | 13.8 young 12.5 old | 0.8 young 1.2 old | Stevenson et al., 1979 |
| Aspirin (in combination with *d*-propoxyphene and antipyrine) | 24–37 (8) [—] | 74–75 (6) [—] | — | — | — | 2.3 young 2.4 old | Melander et al., 1978 |

| | | | | | | | |
|---|---|---|---|---|---|---|---|
| Chlordiazepoxide | 21–30 (28) [25] | 63–74 (8) [69] | — | — | 7.6 young<br>2.1 old | — | Shader et al., 1977 |
| Cimetidine | 28–64 (age as continuous variable) | | NSD in young and old | — | — | — | Somogyi et al., 1980 |
| Digoxin | 34–61 (6) [47] | 72–91 (7) [81] | 0.76 older<br>0.84 younger<br>NSD | — | — | — | Cusack et al., 1979 |
| Practolol | — (13) [27] | — (8) [80] | — | — | 0.8 young<br>0.7 old | 2.8 young<br>3.5 old | Castleden et al., 1977b |
| Propicillin K | 20–30 (10) [—] | 60–80 (16) [—] | — | 53.4% young<br>51.8% old | 1.54 young<br>1.50 old | — | Simon et al., 1972 |
| Propoxyphene (in combination with antipyrine and aspirin) | 24–37 (8) [—] | 74–75 (6) [—] | — | — | — | 1.7 young<br>1.7 old | Melander et al., 1978 |
| Propylthiouracil | — (6) [—] | 74–86 (9) [81] | 83% young<br>71% old | — | young<br>old | — | Kampmann et al., 1979 |
| Sulfamethizole | 22–30 (6) [24] | 73–81 (7) [81] | — | 91% young<br>83% old | — | 1.2 young<br>2.1 old | Triggs et al., 1975 |

[a]Expressed as $t_{1/2}$abs.

The time after oral administration to achieve maximum drug concentrations in plasma has also been found to be similar for acetaminophen, antipyrine, aspirin, practolol, propoxyphene, and sulfamethizole in young and elderly groups.

## Distribution

Age-related changes in drug distribution in the body could result from changes in body composition, in plasma protein and other tissue binding, and in tissue permeability (Crooks et al., 1976; Smith, 1979).

*Plasma Protein Binding*. The total amount of protein in serum does not change significantly with aging, but the albumin/globulin (A/G) ratio decreases with increasing age (Calloway and Dollevoet, 1977; Goldman, 1979; Wallace et al., 1976). In one study, the A/G ratio was 1.61 for those aged 21–30 years and 1.08 for those older than 70 years (Calloway and Dollevoet, 1977). Importantly, most drugs which bind to plasma protein bind to albumin (Gibaldi, 1977). Since the bound fraction of the drug cannot pass through capillary walls, this bound fraction does not distribute to extravascular spaces. Considerable evidence indicates that it is the unbound (free) fraction of drug which is pharmacologically active, which is filtered by the glomeruli, and which in some instances is preferentially metabolized by the liver (Gibaldi, 1977). In contrast, an increase in plasma protein binding may accelerate elimination of certain drugs subject to renal tubular secretion or to rapid hepatic metabolism (Gibaldi, 1977).

Because the age-related decrease in plasma albumin may have important effects on drug distribution, activity, and disposition, the effect of aging on binding of specific drugs to plasma proteins has received considerable attention. As shown in Table 8–3, chlormethiazole, phenylbutazone, and tolbutamide were bound less in the elderly groups than in the younger groups. For chlordiazepoxide, desmethyldiazepam, diazepam, oxazepam, penicillin G, phenobarbital, salicylic acid, and sulfadiazine, there were no significant differences in the extent of binding to plasma of young and old subjects. Results of plasma binding studies on meperidine, phenytoin, and warfarin conflict, that is, for each of these drugs there is one study (two for meperidine) showing no statistically significant age-related difference in binding and another showing decreased binding by plasma of the older subjects. Mather and colleagues (1975) found that meperidine was bound by plasma proteins of the elderly to a significantly lesser degree than observed in the younger group. From the slope developed from their data, they devised a formula for estimation of the proportion of unbound drug (unbound drug = $0.175 + 0.0062 \times$ age). The study of Chan and co-workers (1975) did not show an age-related difference in protein binding of meperidine, perhaps because their study included only five young and four elderly subjects, and perhaps also because a different drug concentration than that of Mather and co-workers was used. Mitchard (1979) repeated the study of Chan and colleagues with 20 subjects and found values in close agreement with the formula proposed by Mather and colleagues (1975).

The extent of plasma binding may also be dependent upon whether or not the patient is receiving drugs at the time of the study. Wallace and co-workers (1976) found no significant difference in binding of salicylic acid in the plasma of their young and old groups who were not receiving drugs; however, plasma from the group of old subjects receiving drugs bound a significantly smaller percent of salicylic acid than did that of the younger drug-free subjects. Similar results were found for sulfadiazine. Highly bound phenylbutazone showed decreased binding with age, and less binding in young and old patients who were receiving drugs than in young volunteers who were drug free.

Wallace and co-workers (1976) also compared the plasma albumin concentrations in the four groups of subjects selected for these experiments. There was significantly less albumin in the two elderly groups ($p < 0.001$). The values were 42 ± 3 g/l for the young controls; 39 ± 5 g/l for the young surgical patients, 36 ± 5 g/l for the elderly group taking no drugs, and 36 ± 3 g/l for the elderly group taking one or more drugs.

Miller and colleagues (1977) determined plasma protein binding of tolbutamide in 18 young patients, 23–46 years old, and in 20 older patients, 61–87 years old. The free fraction of tolbutamide was significantly higher (14 percent) in the elderly group. These data may in part explain why most hypoglycemic reactions associated with sulfonylurea therapy occur in the elderly.

*Volume of Distribution.* With aging the percentage of body weight that is fat increases and the lean body tissue and total body water decrease (Goldman, 1979; Rossman, 1977). Since drugs may preferentially distribute to lean body tissue or to fat, changes in body composition can affect the volume in which drugs are stored in the body and can alter drug concentrations available at receptor sites.

The apparent volume of distribution (Vd) of a drug is a proportionality constant relating the plasma concentration and the total amount of drug in the body (Gibaldi, 1977). Mathematically the Vd may be represented by

$$\text{Vd} = \frac{\text{total amount of drug in body}}{\text{concentration in plasma}} \tag{1}$$

Table 8–3
Effect of Aging on Plasma Protein Binding of Drugs

| Drug | Age group, years Range [mean age] | (n) | % Bound | References |
|---|---|---|---|---|
| Chlordiazepoxide | 16–86 | (27)[a] | 96.5 ± 1.8[b] | Roberts et al., 1978 |
| Chlormethiazole | 25–28 [26] | (6) | 69 | Nation et al., 1977a |
| | 71–86 [76] | (6) | 60[c] | |
| Diazepam | 15–82 | (30)[d] | 97.32 ± 1.2[b] | Klotz et al., 1975 |
| Desmethyldiazepam (a metabolite of some benzodiazepines) | 15–82 | (30)[d] | 97.6 ± 1.3[b] | Klotz et al., 1975 |
| Meperidine | 22–26 [24] | (5) | — | Chan et al., 1975 |
| | 67–87 [78] | (4) | NSD (see text) | |
| Meperidine | 18–73 [Age as a continuous variable] | (19) | Age 30 = 65[e] Age 70 = 35[c,e] | Mather et al., 1975 |
| Meperidine | young [24] | (10) | 55 ± 15.2 | Mitchard, 1979 |
| | elderly [78] | (10) | 40 ± 12.1 | |
| Oxazepam | 14–30 [25] | (8)[f] | 86.69 ± 1.67 | Shull et al., 1976 |
| | 45–84 [54] | (7)[f] | 89.27 ± 1.59 | |

| | | | | |
|---|---|---|---|---|
| Pencillin G potassium | <50 | (5) | 42.4 ± 3.00 | Bender et al., 1975 |
| | >50 | (4) | 45.1 ± 3.62 | |
| Phenobarbital | <50 | (5) | 41.8 ± 1.33 | Bender et al., 1975 |
| | >50 | (3) | 41.9 ± 2.07 | |
| Phenylbutazone | 19–40 [27] | (16)[g] | 96[e] | Wallace et al., 1976 |
| | 14–39 [30] | (15)[h] | 90[e,i] | |
| | 69–85 [79] | (16)[g] | 94[e,i] | |
| | 74–92 [84] | (22)[j] | 92[e,i] | |
| Phenytoin | <50 | (6) | 82.4 ± 0.84 | Bender et al., 1975 |
| | >50 | (3) | 83.6 ± 0.35 | |
| Phenytoin | 20–38 | | 727 μmol/l | Hayes et al., 1975b, cited in Crooks et al., 1976 |
| | 65–90 | | 595 μmol/l[c] | |
| Salicylic acid (salicylate) | 19–40 [27] | (16)[g] | 74[e] | Wallace et al., 1976 |
| | 14–39 [30] | (15)[h] | 72[e] | |
| | 69–85 [79] | (16)[g] | 74[e] | |
| | 74–92 [84] | (22)[j] | 58[e,i] | |

*(Continued)*

| | | | | |
|---|---|---|---|---|
| Sulfadiazine | 19–40 [27] | (16)[g] | 50[e] | Wallace et al., 1976 |
| | 14–39 [30] | (15)[h] | 48[e] | |
| | 69–85 [79] | (16)[g] | 47[e] | |
| | 74–92 [84] | (22)[j] | 34[e,i] | |
| Tolbutamide | 23–46 | (18) | | Miller et al., 1977 |
| | 61–87 | (20) | 14%[c] less in elderly | |
| Warfarin | 17–37 [25] | (13) | 98.6 ± 0.1 | Shepherd et al., 1977 |
| | 68–94 [78] | (15) | 98.5 ± 0.1 | |
| Warfarin | 20–45 | (9) | 561 µmol/l | Hayes et al., 1975a |
| | 65–90 | (12) | 451 µmol/l[c] | |

[a]All nonsmokers.

[b]Constant over both range of concentration and ages studied.

[c]Significant difference between "old" and "young."

[d]13 were heavy smokers (over 20 cigarettes per day); the remainder were nonsmokers.

[e]Estimated from graph.

[f]No drugs or alcohol for at least 3 weeks before the study.

[g]Taking no drugs.

[h]Healthy surgical patients taking sedatives, analgesics, and antibiotics.

[i]Significant difference when compared with young (19–40) group taking no drugs.

[j]Taking one or more drugs.

The Vd of a drug is dependent upon the relative uptake of drug by the tissues and by blood or plasma (Woosley and Shand, 1978); it is a reflection of the degree of distribution of the drug in the body (Gibaldi, 1977).

Since total body water decreases with aging, drugs that are distributed in total body water would be expected to have a smaller Vd in elderly than in young subjects. Antipyrine and ethanol are both distributed into body water, and each of these drugs has a significantly smaller Vd in elderly than in young subjects. The effect of aging on distribution volume is, however, often unpredictable. As shown in Tables 8–4 and 8–5, the volumes of distribution of cimetidine, propicillin, and quinine, as well as antipyrine and alcohol, are less in the elderly than in the young; however, chlordiazepoxide, chlormethiazole, diazepam, gentamicin, kanamycin, lidocaine, nitrazepam, and oxazepam have greater volumes of distribution in the elderly than in younger subjects. The volumes of distribution of acetaminophen, aspirin, desmethyldiazepam, pancuronium, phenylbutazone, propranolol, propylthiouracil, quinidine and sulfamethizole are not significantly different in young and old. Kraus and co-workers (1978) found no significant difference in Vd of lorazepam with aging, but Greenblatt and co-workers (1979) reported a smaller Vd of the drug in subjects aged 60–84 years than in those aged 19–38 years. Digoxin is distributed in lean body tissue and on this basis would be expected to have a smaller Vd in the elderly; Cusack and colleagues (1979) did find a smaller Vd of this drug in their older group, but the difference was not statistically significant on a liter per kilogram (1/kg) body weight basis.

The significance of the Vd of a drug to its half-life ($t_{1/2}$) is clear from formula 2, which relates Vd, drug clearance (Cl) and $t_{1/2}$.

$$t_{1/2} = \frac{0.693 \times Vd}{Cl} \tag{2}$$

Thus, the $t_{1/2}$ of a drug is directly proportional to its Vd and inversely proportional to its Cl. If the Cl of a drug does not change with aging, an age-related increase in Vd will increase drug $t_{1/2}$. Clinically, such an increase in Vd and therefore $t_{1/2}$ would be expected to increase the duration of effect of a drug given intermittently as a single dose and to increase the time needed to reach "steady-state" levels on multiple-dose regimens. Increase in $t_{1/2}$ would also be expected to decrease fluctuations between the minimum and maximum blood levels of a drug administered on a multiple-dose schedule.

A number of drugs have longer half-lives in old than in young subjects (see Tables 8–4 and 8–5 and reviews by Crooks et al., 1976, and by Stevenson et al., 1979); and some authors have assumed that a longer $t_{1/2}$

Table 8–4
Effect of Aging on Half-life, Distribution, and Clearance of Drugs Eliminated Primarily as Unchanged Drugs by the Kidney (Single-Dose Studies)

| *Drug* | *Age group in years range (n) [mean]* | *Mean $t_{1/2}\beta$ (hr)* | *Mean Vd* | *Mean Cl* | *Reference* |
|---|---|---|---|---|---|
| Cimetidine | 20–64 (12) [age as a continuous variable] | age 35 = 1.8<br>age 60 = 2.2 | Vdss:<br>age 35 = 74 l<br>age 60 = 41 l | age 35 = 680 ml/min<br>age 60 = 310 ml/min[a] | Somogyi et al., 1980[b] |
| Cimetidine | 28–45 (5)<br>53–64 (7) | — | — | 702 ml/min<br>347 ml/min[c] | Gugler and Somogyi, 1979 |
| Digoxin | 20–30 (9) [27] | 51 | — | 83 ml/min/1.73m$^2$ | Ewy et al, 1969 |
| | 73–81 (5) [77] | 73[c] | — | 53 ml/min/1.73m$^2$[c] | |
| Digoxin | 34–61 (6) [47] | 37 po<br>38 iv | 339 l<br>5.3 l/kg | 1.7 ml/min/kg | Cusack et al., 1979 |
| | 72–91 (7) [81] | 70 po[a]<br>69 iv[d] | 194 l[a]<br>4.1 l/kg | 0.8 ml/min/kg[a] | |
| Gentamicin | 20–50(12) [—] | 1.5[c] | 15.2% of body wt | — | Lumholtz et al., 1974 |
| | 51–70 (12) [—] | 2.0[c] | 16.2% of body wt | — | |
| | >70 (25) [—] | 3.6[c] | 24.2% of body wt[d] | — | |

| | | | | | |
|---|---|---|---|---|---|
| Kanamycin | 20–50 (13) [—] | 1.8 | 16.7% of body wt | — | Lumholtz et al., 1974 |
| | 51–70 (21) [—] | 2.5 | 16.0% of body wt | — | |
| | >70 (33) [—] | 5.5 | 23.1% of body wt[d] | — | |
| Pancuronium | 20–86 (19) | — | NSD with increasing age | decreased with increasing age | McLeod et al., 1979 |
| Penicillin G | — (9) [31] | 0.4 | — | — | Kampmann et al., 1972 |
| | — (13) | 0.9 | — | — | |
| Propicillin K | 20–30 (10) [—] | 0.57 | 29.1 l | — 0.43 l/kg | Simon et al., 1972 |
| | 60–80 (16) [—] | 0.66 | 18.4[a] 0.26 l/kg[a] | — | |
| Sulfamethizole | 22–30 (6) [24] | 1.75 | 0.345 l/kg | 167 ml/min/1.73 m$^2$ | Triggs et al., 1975 |
| | 73–91 (7) [81] | 3.0[a] | 0.338 l/kg | 90 ml/min/1.73 m$^{2a}$ | |

[a]Significant difference between "old" and "young."

[b]The values for the Somogyi et al. (1980) study were estimated by the reviewers from figures presented in the study. Somogyi et al. reported statistically significant negative correlations of Vdss, Cl, and renal Cl with age, and positive correlation of $t_{1/2}\beta$ with age. The Somogyi et al. (1980) study appears to present a complete analysis of the preliminary report presented earlier (Gugler and Somogyi, 1979).

[c]Statistical analysis of age-related differences not reported.

[d]Significant difference between > 70 and two younger groups.

in the elderly than in the young indicated that the drug was metabolized or excreted more slowly by the older person. However, as shown by formula 2, alteration of $t_{1/2}$ cannot be attributed to change in metabolism or excretion unless the investigators also determined Vd.

## Clearance

Total body clearance is a quantitative measure of body elimination and may be illustrated as the sum of the metabolic and excretion processes shown in Figure 8–1. Pharmacokinetically, total body clearance is the product of the Vd and the apparent first-order elimination rate constant (Gibaldi and Perrier, 1975), which is the rate constant for the sum of systemic drug elimination by urinary excretion of intact drug, by nonrenal excretion, and by drug metabolism. Clearance is also defined in terms of the volume of plasma or blood from which drug is completely removed per unit time, and thus it is expressed in units of flow (Wilkinson and Shand, 1975; Woosley and Shand, 1978).

The concentration of a drug in the plasma at steady state (Css) is directly proportional to the systemically available dose and inversely proportional to the Cl and the dosing interval, as shown by formula 3.

$$\text{Css} = \frac{\text{systemically available dose}}{\text{Cl} \times \text{dosing interval}} \quad (3)$$

Obviously, if Cl of a drug is reduced by aging and if absorption of the drug is quantitatively similar in young and old patients, the elderly will have higher blood levels of the drug than will younger patients given the same dose at the same interval.

*Renal Clearance.* The kidney is by far the most important organ for drug excretion, and an appreciable decline in renal function is a normal event in the aging process. Between the ages of 25 and 85 years the number of nephrons decreases by 30 to 40 percent, and with aging there is decrease in glomerular filtration rate and in maximal tubular secretory and reabsorptive functions (Goldman, 1979).

In a large study of 548 normal men ranging in age from 17 to 96 years, cross-sectional analysis of their creatinine clearances (Clcr), grouped by means of each 10 years of age, showed a progressive, linear decrease in Clcr from a mean of 140 ml/min/1.73 $m^2$ at age 30, to 97 ml/min/1.73 $m^2$ at age 80 (Rowe et al., 1976). Data from a study employing less rigorous health screening showed a mean Clcr of 110 ml/min/1.73 $m^2$ for men aged 20–29 years and a Clcr of 47 ml/min/1.73 $m^2$ for 80–89-year-old men (Siersbaek-Nielsen et al., 1971). In this latter study, serum creatinine (Scr) values were similar in all age groups; in the study by Rowe and colleagues (1976), there was a very slight but statistically significant increase in Scr with age. The decline in Clcr with little or no change in Scr is believed to be secondary to the decreasing muscle mass with increasing age (Rowe et al., 1976). Kampmann and co-workers (1974) determined Scr, Clcr, and urinary excretion of creatinine of 219 women and 149 men whose serum creatinines were <1.4 mg/dl, although many of these individuals were patients with essential hypertension or chronic nephropathy. The investigators found that Scr did not vary significantly with age but that Clcr/1.73 $m^2$ showed decreasing mean values with a fall of about 10 ml per minute per decade from the third to ninth decades. Obviously, estimates of renal function must take age as well as Scr into account. Siersbaek-Nielsen and co-workers (1971) have prepared a useful nomogram that includes the patient's age, sex, weight, and Scr in the estimation of Clcr.

Kampmann and Hansen (1979) reviewed a number of studies in which the kinetics of renally eliminated drugs were compared in elderly and young subjects. Most of these studies were incomplete in that the investigators determined only drug $t_{1/2}$ or serum level; Kampmann and Hansen pointed out that without Vd or Cl data, conclusions could not be drawn about the effect of aging on the drug's elimination by the kidney. In their review, Kampmann and Hansen stated that the total renal Cl of most drugs excreted by the kidney parallels the glomerular filtration rate even when the main route of excretion is tabular secretion.

Table 8–4 includes several recent, as well as some older, studies comparing age-related pharmacokinetics of drugs excreted unchanged by the kidney. The Cl of cimetidine, digoxin, pancuronium, and sulfamethizole decreases with increased age. The other studies included in Table 8–4 did not report data on drug Cl. However, the larger increases in $t_{1/2}$ than in Vd shown for gentamicin and kanamycin by Lumholtz and colleagues (1974) suggest that Cl of these drugs was reduced at advanced age. And although the $t_{1/2}$ of propicillin was similar in the old and young groups, the Vd was significantly smaller in the older subjects, suggesting that Cl must also have been reduced by aging. Penicillin G was found by Kampmann and co-workers (1972) to have a longer $t_{1/2}$ in older than in younger subjects; however, no conclusions regarding comparative Cl of the drug can be drawn since Vd was not determined. Thus, although we have found few studies in which the pharmacokinetics of renally excreted drugs had been adequately compared in young and old subjects, the information which is available strongly supports the idea that for drugs excreted intact by the kidney, the rate of excretion decreases with increasing age.

Kampmann and Hansen (1979) listed a group of renally excreted drugs for which dosage should be reduced for the elderly, and they proposed practical guidelines for adjusting dosage based on a "dosage-adjustment" factor.

Another clinical implication of reduced renal excretion of drugs by elderly patients is pointed out by Mitchard (1979). Studies by his group have shown that corresponding to a longer $t_{1/2}$ of two antibiotics in elderly patients than in a young control group, the antibiotic concentrations in the urine were lower in the elderly. These low concentrations were associated with failure to clear the infection.

*Drug Metabolism.* The effects of aging on drug metabolism are not yet sufficiently defined to permit generalizations. The weight of the liver decreases with age at a rate consistent with total body weight until the seventh decade and then declines more rapidly than does body weight (Goldman, 1979). Bilirubin Cl, total serum bilirubin, SGOT, SGTP, and alkaline phosphatase are not significantly different in healthy old and healthy young persons (Goldman, 1979).

Alterations of hepatic Cl of drugs could result from change in liver blood flow, change in "intrinsic free clearance" (the inherent activity of the removal process including the activity of the liver enzymes) or change in the extent of drug binding to plasma (Wood et al., 1979). Hepatic blood flow declines with aging but available data are conflicting as to whether the fractional decrease is less or greater than the decline corresponding to decrease in total cardiac output (Goldman, 1979). Gillette and Hinson (1978), Gillette (1979), and Stevenson and colleagues (1979) have summarized results of early studies by Kato and co-workers of hepatic enzymatic activity, indicating that in rats aging is associated with decreased ability of liver microsomal enzymes to metabolize certain barbiturates. No studies on the relationship of age to drug-metabolizing ability of human liver biopsy samples have been reported (Stevenson et al., 1979).

As shown in Table 8–5, a number of drugs that are eliminated primarily by metabolism have longer half-lives in the elderly than in the young. However, the prolongation of half-lives of diazepam, lidocaine, and nitrazepam appears to be a result of increased Vd rather than reduced Cl in the elderly; and increased Vd appears to contribute to the longer $t_{1/2}$ of aspirin and chlormethiazole. Examination of the data shown in Table 8–5 on the benzodiazepines illustrates the complexity of attempting to generalize about the effects of aging on the pharmacokinetics of drugs eliminated by metabolism. The half-lives of chlordiazepoxide, diazepam, and nitrazepam are increased with age. The increase in $t_{1/2}$ of chlordiazepoxide results from increased Vd and decreased Cl, whereas the volumes of distribution of diazepam and nitrazepam are greater in the elderly than in the young, but Cl of these drugs does not decrease with age. The half-lives of oxazepam and lorazepam do not change with aging, and although one of the two studies of lorazepam showed slightly smaller Vd and Cl of the drug in the older subjects, when data from the smokers were excluded from the study analysis, there was no significant difference in Cl in the two age groups. Shader and Greenblatt (1979) outline the initial steps in the metabolism of the various benzodiazepines, stating that the variability of the influence of age on the pharmacokinetics of these drugs results from differences in the initial biotransformation reactions for their degradation.

Several reviewers have concluded that whereas there is some evidence for an age-related decrease in the hepatic microsomal enzyme metabolism of certain drugs, relatively little is known about age-related changes in drug metabolizing capacity (Crooks et al., 1976; O'Malley et al., 1980; Smith, 1979; Swift, 1979; Vestal, 1978). As mentioned above in regard to lorazepam, and as discussed below in the descriptions of antipyrine and of propranolol pharmacokinetics, aging decreases smoking-induced drug metabolizing enzymes. This fact further complicates interpretation of metabolism data and strongly suggests that smoking habits must be considered in designing studies of drug metabolism.

Vestal (1978) suggested that aging may not affect non-microsomal enzyme pathways of drug metabolism. Ethanol is oxidized primarily by alcohol dehydrogenase, an enzyme in the soluble fraction of liver homogenates. Vestal and colleagues (1977) studied ethanol distribution and metabolism in 50 healthy men aged 21–81 years and found that rates of ethanol elimination were not affected by age (peak ethanol concentrations in blood water at the end of the infusion period correlated positively with age, however, and Vd correlated negatively with age). Farah and co-workers (1977) measured the $t_{1/2}$ of acetanilid, as a "model substrate" for oxidation, and the $t_{1/2}$ of isoniazid, as a "model substrate" for acetylation, in a group of young and a group of elderly subjects. The mean $t_{1/2}$ of acetanilid was significantly longer in the older group. With isoniazid the half-lives showed bimodal distribution in both age groups, and mean half-lives did not differ with age. Although Vd was not determined in the study, the investigators stated that their findings confirmed an age-related decrease in microsomal oxidation rates and showed that in the same population acetylation did not change with age. These investigators' interpretation of their data on isoniazid has been cited by some reviewers.

The following section on pharmacokinetics of some specific drugs includes additional discussion of the effects of age on drug metabolism.

*Antipyrine.* Antipyrine, a drug formerly in wide use as an antipyretic and mild analgesic, has several properties that have made it valuable as a pharmacokinetic tool (Stevenson, 1977; Vestal et al., 1975; Wood et al., 1979). The drug is rapidly absorbed and distributed throughout total body

Table 8–5.
Effects of Aging on Half-Life, Distribution, and Clearance of Drugs Eliminated Primarily by Metabolism (Single-Dose Studies)

| *Drug* | *Age group in years range (n) [mean]* | | *Mean* $t_{1/2}\beta$(hr) | *Mean Vd* | *Mean Cl* | *Reference* |
|---|---|---|---|---|---|---|
| Acetaminophen | 22–30 [24] | (6) | 1.8 | 1.03 1/kg | 477 ml/min/1.73 $m^2$ | Triggs et al., 1975 |
| | 73–91 [81] | (7) | 2.2[a] | 1.05 1/kg | 379 ml/min/1.73 $m^2$ | |
| Acetaminophen | — [24] | (11) | — | — | 364 ml/min | Fulton et al., 1979 |
| | — [76] | (12) | — | — | 241 ml/min | |
| Acetanilid | 20–35 [—] | (19) | 1.45 | — | — | Farah et al., 1977 |
| | > 65 [—] | (24) | 2.1[a] | — | — | |
| Alcohol | 21–81 [age as a continuous variable] | (50) | — | decreased with increasing age | not age related | Vestal et al., 1977 |
| Antipyrine | 18–39 [33] | (73) | 12.7 | 0.573 1/kg[b] | 34.6 ml/hr/kg[b] | Vestal et al., 1975 |
| | 40–59 [50] | (150) | 13.8 | 0.537 l/kg | 30.9 ml/hr/kg[b] | |
| | 60–92 [69] | (84) | 14.8[b] | 0.536 l/kg | 28.2 ml/hr/kg[b] | |
| Aspirin | 20–40 [—] | (6) | 2.3 | 0.078 l/kg | 24 ml/hr/kg | Stevenson et al., 1979 |
| | > 65 [—] | (5) | 5.2[a] | 0.106 l/kg | 17 ml/hr/kg | |

| | | | | | | |
|---|---|---|---|---|---|---|
| Chlordiazepoxide | 21–30 [25] | (28) | 10.1 | 0.42 l/kg | 46 ml/min<br>0.61 ml/min/kg | Shader et al., 1977 |
| | 63–74 [69] | (8) | 18.2[a] | 0.52 l/kg[a] | 27 ml/min[a]<br>0.345 ml/min/kg[a] | |
| Chlordiazepoxide | 16–86 [age as a continuous variable] | (27) | 20 yr = 6[c]<br>80 yr = 34[a,c] | 20 yr = 0.26 l/kg[c]<br>80 yr = 0.38 l/kg[c,a] | 20 yr = 30 ml/min[c]<br>80 yr = 8 ml/min[c,a] | Roberts et al., 1978 |
| Chlormethiazole (iv) | 20–27 [23] | (6) | 4.05 | 7.9 l/kg | 23 ml/min/kg | Triggs, 1979 |
| | 69–91 [75] | (8) | 8.5[a] | 11.2 l/kg[a] | 16.1 ml/min/kg[a] | |
| Chlormethiazole (po) | 25–28 [27] | (3) | 6.15 | — | 14 l/min<br>222 ml/min/kg | Nation et al., 1977a |
| | 68–71 [70] | (3) | 6.3 | — | 1.8 l/min[a]<br>35 ml/min/kg[a] | |
| Desmethyldiazepam[d] | 29–34 [—] | (4) | 51 | 0.64 l/kg | 11.3 ml/min | Klotz and Müller-Seydlitz, 1979 |
| | 65–85 [—] | (4) | 151[a] | 0.85 l/kg | 4.3 ml/min[a] | |
| Diazepam | 15–82 [age as a continuous variable] | (33) | 20 yr = 20<br>80 yr = 90[a] | initial distribution space and Vdss increased with age[a] | NSD with age | Klotz et al., 1975 |
| Diazepam | 21–30 [26][e] | (9) | 32 | 76.1 1[e] | 27.6 ml/min[e] | MacLeod et al., 1979 |
| | 70–88 [82][e] | (10) | 41.7[e] | 103.2 1[e] | 24.9 ml/min[e] | |
| Lidocaine | 22–26 [24] | (4) | 1.3 | 0.895 l/kg | 543.1 ml/min<br>7.6 ml/min/kg | Nation et al., 1977b |
| | 61–71 [65] | (6) | 2.3[a] | 1.586 l/kg[a] | 556 ml/min<br>8.1 ml/min/kg | |
| Lorazepam | 15–73 [age as a continuous variable] | (11) | 22<br>NSD with aging | 1.28 l/kg<br>NSD with aging | 0.75 ml/min/kg<br>NSD with aging | Kraus et al., 1978 |

*(Continued)*

| | | | | | | |
|---|---|---|---|---|---|---|
| Lorazepam | 19–38 [—] | (15) | 14.1 | 1.11 l/kg | 0.99 ml/min/kg | Greenblatt et al., 1979 |
| | 60–84 [—] | (75) | 15.9 | 0.99 l/kg[a] | 0.77 ml/min/kg[a,f] | |
| Nitrazepam | 18–38 [24] | (25) | 28.9 | 2.4 l/kg | 4.1 1/hr | Kangas et al., 1979[g] |
| | 66–89 [77] | (12) | 40.4[a] | 4.8 l/kg[a] | 4.7 1/hr | |
| Oxazepam | 14–30 [25] | (8) | 5.1 | $V_d$(extrap.) 52.5 l<br>$V_d\beta$ 47.7 l | 113.5 ml/min | Shull et al., 1976 |
| | 45–84 [54] | (8) | 5.6 | $V_d$(extrap.) 70.6 l<br>$V_d\beta$ 61.2 l[a] | 136.0 ml/min | |
| Phenylbutazone | 22–30 [24] | (8)[h] | 110 | 172 ml/kg | — | Triggs et al., 1975 |
| | 73–91 [81] | (7) | 87 | 165 ml/kg | — | |
| Propranolol[i] | — [approx. 29] | (6) | 2.5 | 3.0 l/kg | 13.2 ml/min/kg | Castleden and George, 1979a |
| | — [78] | (8) | 4.2[a] | 2.7 l/kg | 7.8 ml/min/kg[a] | |
| Propranolol[j] | 21–73 [age as a continuous variable] | (27) | increased with age | NSD with age | for nonsmokers, NSD with age<br>for smokers and total group, Cl decreased with age[j] | Vestal et al., 1979a |
| Propylthiouracil | "younger" | (6) | — | Vdβ 0.35 l/kg | 122 ml/min/m$^2$ | Kampmann et al., 1979 |
| | 74–86 [80] | (9) | — | Vdβ 0.37 l/kg | 105 ml/min/m$^2$ | |
| Quinidine | 23–34 [29] | (14) | 7.3 | 2.39 l/kg | 4.04 ml/min/kg | Ochs et al., 1978 |
| | 60–69 [66] | (8) | 9.7[a] | 2.18 1/kg | 2.64 ml/min/kg[a,k] | |

| | | | | | | |
|---|---|---|---|---|---|---|
| Quinine | 20–40 [—] | (6) | 5.7 | 3.17 l/kg | 0.397 1/hr/kg | Stevenson et al., 1979 |
| | > 65 [–] | (5) | 6.6 | 1.74 l/kg[a] | 0.193 1/hr/kg[a] | |
| Warfarin | — [24] | (18) | 34[m] | 0.16 l/kg[m] | 3.45 ml/hr/kg | Shepherd et al., 1979 |
| | — [85] | (20) | 41[m] | 0.19 l/kg[m,a] | 3.4 ml/hr/kg | |

[a]Significant difference between "old" and "young."

[b]$t_{1/2}\beta$ greater in "old" than "young" group; other group differences in $t_{1/2}\beta$ NSD in this study; Vd significantly greater in "young" than other two groups; clearance differences among groups in this study all statistically significant [see text and Vestal et al.(1975) and Wood et al. (1979) for effect of smoking on clearance of antipyrine].

[c]Values estimated from plots of correlation. Aging was associated with increasing $t_{1/2}\beta$ and Vdss and decreasing plasma clearance.

[d]Desmethyldiazepam is not a drug per se but is an active metabolite of chlorazepate, chlordiazepoxide, diazepam, and prazepam (Anderson, 1980).

[e]Median rather than mean. In this study, men showed statistically higher Cl values and lower $t_{1/2}\beta$ of diazepam than did women.

[f]Greenblatt et al. (1979) note that when only data from nonsmokers were included in the analysis, mean lorazepam clearances of young and old subjects did not differ statistically.

[g]Kangas et al. (1979) study compared healthy group volunteers with elderly hospitalized patients.

[h]Seven of the subjects' ages ranged from 22 to 30 with a mean of 24; the age of the eighth young subject was not stated. In this study, two to ten blood samples were taken on day one, followed by at least one sample per day to the fifth day after administration. There was a significant negative correlation between β and the concentration of serum albumin of the subjects.

[i]Data shown are with iv administration; the drug was also given orally to the same subjects and first-pass extraction and metabolism was found to be significantly less in the elderly group than the young group.

[j]In this study, simultaneous oral and intravenous kinetics of propranolol at steady state were investigated. See text for discussion of this paper and the effects of smoking on propranolol disposition.

[k]Renal clearance was also significantly lower in the elderly group.

[l]Decreased clearance of propranolol with aging was also reported by Drayer et al. (1980).

[m]Values estimated from a figure. Vd data may have been obtained by extrapolation to zero time following oral administration.

water; and less than 10 percent of the antipyrine in blood is bound to plasma proteins. Antipyrine's plasma disappearance follows first-order kinetics with the drug being extensively metabolized by cytochrome P-450-dependent liver microsomal enzymes; and only about 5 percent is excreted unchanged in the urine (Stevenson 1977; Vestal et al., 1975). Because of these properties, $t_{1/2}$ of antipyrine has been used as a measure of its metabolism. In an early study, O'Malley and co-workers (1971) reported a longer $t_{1/2}$ of orally administered antipyrine in elderly patients than in young volunteers; this study has been frequently cited in statements that the rate of hepatic drug metabolism is decreased in the elderly.

As has been noted above, and as Wood and co-workers (1979) point out in their study of the effects of aging and cigarette smoking on elimination of antipyrine, hepatic Cl is a preferable measure of liver metabolic efficiency than is $t_{1/2}$ since the former is independent of changes in Vd. Vestal and colleagues (1975) determined the pharmacokinetics of intravenous antipyrine in 307 healthy men ranging in age from 18 to 92 years and found that $t_{1/2}$ increased and Vd and Cl decreased with age. Multiple regression analysis of data showed, however, that 12 percent of the variance in metabolic Cl was explained by cigarette smoking and only 3 percent was explained by age.

Wood and colleagues (1979) note that mechanisms of altering hepatic Cl could involve change in liver blood flow, in "intrinsic free Cl," or in the extent of drug binding to plasma. In studying the effects of aging on hepatic drug Cl, these authors compared the elimination of antipyrine, the Cl of which is rate limited by activity of liver enzymes and not appreciably influenced by volume of blood flow, with the elimination of idocyanine green, which has an intrinsic Cl so high that its Cl is largely dependent upon liver blood flow. Antipyrine was administered intravenously to 20 normal men between the ages of 22 and 72 years, and indocyanine green was given intravenously to these same subjects plus four others. Results showed that antipyrine Cl decreased with age in the group as a whole and in cigarette smokers, but there was no significant correlation with age in nonsmokers. For the group less than 40 years old, but not for the group older than 40, Cl of antipyrine was greater in smokers than in nonsmokers, suggesting that the enzyme-induction effect of smoking decreases with aging. The Cl of indocyanine green decreased with age in both smokers and nonsmokers, a result consistent with a decrease in cardiac output and therefore decreased liver blood flow with increased age (Wood et al., 1979).

*Propranolol.* The effects of aging on propranolol pharmacokinetics are complex and are further complicated by the effects of cigarette smoking on metabolism of the drug. With single-dose oral administration of propranolol (Castleden and George, 1979a; Castleden et al., 1975), and in multiple-dose studies (Castleden and George, 1979a; Feely and Stevenson, 1978; Vestal et al., 1979a), blood levels were higher in older than in younger subjects given the same dosage. When Vestal and colleagues (1979a) divided their group of 27 normal men, aged 21–73 years, into those who were cigarette smokers and those who were nonsmokers, the propranolol blood levels were almost twice as high in the nonsmokers as in the smokers. Although there was a tendency for propranolol blood levels to increase with age in the smokers, age-related differences in smokers' propranolol blood levels were not statistically significant; and propranolol blood levels did not appear to increase with aging in nonsmokers.

The studies of Castleden and George (1979a) and Vestal and co-workers (1979a) showed that following intravenous administration of propranolol, the Vd of the drug was similar in young and old subjects, but that Cl decreased and therefore $t_{1/2}\beta$ increased with aging. Castleden and George (1979a) concluded from their study that first-pass extraction and metabolism of propranolol were less in the elderly than in the young. Vestal and co-workers (1979a) showed that liver blood flow decreased with age to the same extent in smokers and non-smokers, and that intrinsic total Cl of propranolol decreased with age only in smokers. Systemic Cl, which depends quantitatively on liver blood flow and on intrinsic Cl, decreased significantly with age for the group as a whole and for the smokers, but not for the nonsmokers. Since cigarette smoke contains inducers of drug-metabolizing enzymes, the investigators suggested that the smokers' decrease in intrinsic Cl of propranolol with aging was a result of a decrease in drug-metabolizing enzymes with increasing age.

*Amobarbital.* Following administration of a single dose of amobarbital to two groups of clinically healthy male subjects, one group aged 20–40 years and the other group older than 65 years, amobarbital plasma levels at four and 24 hours after administration were measured (Irvine et al., 1974). The urinary excretion of the 3-hydroxy metabolite was also determined. The 24-hour plasma level of amobarbital was significantly higher in the older group; and at 24 and 48 hours after administration, the younger group had excreted a significantly higher percent of the dose as the metabolite in the urine. The authors concluded that the rate of hydroxylation of amobarbital decreases with age. Ritschel (1978) used an analog computer to analyze the data reported in the study of Irvine and colleagues. The computer-generated analysis indicated that the Vd of the drug did not change with age but that the biologic $t_{1/2}$ increased from approximately 23 hours in the younger group to about 87 hours in the elderly group, thus indicating a slower rate of metabolism in the older subjects. Using the one-point method, Ritschel suggested that a nightly dose of 50 mg of amobarbital for the older group would result in the same steady-state levels as would 200 mg in the 20–40-year-olds.

*Methaqualone.* Reynolds and co-workers (1978) determined the 24-hour urinary excretion of six metabolites of methaqualone following administration of a single oral dose to 11 geriatric patients aged 71–90 years. The total 24-hour excretion of the six metabolites was approximately one-half that of a group of 19 young adults studied previously by the same investigators.

*Phenytoin.* In their study of the effects of age on the pharmacokinetics of phenytoin, Hayes and colleagues (1975b) found lower plasma binding and a higher mean Cl rate of the drug in their old (67–95 years) than in their young (20–43 years) group. Taking into account the low serum albumin of the olders subjects in the study by Hayes and co-workers, Shader and Greenblatt (1979) analyzed the Hayes group's data using a covariance adjustment of means in which each patient's albumin level was used as a covariate. Analyzed in this way, there was no significant difference in phenytoin clearance of the older and younger groups, which suggests that the greater rate of Cl in the older group resulted from their decreased binding of phenytoin rather than a higher rate of intrinsic metabolism of the drug.

Houghton and co-workers (1975) studied the effect of age and other factors on the serum phenytoin concentrations of 170 adult epilepsy patients who were receiving 300 mg of phenytoin daily (many of whom were also receiving other anticonvulsant drugs). There was a statistically significant positive correlation of serum levels with age, but the correlation coefficient was low, and the authors suggested that other variables are more important than age in determining serum concentrations. There was a statistically significant negative correlation of serum phenytoin concentrations with patient weight. However, the authors conclude that the magnitude of the correlation coefficients of age and weight indicated that these factors accounted for only a small amount of the patient variability, and that genetic differences, "exaggerated by enzyme saturation," were much more important than age, weight, and height in determining a patient's steady-state plasma phenytoin level.

*Tricyclic Antidepressants.* Steady-state plasma levels of the tricyclic antidepressants (TCAs) show very wide interpatient variability. Nies and colleagues (1977) determined steady-state blood levels of amitriptyline and its metabolite nortriptyline in 35 patients aged 21–68 years who received 150 mg of amitriptyline daily for four weeks or more. Plasma levels of amitriptyline, but not of the metabolite, correlated positively with age. In a similar study, these investigators determined steady-state plasma levels of imipramine and its metabolite, desipramine, in 18 patients of various ages who received imipramine daily for at least three weeks. Plasma levels of both the parent compound and the metabolite correlated positively with age. These authors also reported a longer plasma $t_{1/2}\beta$ of desipramine in patients over 65 years of age than in "young" patients, but few data are given.

Norman and colleagues (1977) studied steady-state plasma levels of nortriptyline in 53 depressed patients aged 18–66 who were given a standard dose of the drug. Although there appeared to be a positive correlation of patient age with drug plasma level, the correlation was not significant when corrected for sex and smoking status. Braithwaite and co-workers (1979) found that in 36 patients given 100 mg of nortriptyline daily, steady-state plasma levels of the drug ranged from 36 to 381 μg/ml. Plasma levels appeared to correlate with age but the correlation did not reach statistical significance. Similar to the results of Nies and co-workers, Braithwaite and his colleagues found a positive correlation of amitriptyline steady-state blood levels with patients' ages, and lack of correlation of the drug's nortriptyline metabolite levels with patient age. Braithwaite and co-workers compared data on plasma nortriptyline $t_{1/2}\beta$ and Cl following single oral doses as reported in five different studies. When data from the five studies were combined, a positive correlation was shown between age and plasma $t_{1/2}$. Clearance values were lower in depressed patients than in volunteers; these findings are discussed by the investigators.

Norman and colleagues (1979) briefly summarized studies of the effects of aging on pharmacokinetics of TCAs. They concluded that although it appears that the elderly may have a slower rate of elimination of TCAs than have younger people, the effects of age on plasma concentrations are not pronounced with nortriptyline, doxepin, and maprotiline.

*Lithium.* Lithium is excreted unchanged, almost entirely in the urine (Hewick et al., 1977). It would be expected therefore that lithium Cl would be reduced by aging and that lower doses would be needed by elderly than by young patients. Hewick and colleagues (1977) noted that information published between 1968 and 1974, relating dosage of lithium to patient age, was fragmented and sometimes contradictory. In a preliminary report, Hewick and Newbury (1976) analyzed case records of 82 patients receiving lithium and plotted the dosage calculated to give a lithium plasma concentration of 1 mmol/l against patient age. Their results showed that in order to achieve the same plasma level, an 80-year-old would require two-thirds of the dose needed by a 20-year-old. In a more complete study, Hewick and co-workers (1977) reported on the same 82 psychiatric outpatients, aged 21–84 years, who were receiving prophylactic lithium and who had relatively stable plasma lithium levels. The researchers found that the calculated daily doses of lithium in millimoles per kilogram required to give one millimole lithium per liter of plasma remained constant from the third to fifth decades and then declined over the next three decades. For comparable plasma levels, patients aged 70–79 years required 31 percent lower dosage than patients under 50 years; and interindividual variation was large. It was estimated that age contributed only about 14 percent to total interpatient variation. The mean daily, weight-related doses actually prescribed declined with patient age, decreasing by about 50 percent between the third and eighth decades. This age-related dose reduction appeared necessary to accommodate reduced renal excretion and reduced tolerance to lithium by the older patients.

*Theophylline.* Therapy with theophylline is complicated both by a narrow range of therapeutic serum concentrations between levels that are ineffective and those that cause toxicity, and by variability in rates of theophylline metabolism among patients (Koup et al., 1976). Although it is widely assumed that the elderly metabolize theophylline at a somewhat slower rate than younger individuals, further study is needed.

In studying theophylline kinetics in acute pulmonary edema, Piafsky and co-workers (1977) included a control group of 19 men who ranged in age from the early 20s to approximately 80 years and who had apparently normal renal, hepatic, and pulmonary functions. Results showed that among the controls there was NSD in either $t_{1/2}\beta$ or Vdss with age. There was a four-fold variation in $t_{1/2}\beta$ among controls and a 20-fold interpatient variation in $t_{1/2}\beta$ among the nine patients with acute cardiogenic pulmonary edema.

Based upon preliminary pharmacokinetic studies in five patients and on Cl data from the literature, Koup and colleagues (1976) designed a dosage regimen nomogram for selecting theophylline dosage. The nomogram provides for a loading dose based on body weight and for maintenance dosage based on body weight, age, cardiac function, and hepatic function. With use of the nomogram, a "typical" older patient receives maintenance dosage 25 percent less than that used for "relatively young, reasonably healthy adults who were expected to be rapid metabolizers of the drug." The usefulness of the nomogram was prospectively studied by Koup and co-workers (1976) in 72 patients hospitalized primarily with moderate to severe respiratory disease. With nomogram-indicated dosage, 29 of the 40 patients categorized by their physicians to be in the typical older patient group had serum levels within the therapeutic range (8–20 μg/ml) 24 hours from onset of therapy. Some of the other 11 typical older patients had lower and some had higher blood levels than the usual therapeutic range. Asked to describe what was meant by a "typical" older patient in this study (Majerus and Feroli, 1977), Jusko and colleagues (1977) replied, in part, that assignment of patients to this category was based on subjective assessment of physiologic and chronologic aging.

In preparation for a large clinical trial on use of aminophylline in patients suffering from symptoms of acute cerebral ischemia, Nielsen-Kudsk and co-workers (1978) studied theophylline kinetics in 10 hospitalized patients aged 60–77 years who had apparently normal renal, hepatic, and cardiopulmonary functions. The investigators found less variability among individuals than would have been expected from other studies. Half-lives ranged from 5.4 to 9 hours, Cl from 28 to 42 ml/kg/hr, and apparent Vd from 0.33 to 0.43 l/kg. The investigators concluded that in this elderly group of patients, a therapeutic serum concentration of 10 μg theophylline/ml could be established by an IV loading dose of 3.7 mg/kg of body weight followed by a continuous infusion of 0.35 mg/kg/hr. However, they advised monitoring of theophylline levels because of the variable $t_{1/2}$ reported in other studies.

*Warfarin.* As noted above, the data on the effects of aging on plasma protein binding of warfarin are conflicting, that is, Hayes and colleagues (1975a) found warfarin to be less protein bound in the plasma of elderly than young subjects, whereas Shepherd and colleagues (1977) reported almost identical warfarin binding in plasma obtained from young and old. Shepherd and co-workers (1977) suggest that this variation in findings may result from use of higher warfarin/plasma albumin concentrations in the earlier study.

Shepherd and colleagues (1977) studied the pharmacokinetics of warfarin in 13 healthy young persons and 13 healthy elderly. Each subject was given 1.5 mg of oral racemic warfarin per kilogram of body weight with 50 mg of oral vitamin $k_1$, and, where necessary, further vitamin $k_1$ to maintain a normal Thrombotest value. The mean $t_{1/2}$ was longer in the older group, but the difference was not statistically significant. Although the Vd and Cl were reported not to differ significantly between the two groups, unfortunately the method of calculation of these values was not appropriate for a drug administered by mouth.

In a later report, Shepherd and colleagues (1979) compared the pharmacokinetics of warfarin in 18 young and 20 elderly subjects following a single oral dose. As shown in Table 8–5, both $t_{1/2}$ and Vd were greater in the elderly than in the young; and Cl was almost identical in the two groups. The method of calculating these data from the plasma levels is not reported.

## AGING AND RESPONSIVENESS TO DRUG ACTION

As described above, changes in pharmacokinetics with aging can alter the amount of drug available to receptors and the duration of contact of a threshold concentration of the drug at receptor sites. Aging may also affect the numbers of receptors and the affinity of the receptors for the drug. Response to drugs is also affected by age-related physiologic changes such as neurotransmitter concentrations and by underlying disease processes, which are more likely to be present in the elderly than in younger individuals. Efficiency of homeostatic mechanisms also decreases with aging.

In a recent review, Bender (1979) traced interest in the effects of aging on drug activity to research in the 1940s showing increased sensitivity to certain drugs in older experimental animals. Bender noted that in 1949 Leake presented a paper at a symposium on geriatrics summarizing the state of knowledge of drug sensitivity in the aged. Leake (1949) stated that alcohol, digitalis, and morphine were apparently more toxic in old people than in "healthy adults," and that sulfa drugs were better tolerated by young people than by the elderly. Despite this early interest, however, as Bender (1979) notes, "The subject of geriatric pharmacology has only been approached in earnest over the past 10 years" (p. 148).

Research concerned with the effects of aging on susceptibility to drug effects has been focused primarily on two broad categories of pharmacologic-therapeutic agents—CNS depressants and cardiovascular drugs. Much of the age-related research on sensitivity to CNS agents has been epidemiologic, documenting adverse reaction rates in patients of various ages. Some recent cardiovascular-drug research relates to receptor sensitivity as a function of age. The following section of this chapter is divided into discussion of the effects of age on responsiveness to CNS drugs, to warfarin, and to certain agents acting on autonomic receptors.

### Aging and Responsiveness to CNS Drugs

Castleden and colleagues (1979) reviewed evidence that adverse reactions to hypnotics occur more commonly in the elderly than in younger people and cited as one mechanism that there is evidence that the brain becomes more responsive to hypnotics as age advances.

Castleden and colleagues (1977a) and Castleden and George (1979b) reported on increased sensitivity to a benzodiazepine hypnotic, nitrazepam, in the elderly. Their study involved ten healthy young and ten healthy elderly subjects in a double-blind, cross-over comparison of a single 10 mg dose of nitrazepam with placebo. Twelve, 36, and 60 hours after dosing, each subject had blood drawn for plasma drug estimation, completed a psychomotor test, and indicated on an analogous scale how well he or she had slept. The investigators reported that their pharmacokinetic studies on these subjects showed there was NSD between elderly and young in plasma concentrations at the specified times, and that

$t_{1/2}$ and Vd of nitrazepam were not significantly different in the two groups. [Note: Castleden et al. (1977a) based these conclusions on the three blood level determinations indicated above, which precludes accurate estimation of Vd and probably of $t_{1/2}$. The Kangas et al. (1979) study of nitrazepam pharmacokinetics (see Table 8–5) showed smaller Vd and shorter $t_{1/2}$ in healthy young volunteers than in elderly hospitalized patients.] In the psychomotor test the elderly made more mistakes than the young, even on testing with placebo. The young seemed to be less accurate at 12 and 36 hours after nitrazepam than they were after placebo, but the difference was not statistically significant. The elderly subjects were less accurate after nitrazepam than after placebo at 12 and 36 hours, and even at 60 hours, although the difference at 60 hours was not statistically significant. All subjects, young and elderly, took longer to complete the test at 12 and 36 hours after nitrazepam than after placebo, but at 60 hours there was NSD in time required. These data point out that nitrazepam depressed motor function regardless of age; and the drug affected cognitive function to a greater degree in the elderly than it did in the young. Because the pharmacokinetic methods used make the reported lack of age-related differences in Vd and $t_{1/2}$ questionable, it is possible that the observed differences in cognitive function were due to differences in concentration of nitrazepam at receptor sites.

The Boston Collaborative Drug Surveillance Program (1973) reported on clinical CNS depression due to diazepam, chlordiazepoxide, and phenobarbital in relation to cigarette smoking and to age. Of 2,274 hospitalized patients who received one of the drugs for anxiety, 154 were reported to have developed drowsiness, which was severe enough in 128 patients to cause the physician to discontinue treatment. Among the patients receiving benzodiazepines, the incidence of drowsiness increased with age from 4.4 percent of 428 patients under 40 years of age to 10.9 percent of 248 patients over 70 years of age. These data were analyzed with smoking habits taken into account and the age-related effects were found to be highly significant ($p < 0.002$). The authors reported that incidence of drowsiness did not increase with age in the phenobarbital recipients. More recent studies have shown an age-related increase in $t_{1/2}$ of chlordiazepoxide and diazepam, as well as an age-related decrease in Cl of chlordiazepoxide (see Table 8–5 and discussion under Drug Metabolism, above).

In a survey of 12,577 hospitalized medical patients (Greenblatt et al., 1977), 78 (3.1 percent) of the 2,542 patients who received flurazepam suffered adverse reactions, primarily unwanted CNS depression. The frequency of adverse effects increased with the average daily dose, ranging from 1.3 percent among those receiving less than 15 mg flurazepam per day to 12.3 percent for those receiving doses of 30 mg or more per day. Adverse reactions increased with age from 1.9 percent among those under age 60 to 7.1 percent among those age 80 or over. Only 2 percent of those 70 or older experienced adverse reactions at doses less than 15 mg per day, but 39 percent of these patients had reactions at 30 mg or more per day.

Sensitivity of the CNS to depressant effects of flurazepam may be greater in the elderly than in young patients (Greenblatt et al., 1977), but other factors may also be involved. An active metabolite of flurazepam has a $t_{1/2}$ of 50 to 100 hours, and with chronic dosing the impact of this metabolite might not be known for 10–21 days (Martilla et al., 1977). Martilla and his group surveyed the use of flurazepam in 750 nursing home patients and found that 195 of these patients had received the drug one or more times in the past year and that 26 percent of those who took the drug had experienced reported adverse reactions.

MacDonald and MacDonald (1977) surveyed 390 patients over 65 years of age who were admitted to a Nottingham hospital with femoral fractures. They found that of the 98 patients who suffered nocturnal fractures, 93 percent were taking barbiturate hypnotics; only 6 percent of those with morning fractures and none of those with afternoon fractures were taking barbiturate hypnotics. Additionally, whereas 45 percent of the 103 patients taking barbiturates had a history of frequent falls (over four per week), only 22 percent of those (287) not taking barbiturates had had frequent falls. The association between barbiturate use and frequent falls was significant ($p < 0.001$).

Raskind and colleagues (1978) reviewed case histories of four patients (aged 67–84) with dysfunction of the CNS secondary to bromide intoxication. Known sources of the bromides were Miles Nervine® (which no longer contains bromide) and Carbrital®. After treatment for bromism, three of the patients were able to function at home; the fourth, discharged with markedly improved mental status, was lost to follow-up. The serum bromide levels in these four patients were initially 22–65 mg/dl, considerably lower than threshold levels of 80 mg/dl considered necessary for the development of bromide intoxication (Raskind et al., 1978). Three of these patients had been referred because of symptoms of senility and the fourth was disoriented and confused, illustrating the tendency of elderly patients to manifest CNS toxicity at levels below the usual textbook standard, which is probably accurate for young patients. Bromide has a long $t_{1/2}$ (12 days), which is even longer in patients with the decreased renal function accompanying normal aging.

Aging may increase response to strong analgesics. In a large double-blind study, Bellville and co-workers (1971) evaluated standard doses of morphine (10 mg) and pentazocine (20 mg) for relief of acute postoperative pain. Results showed that with increasing age there was a progressive increase in analgesic effectiveness of the drugs as measured by relief of pain intensity. Vestal (1978) suggested that increased responsiveness to these drugs was most likely due to decreased pain perception in older patients. Berkowitz and co-workers (1975) studied the disposition of morphine following IV injection in anesthetized surgical patients ranging in age from 23 to 75 years. Morphine serum levels two minutes following administration were correlated positively with age, but this effect was only transient since serum levels ten minutes after administration and $t_{1/2}$ were independent of age. These results suggest that increased analgesic effectiveness of morphine in older people is not due to age-related differences in pharmacokinetics. Chan and colleagues (1975), however, found with meperidine considerably higher plasma levels following intramuscular administration of the drug to ten patients older than 70 years than following the same seven milligram per kilogram of body weight dose to patients younger than 30 years. Available evidence suggests that meperidine is probably less protein bound in the elderly (see discussion under Plasma Protein Binding, above). Pharmacokinetic age-related differences may therefore account for the observation of Mather and co-workers (1975) that clinically, reduction of meperidine dosage is necessary for the elderly because these patients are more sentivite to the respiratory depressant effects of the drug.

In reviewing drugs used in anesthesiology, Dundee (1979) stated that although most examples of sensitivity to anesthetic drugs in the elderly could be explained by alterations in pharmacokinetics, nevertheless there are important changes in organ responsiveness to drugs as the individual ages. One example cited was the profound hypotension that may follow the use of thiopental in the elderly, due in part to increased sensitivity of the myocardium to depressants and to decreased ability to compensate for peripheral vasodilation. Dundee reported that sensitivity to this hypotensive effect is also seen with some opiates, with meperidine, and occasionally with the histamine-releasing tubocurarine. He noted that phenothiazines, droperidol, and other drugs producing vasodilatation may produce marked hypotension in elderly individuals.

Cumming (1980) reviewed age-dependent changes in four organ systems of particular interest in the administration of anesthetics to elderly people—CNS, respiratory system, cardiovascular system, and renal system. He suggested that loss of brain cells and reduction in neuron reserve with aging may partly explain the elderly person's reduced tolerance to alcohol and other CNS depressants including anesthetics. He noted that reduction in respiratory functional ability in the elderly may not cause a problem during anesthesia but post-anesthetic pneumonia is more frequent in elderly than in young patients; and administration of anesthetics is likely to cause greater reduction in blood pressure and organ perfusion in the elderly than in the young. Cumming also discussed anesthesia in relationship to chronic therapy with drugs frequently use by older adults.

A number of reports have indicated that tricyclic antidepressants (TCAs) should be given cautiously to elderly persons because these drugs are apt to produce adverse cardiovascular effects (Hollister, 1978; Rodstein and Oei, 1979; Salzman et al., 1975). Rodstein and Oei (1979) followed the long-term therapy of 31 geriatric patients (70–91 years of age) receiving TCAs. Two of the ten who took amitriptyline developed minor cardiac side effects. Of the 21 patients given imipramine, four developed cardiac side effects. The authors stated that the group studied was composed of elderly individuals who had a high prevalence of heart disease and who were taking other drugs that might induce cardiac side effects. It was therefore difficult to determine whether or not the TCAs were responsible for toxic effects; however, after a review of "before-and-after clinical and ECG findings" (p.233), it was concluded that the TCAs were largely responsible for the adverse effects.

The elderly are particularly sensitive to the delirium-producing effects of centrally acting anticholinergic drugs, including TCAs, antipsychotics, and the anticholinergics used in Parkinson's disease (Hollister, 1978).

Tepper and Haas (1979), in critically evaluating 44 epidemiologic studies on tardive dyskinesia, verified previous observations that a consistently higher prevalence of this adverse reaction to neuroleptics occurs in the elderly and in women. These authors also reported that studies which included many elderly patients tended to report high rates of spontaneous dyskinesias and that it is therefore possible that the greater risk of neuroleptic-induced tardive dyskinesia in the elderly could partially reflect an increased rate of the spontaneous disorder.

Equivalent blood levels of ethanol in young and elderly subjects caused greater decrease in reaction time, memory, and auditory attention in the older persons (Robertson-Tchabo et al., 1975). This is of particular importance since a comparable dosage of ethanol produces higher peak blood levels in the elderly (Vestal et al., 1977), increasing the likelihood of clinical alcohol toxicity with aging.

Grad and colleagues (1974) studied the effects of long-term levodopa on the blood pressures and pulse rates of 51 patients with Parkinson's disease. The dosage of levodopa was adjusted to produce a "clinically significant therapeutic effect" (p.492) with minimum side effects; each patient was followed for 36 to 1,092 days. Five patients developed hypotension and syncope, and their treatment with the drug was discontinued. For data analysis the 46 remaining patients were divided into two age groups—70 or younger, and older than 70 years. It was observed that younger patients tolerated a higher dose than the older patients. The influence of lower body weight in the older group was removed by analysis of covariance and the older group still received lower doses of levodopa with "a probability close to the 5 percent level" (p.493). It was also noteworthy that the lower tolerance for levodopa in the older group was more apparent in women than in men. During the fourth interval of the study (therapy continued for more than 180 days), younger women tolerated levodopa dosage 55 percent higher than older women, while in men the comparable difference was only 14 percent.

Wener and co-workers (1976) reported on the cardiovascular effects of prolonged administration of 2.5–3.0 g of levodopa per day to 23 patients under 70 and 31 patients over 70. They concluded that the administrations of levodopa to elderly persons, even those with heart disease, is relatively safe, with the exception of those patients over 70 who have previous histories of myocardial infarction. In this group they found a higher incidence of hypotension with levodopa therapy and recommended caution with use of this drug.

## Aging and Responsiveness to Warfarin

In a retrospective study of 177 patients aged 30–83 years, O'Malley and co-workers (1977) plotted the mean daily warfarin dosage and the anticoagulant control achieved (Thrombotest %) against patient age. Although warfarin dosages decreased progressively after the fifth decade, there was a progressive increase in anticoagulant effect after that age, indicating markedly increased sensitivity to warfarin in the elderly.

In a prospective study Shepherd and colleagues (1977) determined the anticoagulant response of four young (mean age 31 years) and four elderly (mean age 76 years) patients to a loading dose of racemic warfarin. Although the elderly received smaller doses than than younger patients, the anticoagulant response of the older patients was greater. These investigators also compared the sensitivity of clotting factor synthesis to effects of warfarin in six young and six elderly patients. By plotting the rate of synthesis of clotting factors against the logarithm of the patients' warfarin plasma concentrations, they found that at the same plasma warfarin levels there was greater inhibition of vitamin K-dependent clotting factors in the elderly than in the young patients.

Further details on apparently the same study (Shepherd et al., 1979) showed that at comparable warfarin levels, the synthesis rate of the clotting factors was depressed about twice as much in the six elderly (mean age 76 years) as in the six young (mean age 31 years) patients. However, this later report includes data showing that this age difference in synthesis rate of clotting factors also occurred in absence of warfarin. The authors suggested the differences in synthesis rate could be due to differences in vitamin K metabolism or effect rather than to differences in warfarin pharmacokinetics or effect. When these investigators compared the kinetics of vitamin $K_1$ in small groups of young and elderly subjects, clearance of the vitamin, in the absence of warfarin, appeared to be more rapid in the elderly. If the subjects were anticoagulated with warfarin and then given vitamin $K_1$, there was greater accumulation of vitamin $K_1$ oxide in the elderly than in the young. [Vitamin $K_1$ oxide is a metabolite of the vitamin; reduction of the metabolite to regenerate vitamin $K_1$ is blocked by warfarin (Shepherd et al., 1979)]. The investigators suggested that aging may decrease receptor sensitivity to vitamin K, concluding that "the observed increase in sensitivity to warfarin in the elderly is complex and perhaps is multifactorial in origin" (p.208).

### Aging and Responsiveness to Certain Autonomic Neuroeffectors

Vestal (1978) reviewed several studies published between 1971 and 1977 which indicate that aging affects the pharmacology of the autonomic nervous system. He noted that there is evidence that the number of β-adrenergic receptors in membrane fractions decreases with aging but that the affinity of the receptors apparently is not age-related; that resistance to the chronotropic effect of isoproterenol increases with age; and that propranolol affects exercise-induced increase in heart rate and cardiac output to a lesser extent in older than in younger subjects.

Vestal and colleagues (1979b) studied the effect of age on sensitivity to both isoproterenol and propranolol in 27 subjects 21–73 years of age, some of whom were smokers. The dose of isoproterenol required to increase resting heart rate by 25 beats per minute increased with age, showing progressive increase in isoproterenol resistance as age increased, irrespective of smoking habits. Then during propranolol infusions, a second dose-response curve to isoproterenol was determined. Propranolol resistance values were calculated, showing that resistance to propranolol also increased with age. The investigators concluded that the chronotropic effects of single intravenous doses of isoproterenol decreases with aging in adults, and that the effects of a given free drug concentration of propranolol decrease progressively with age. They stated that their results were consistent with a decreased responsiveness of β-adrenoreceptors to both agonist and antagonist drugs with aging. The study of Bertel and colleagues (1980) confirmed a decrease in isoproterenol sensitivity with aging in normal subjects and showed that the decrease was more pronounced in patients with essential hypertension.

Although sensitivity to propranolol decreases with aging, Vestal (1978) notes that the incidence of propranolol toxicity has been shown to be higher in patients 60 years of age or older than in younger patients, and that this higher toxicity rate is probably related to more extensive cardiovascular disease, decreased renal function, and use of multiple cardiovascular drugs in older patients.

Freed and co-workers (1978) reported on four patients aged 72–87 years for whom dopamine was used as an adjunct in treating shock associated with abdominal catastrophe. All four patients responded, but when attempts were made to discontinue the dopamine, a serious degree of hypotension resulted. The authors reported that although the vasoactivity of dopamine is dose-dependent (in low doses causing vasodilation and in higher doses causing vasoconstriction), in the elderly the drug appears to produce some vasoconstriction in any dosage. It was recommended that in order to prevent a hypotensive response upon withdrawal of the drug in elderly patients, additional volume loading and tapered withdrawal of dopamine were necessary.

Not all studies have shown age-related differences in response to autonomic agents. Chmielewski and co-workers (1978) compared recovery from neuromuscular blockade in a group of 13 elderly (mean age 80 years) and a group of 13 young (mean age 21 years) patients receiving tubocurarine for muscle relaxation in elective surgery. Following reversal with neostigmine, the time taken to recover from neuromuscular blockade was measured. Results showed similar reversal patterns in young and elderly patients and the investigators concluded that when reversal of a neuromuscular drug was inadequate in an elderly patient, an explanation other than increased sensitivity due to age should be sought.

## CONCLUSIONS

In this chapter we have cited considerable recent research concerning the effects of age on pharmacokinetics of specific drugs. This research has increased in quantity and often in sophistication over the past five or six years. Recent research on aging and responsiveness to drug action has also yielded data of much importance to ways drugs should be prescribed. Fortunately, interest in the complex relationships of aging and drug therapy is still rapidly accelerating. Fortunately, also, this interest is shared by increasing numbers of investigators and enlightened clinicians.

## REFERENCES

Anderson, G. D. Benzodiazepines. *The Nurse Practitioner,* 1980, *5,* 47, 50–51, 60.

Bellville, J. W., Forrest, W. H., Miller, E., and Brown, B. W. Influence of age on pain relief from analgesics. *Journal of the American Medical Association,* 1971, *217,* 1835–1841.

Bender, A. D. Drug sensitivity in the elderly. In J. Crooks and I. H. Stevenson (Eds.), *Drugs and the Elderly.* Baltimore: University Park Press, 1979.

Bender, A. D., Post, A., Meier, J. P., Higson, J. E., and Reichard, G. Plasma protein binding of drugs as a function of age in adult human subjects. *Journal of Pharmaceutical Sciences,* 1975, *64,* 1711–1713.

Berkowitz, B. A., Ngai, S. H., Yang, J. C., Hempstead, J. and Spector, S. The disposition of morphine in surgical patients. *Clinical Pharmacology and Therapeutics,* 1975, *17,* 629–635.

Bertel, O., Bühler, F. R., Kiowski, W., and Lütold, B. E. Decreased beta-adrenoreceptor responsiveness as related to age, blood pressure and plasma catecholamines in patients with essential hypertension. *Hypertension,* 1980, *2,* 130–138.

Bhanthumnavin, K., and Schuster, M. M. Aging and gastrointestinal function. In C. E. Finch and L. Hayflick (Eds.), *Handbook of the Biology of Aging.* New York: Van Nostrand Reinhold, 1977.

Boston Collaborative Drug Surveillance Program, Boston University Medical Center. Clinical depression of the central nervous system due to diazepam and chlordiazepoxide in relation to cigarette smoking and age. *New England Journal of Medicine,* 1973, *288,* 277–280.

Braithwaite, R., Montgomery, S., and Dawling, S. Age, depression and tricyclic antidepressant levels. In J. Crooks and I. H. Stevenson (Eds.), *Drugs and the Elderly.* Baltimore: University Park Press, 1979.

Butler, R. N. Pharmacological interventions of the aging process. *Advances in Experimental Medicine and Biology,* 1978, *97,* 231–241.

Calloway, N. O., and Dollevoet, P. L. Selected tabular material on aging. In C. E. Finch and L. Hayflick (Eds.), *Handbook of the Biology of Aging.* New York: Van Nostrand Reinhold, 1977.

Castleden, C. M., and George, C. F. The effect of ageing on the hepatic clearance of propranolol. *British Journal of Clinical Pharmacology,* 1979a, *7,* 49–54.

Castleden, C. M., and George, C. F. Increased sensitivity to benzodiazepines in the elderly. In J. Crooks and I. H. Stevenson (Eds.), *Drugs and the Elderly.* Baltimore: University Park Press, 1979b.

Castleden, C. M., Kaye, C. M., and Parsons, R. L. The effect of age on plasma levels of propranolol and practolol in man. *British Journal of Clinical Pharmacology,* 1975, *2,* 303–306.

Castleden, C. M., George, C. F., Marcer, D., and Hallett, C. Increased sensitivity to nitrazepam in old age. *British Medical Journal,* January 1, 1977a, *1,* 10–12.

Castleden, C. M., Volans, C. N., and Raymond, K. The effect of ageing on drug absorption from the gut. *Age and Ageing,* 1977b, *6,* 138–143.

Castleden, C. M., Houston, A., and George, C. F. Are hypnotics helpful or harmful to elderly patients? *Journal of Drug Issues,* 1979, *9*(1), 55–61.

Chan, K., Kendall, M. J., Mitchard, M., Wells, W. D. E., and Vickers, M. D.

The effect of ageing on plasma pethidine concentration. *British Journal of Clinical Pharmacology*, 1975, *2*, 297–302.

Chmielewski, A. T., Pybus, D. A., Loach, A. B., and Goat, V. A. Recovery from neuromuscular blockade: a comparison between old and young patients. *Anaesthesia*, 1978, *33*, 539–542.

Crooks, J., O'Malley, K., and Stevenson, I. H. Pharmacokinetics in the elderly. *Clinical Pharmacokinetics*, 1976, *1*, 280–296.

Cumming, J. F. Choice of an anesthetic for the elderly. *Hospital Formulary*, 1980, *15*(1), 52–54.

Cuny, G., Royer, R. J., Mur, J. M., Serot, J. M., Faure, G., Netter, P., Maillard, A., and Penin, F. Pharmacokinetics of salicylates in elderly. *Gerontology*, 1979, *25*, 49–55.

Cusack, B., Kelly, J., O'Malley, K., Noel, J., Lavan, J., and Horgan, J. Digoxin in the elderly: pharmacokinetic consequences of old age. *Clinical Pharmacology and Therapeutics*, 1979, *25*, 772–776.

Drayer, D. E., Hughes, M., Lorenzo, B., and Reidenberg, M. M. Prevalence of high (3S)-3-hydroxyquinidine/quinidine ratios in serum, and clearance of quindine in cardiac patients with age. *Clinical Pharmacology and Therapeutics*, 1980, *27*, 72–75.

Dundee, J. W. Response to anaesthetic drugs in the elderly. In J. Crooks and I. H. Stevenson (Eds.), *Drugs and the Elderly*. Baltimore: University Park Press, 1979.

Ewy, G. A., Kapadia, G. G., Yao, L., Lullin, M., and Marcus, F. I. Digoxin metabolism in the elderly. *Circulation*, 1969, *34*, 449–453.

Farah, F., Taylor, W., Rawlins, M. D., and James, O. Hepatic drug acetylation and oxidation: effects of aging in man. *British Medical Journal*, July 16, 1977, *2*, 155–156.

Feely, J., and Stevenson, I. H. The effect of age and hyperthyroidism on plasma propranolol steady-state concentration. *British Journal of Clinical Pharmacology*, 1978, 446P (Abstract).

Freed, J. S., Kaynan, A., and Szuchmacher, P. H. Dopamine and the aged. *Journal of the American Geriatrics Society*, 1978, *26*, 524–525.

Fulton, B., James, O., and Rawlins, M. D. The influence of age on the pharmacokinetics of paracetamol. *British Journal of Clinical Pharmacology*, 1979, *7*, 418P.

Gibaldi, M. *Biopharmaceutics and Clinical Pharmacokinetics*. Philadelphia: Lea and Febiger, 1977.

Gibaldi, M., and Perrier, D. *Pharmacokinetics*. New York: Marcel Dekker, 1975.

Gillette, J. R. Biotransformation of drugs during aging. *Federation Proceedings*, 1979, *38*, 1900–1909.

Gillette, J. R., and Hinson, J. A. Biotransformation of drugs. *Advances in Experimental Medicine and Biology*, 1978, *97*, 5–25.

Goldman, R. Decline in organ function with aging. In I. Rossman (Ed.), *Clinical Geriatrics*, 2nd ed. Philadelphia: J. B. Lippincott, 1979.

Grad, B., Wener, J., Rosenberg, G., and Wener, S. W. Effects of levodopa therapy in patients with Parkinson's disease: statistical evidence for reduced tolerance to levodopa in the elderly. *Journal of the American Geriatrics Society*, 1974, *22*, 489–494.

Greenblatt, D. J., Allen, M. D., and Shader, R. I. Toxicity of high-dose flurazepam in the elderly. *Clinical Pharmacology and Therapeutics*, 1977, *21*, 355–361.

Greenblatt, D. J., Allen, M. D., Locniskar, A., Harmatz, J. S., and Shader, R. I. Lorazepam kinetics in the elderly. *Clincial Pharmacology and Therapeutics,* 1979, *26,* 103–113.

Gugler, R., and Somogyi, A. Reduced cimetidine clearance with age. *New England Journal of Medicine,* 1979, *301,* 435.

Hayes, M. J., Langman, M. J. S., and Short, A. H. Changes in drug metabolism with increasing age: 1. Warfarin binding and plasma proteins. *British Journal of Clinical Pharmacology,* 1975a, *2,* 69–72.

Hayes, M. J., Langman, M. J. S., and Short, A. H. Changes in drug metabolism with increasing age: 2. Phenytoin clearance and protein binding. *British Journal of Clinical Pharmacology,* 1975b, *2,* 73–79.

Hewick, D. S., and Newbury, P. A. Age: its influence on lithium dosage and plasma levels. *British Journal of Clinical Pharmacology,* 1976, *3,* 345P.

Hewick, D. S., Newbury, P., Hopwood, S., Naylor, G., and Moody, J. Age as a factor affecting lithium therapy. *British Journal of Clinical Pharmacology,* 1977, *4,* 201–205.

Hollister, L. E. Treatment of depression with drugs. *Annals of Internal Medicine,* 1978, *89,* 78–84.

Houghton, G. W., Richens, A., and Leighton, M. Effect of age, height, weight, and sex on serum phenytoin concentration in epileptic patients. *British Journal of Clinical Pharmacology,* 1975, *2,* 251–256.

Irvine, R. E., Grove, J., Toseland, P. A., and Trounce, J. R. The effect of age on the hydroxylation of amylobarbitone sodium in man. *British Journal of Clinical Pharmacology,* 1974, *1,* 41–43.

Jusko, W. J., Schentag, J. J., and Koup, J. R. Pharmacokinetics of theophylline therapy. *American Journal of Hospital Pharmacy,* 1977, *34,* 332.

Kampmann, J. P., and Hansen, J. E. M. Renal excretion of drugs. In J. Crooks, and I. H. Stevenson (Eds.), *Drugs and the Elderly.* Baltimore: University Park Press, 1979.

Kampmann, J., Hansen, J. M., Siersbaek-Nielsen, K., and Laursen, H. Effect of some drugs on penicillin half-life in blood. *Clinical Pharmacology and Therapeutics,* 1972, *13,* 516–519.

Kampmann, J., Siersbaek-Nielsen, K., Kristensen, M., and Hansen, J. M. Rapid evaluation of creatinine clearance. *Acta Medica Scandinavica,* 1974, *196,* 517–520.

Kampmann, J. P., Mortensen, H. B., Bach, B., Waldorff, S., Kristensen, M. B., and Hansen, J. M. Kinetics of propylthiouracil in the elderly. *Acta Medica Scandinavica,* 1979, Supplement 624, 93–98.

Kangas, L., Iisalo, E., Kanto, J., Lehtinen, V., Pynnönen, S., Ruikka, I., Salminen, J., Sillanpää, M., and Syvälahti, E. Human pharmacokinetics of nitrazepam: effect of age and diseases. *European Journal of Clinical Pharmacology,* 1979, *15,* 163–170.

Klotz, U., and Müller-Seydlitz, P. Altered elimination of desmethyldiazepam in the elderly. *British Journal of Clinical Pharmacology,* 1979, *7,* 119–120.

Klotz, U., Avant, G. R., Hoyumpa, A., Schenker, S., and Wilkinson, G. R. The effects of age and liver disease on the disposition and elimination of diazepam in adult man. *The Journal of Clinical Investigation,* 1975, *55,* 347–359.

Koup, J. R., Schentag, J. J., Vance, J. W., Kuritzky, P. M., Pyszczynski, D. R., and Jusko, W. J. System for clinical pharmacokinetic monitoring of theophylline therapy. *American Journal of Hospital Pharmacy,* 1976, *33,* 949–956.

Kraus, J. W., Desmond, P. V., Marshall, J. P., Johnson, R. F., Schenker, S., and Wilkinson, G. R. Effects on aging and liver disease on disposition of lorazepam. *Clinical Pharmacology and Therapeutics*, 1978, *24*, 411–419.

Leake, C. D. Outlook for improved drug therapy in geriatrics. *Texas Reports in Biology and Medicine*, 1949, *7*, 336–349.

Lumholtz, B., Kampmann, J., Siersbaek-Nielsen, K., and Hansen, J. M. Dose regimen of kanamycin and gentamicin. *Acta Medica Scandinavica*, 1974, *196*, 521–524.

MacDonald, J. B., and MacDonald, E. T. Nocturnal femoral fracture and continuing widespread use of barbiturate hypnotics. *British Medical Journal*, 1977, *2*, 483–485.

Macleod, S. M., Giles, H. G., Bengert, B., Liu, F. F., and Sellers, E. M. Age and gender-related differences in diazepam pharmacokinetics. *Journal of Clinical Pharmacology*, 1979, *19*, 15–19.

Marttila, J. K., Hammel, R. J., Alexander, B., and Zustiak, R. Potential untoward effects of long-term use of flurazepam in geriatric patients. *Journal of the American Pharmaceutical Association*, 1977, *NS17*, 692–695.

Mather, L. E., Tucker, G. T., Pflug, A. E., Lindop, M. J., and Wilkerson, C. Meperidine kinetics in man. *Clinical Pharmacology and Therapeutics*, 1975, *17*, 21–30.

Majerus, T. C., and Feroli, E. R. Pharmacokinetics of theophylline therapy. *American Journal of Hospital Pharmacy*, 1977, *34*, 332.

McLeod, K., Hull, C. J., and Watson, M. J. Effects of ageing on the pharmacokinetics of pancuronium. *British Journal of Anaesthesia*, 1979, *51*, 435–438.

Melander, A., Bodin, N.-O., Danielson, K., Gustafsson, B., Haglund, G., and Westerlund, D. Absorption and elimination of *d*-propoxyphene acetylsalicylic acid, and phenazone in a combination tablet (Doloron®): comparison between young and elderly subjects. *Acta Medica Scandinavica*, 1978, *203*, 121–124.

Miller, A. K., Adir, J., and Vestal, R. E. Effect of age on the pharmacokinetics of tolbutamide in man. *The Pharmacologist*, 1977, *19*, 128 (Abstract).

Mitchard, M. Drug distribution in the elderly. In J. Crooks and I. H. Stevenson (Eds.), *Drugs and the Elderly*. Baltimore: University Park Press, 1979.

Nation, R. L., Vine, J., Triggs, E. J., and Learoyd, B. Plasma levels of unchanged drug and two metabolites after oral administration of chlormethiazole to young and aged human subjects. *European Journal of Clinical Pharmacology*, 1977a, *12*, 137–145.

Nation, R. L., Triggs, E. J., and Selig, M. Lignocaine kinetics in cardiac patients and aged subjects. *British Journal of Clinical Pharmacology*, 1977b, *4*, 439–448.

Nielsen-Kudsk, F., Magnussen, I., and Jakobsen, P. Pharmacokinetics of theophylline in ten elderly patients. *Acta Pharmacologica et Toxicologica*, 1978, *42*, 226–234.

Nies, A., Robinson, D. W., Friedman, M. J., Green, R., Cooper, T. B., Ravaris, C. L., and Ives, J. O. Relationship between age and tricyclic antidepressant plasma levels. *American Journal of Psychiatry*, 1977, *134*, 790–793.

Norman, T. R., Burrows, G. D., Maguire, K. P., Rubinstein, G., Scoggins, B. A., and Davies, B. Cigarette smoking and plasma nortriptyline levels. *Clinical Pharmacology and Therapeutics*, 1977, *21*, 453–456.

Norman, T. R., Burrows, G. D., Scoggins, B. A., and Davies, B. Pharmacokinetics and plasma levels of antidepressants in the elderly. *The Medical Journal of Australia*, 1979, *1*, 273–274.

Ochs, H. R., Greenblatt, D. J., Woo, E., and Smith, T. W. Reduced quinidine clearance in elderly persons. *The American Journal of Cardiology,* 1978, *42,* 481–485.

O'Malley, K., Crooks, J., Duke, E., and Stevenson, I. H. Effect of age and sex on human drug metabolism. *British Medical Journal,* 1971, *3,* 607–609.

O'Malley, K., Stevenson, I. H., Ward, C. A., Wood, A. J. J., and Crooks, J. Determinants of anticoagulant control in patients receiving warfarin. *British Journal of Clinical Pharmacology,* 1977, *4,* 309–314.

O'Malley, K., Judge, T. G., and Crooks, J. Geriatric clinical pharmacology and therapeutics. In G. S Avery (Ed.), *Drug Treatment,* 2nd ed. New York: Adis Press, 1980.

Piafsky, K. M., Sitar, D. S., Rangno, R. E., and Ogilvie, R. I. Theophylline kinetics in acute pulmonary edema. *Clinical Pharmacology and Therapeutics,* 1977, *21,* 310–316.

Raskind, M. A., Kitchell, M., and Alavarez, C. Bromide intoxication in the elderly. *Journal of the American Geriatrics Society,* 1978, *26,* 222–224.

Reynolds, C. N., Wilson, K., and Burnett, D. Metabolism of methaqualone in geriatric patients. *European Journal of Clinical Pharmacology,* 1978, *13,* 285–289.

Ritschel, W. A. Age-dependent disposition of amobarbital: analog computer evaluation. *Journal of the American Geriatrics Society,* 1978, *26,* 540–543.

Roberts, R. K., Wilkinson, G. R., Branch, R. A., and Schenker, S. Effect of age and parenchymal liver disease on the disposition and elimination of chlordiazepoxide (librium). *Gastroenterology,* 1978, *75,* 479–485.

Robertson-Tchabo, E. A., Arenberg, D., and Vestal, R. E. Age differences in memory performance following ethanol infusion (Abst. 455). *Proceedings of the 10th International Congress of Gerontology,* Jerusalem, Israel, 1975, *2,* 62.

Rodstein, M., and Oei, L. S. Cardiovascular side effects of long-term therapy with tricyclic antidepressants in the aged. *Journal of the American Geriatrics Society,* 1979, *27,* 231–234.

Rossman, I. Anatomic and body composition changes with aging. In C. E. Finch and L. Hayflick (Eds.), *Handbook of the Biology of Aging.* New York: Van Nostrand Reinhold, 1977.

Rowe, J. W., Andres, R., Tobin, J. D., Norris, A. H., and Shock, N. W. The effect of age on creatinine clearance in man: a cross-sectional and longitudinal study. *Journal of Gerontology,* 1976, *31,* 155–163.

Salzman, C., van der Kolk, B., and Shader, R. I. Psychopharmacology and the geriatric patient. In R. I. Shader (Ed.), *Manual of Psychiatric Therapeutics.* Boston: Little, Brown, 1975.

Shader, R. I., and Greenblatt, D. J. Pharmacokinetics and clinical drug effects in the elderly. *Psychopharmacology Bulletin,* 1979, *15*(2), 8–14.

Shader, R. I., Greenblatt, D. J., Harmatz, J. S., Franke, K., and Koch-Weser, J. Absorption and disposition of chlordiazepoxide in young and elderly male volunteers. *Journal of Clinical Pharmacology,* 1977, *17,* 709–718.

Shepherd, A. M. M., Hewick, D. S., Moreland, T. A., and Stevenson, I. H. Age as a determinant of sensitivity to warfarin. *British Journal of Clinical Pharmacology,* 1977, *4,* 315–320.

Shepherd, A. M. M., Wilson, N., and Stevenson, I. H. Warfarin sensitivity and the elderly. In J. Crooks, and I. H. Stevenson (Eds.), *Drugs and the Elderly.* Baltimore: University Park Press, 1979.

Shull, H. J., Wilkinson, G. R., Johnson, R., and Schenker, S. Normal disposition of oxazepam in acute viral hepatitis and cirrhosis. *Annals of Internal Medicine*, 1976, *84*, 420–425.

Siersbaek-Nielsen, K., Hansen, J. M., Kampmann, J., and Kristensen, M. Rapid evaluation of creatinine clearance. *The Lancet*, May 29, 1971, 1133–1134.

Simon, C., Malerezyk, V., Müller, U., and Müller, G. Zur pharmakokinetik von propicillin bei geriatrischen patienten im vergleich zu jüngeren erwachsenen. *Deutsche Medizinische Wochenschrift*, 1972, *97*, 1999–2003.

Smith, C. R. Use of drugs in the aged. *The John Hopkins Medical Journal*, 1979, *145*(2), 61–64.

Somogyi, A., Rohner, H.-G., and Gugler, R. Pharmacokinetics and bioavailability of cimetidine in gastric and duodenal ulcer patients. *Clinical Pharmacokinetics*, 1980, *5*, 84–94.

Stevenson, I. H. Factors influencing antipyrine elimination. *British Journal of Clinical Pharmacology*, 1977, *4*, 261–265.

Stevenson, I. H., Salem, S. A. M., and Shepherd, A. M. M. Studies on drug absorption and metabolism in the elderly. In J. Crooks and I. H. Stevenson (Eds.), *Drugs and the Elderly*. Baltimore: University Park Press, 1979.

Swift, C. G. Clinical pharmacology in the elderly. *Scottish Medical Journal*, 1979, *24*, 221–225.

Tepper, S. J., and Haas, J. F. Prevalence of tardive dyskinesia. *Journal of Clinical Psychiatry*, 1979, *40*, 508–516.

Triggs, E. J. Pharmacokinetics of lignocaine and chlormethiazole in the elderly; with some preliminary observations on other drugs. In J. Crooks and I. H. Stevenson (Eds.), *Drugs and the Elderly*. Baltimore: University Park Press, 1979.

Triggs, E. J., and Nation, R. L. Pharmacokinetics in the aged: a review. *Journal of Pharmacokinetics and Biopharmaceutics*, 1975, *3*, 387–418.

Triggs, E. J., Nation, R. L., Long, A., and Ashley, J. J. Pharmacokinetics in the elderly. *European Journal of Clinical Pharmacology*, 1975, *8*, 55–62.

Vestal, R. E., Drug use in the elderly: a review of problems and special considerations. *Drugs*, 1978, *16*, 358–382.

Vestal, R. E., Norris, A. H., Tobin, J. D., Cohen, B. H., Shock, N. W., and Andres, R. Antipyrine metabolism in man: influence of age, alcohol, caffeine and smoking. *Clinical Pharmacology and Therapeutics*, 1975, *18*, 425–432.

Vestal, R. E., McGuire, E. A., Tobin, J. D., Andres, R., Norris, A. H., and Mezey, E. Aging and ethanol metabolism. *Clinical Pharmacology and Therapeutics*, 1977, *21*, 343–354.

Vestal, R. E., Wood, A. J. J., Branch, R. A., Shand, D. G., and Wilkinson, G. R. Effects of age and cigarette smoking on propranolol disposition. *Clinical Pharmacology and Therapeutics*, 1979a, *26*, 8–15.

Vestal, R. E., Wood, A. J. J., and Shand, D. G. Reduced β-adrenoceptor sensitivity in the elderly. *Clinical Pharmacology and Therapeutics*, 1979b, *26*, 181–186.

Wallace, S., Whiting, B., and Runcie, J. Factors affecting drug binding in plasma of elderly patients. *British Journal of Clinical Pharmacology*, 1976, *3*, 327–330.

Wener, J., Rosenberg, G., Grad, B., and Wener, S. Cardiovascular effects of levodopa in aged versus younger patients with Parkinson's disease. *Journal of the American Geriatrics Society*, 1976, *24*, 185–188.

Wilkinson, G. R., and Shand, D. G. A physiological approach to hepatic drug clearance. *Clinical Pharmacology and Therapeutics*, 1975, *18*, 377–390.

Wood, A. J. J., Vestal, R. E., Wilkinson, G. R., Branch, R. A., and Shand, D. G. Effect of aging and cigarette smoking on antipyrine and indocyanine green elimination. *Clinical Pharmacology and Therapeutics*, 1979, *26*, 16–20.

Woosley, R. L., and Shand, D. G. Pharmacokinetics of antiarrhythmic drugs. *The American Journal of Cardiology*, 1978, *41*, 986–995.

## SELECTED READINGS

Beattie, B. L., and Seller, E. M. Psychoactive drug use in the elderly: the pharmacokinetics. *Psychosomatics*, 1979, *20*, 474–479.

Freidel, R. O., and Raskind, M. D. Psychopharmacology of aging. In M. F. Elias, B. E. Eleftherion, and P. K. Elias (Eds.), *Special Review of Experimental Aging Research, Progress in Biology*. Bar Harbor, Maine: EAR, Inc. 1976.

Plein, J. B. Drug dosing for geriatric patients. *The Nurse Practitioner*, 1979, *4*, 30–31, 38, 46.

Raskind, M., and Eisdorfer, C. Psychopharmacology of the aged. In L. L. Simpson (Ed.), *Drug Treatment of Mental Disorders*. New York: Raven Press, 1976.

Richey, D. P., and Bender, A. D. Pharmacokinetic consequences of aging. *Annual Review Pharmacology and Toxicology*, 1977, *17*, 49–65.

Salzman, C. Update on geriatric psychopharmacology. *Geriatrics*, 1979, *34*, 87–90.

Schmucker, D. L. Age-related changes in drug disposition. *Pharmacological Reviews*, 1978, *30*, 445–456.

Schumacher, G. E. Using pharmacokinetics in drug therapy. VII. Pharmacokinetic factors influencing drug therapy in the aged. *American Journal of Hospital Pharmacy*, 1980, *37*, 559–562.

Steinberg, S.K. A rational approach to the use of drugs in the elderly. *Canadian Pharmaceutical Journal*, 1978, *111* (March), 10–16.

Wallace, D. E., and Watanabe, A. S. Drug effects in geratric patients. *Drug Intelligence and Clinical Pharmacy*, 1977, *11*, 597–603.

Witts, D. J., Bowhay, A. A., Garland, M., McLean, A. E. M., and Exton-Smith, A. N. Studies of chlormethiazole in the elderly: pharmacokinetic aspects. *Age and Ageing*, 1979, *8*, 271–284.

CHAPTER 9

# Alcoholism and Over-the-Counter and Prescription Drug Misuse in the Elderly

JOSEPH H. ATKINSON, JR., M.D. MARC A. SCHUCKIT, M.D.

DEPARTMENT OF PSYCHIATRY
UNIVERSITY OF CALIFORNIA, SAN DIEGO
SCHOOL OF MEDICINE
LA JOLLA, CALIFORNIA

## INTRODUCTION AND OVERVIEW

This chapter summarizes the prominent characteristics of alcoholism and over-the-counter and prescription drug misuse in the elderly. We will cover the pharmacologic effects of alcohol in the elderly, define alcoholism, explore the problems in its diagnosis, outline the epidemiology and natural histories of geriatric alcoholism, and recommend treatments for this special group. The epidemiology and the psychologic, medical, and social factors associated with prescription and over-the-counter drug misuse will be presented, and the most commonly misused agents will be identified. We hope by presenting this survey of alcohol and medication misuse to alert health care professionals to an important problem, provide clinically useful information, and clarify areas needing further research.

### The Elderly Are an Increasingly Important Group

In the past, health care professionals have addressed the problems of the elderly as if everyone over 65 years of age were similar. Yet risk factors for illness, disability, cognitive dysfunction, social isolation, poverty, and frailty increase past age 75 (Butler, 1976; Kovar, 1977). We therefore need to distinguish between the "young" old, those aged 60 to approximately 74 years, and the "old" old, those 75 years old and beyond. It is worth observing that the proportion of the elderly 75 and above is now increasing at a rate approximately one-third faster than the overall growth of the population over 65.

Aging is not a purely physical process but a biopsychosocial process. Some individuals may be considered physiologically or psychologically "aged" at 55 or 60. If "aged" as a social definition applies to retired persons, it also includes many 60-year-olds and younger—the "older worker" in Federal and State programs is defined as over 45.

### The Elderly Are Vulnerable to Alcohol and Drugs

Alcohol and drug use, misuse, and effect depend upon many factors including access to the substance; pattern of use; the physical state of the individual at the time of use; use of other interactive substances; and, finally, the pharmacodynamics and the pharmacokinetics of the substance taken. Pharmacodynamics refers to the effects of drugs at their site of action. Pharmacokinetics describe the rate of drug absorption, its differential disposition into particular kinds of tissue (such as fat), the blood levels reached by a given amount of the substance, and the metabolism and route of excretion of the drug.

A major fact, one that affects nonalcoholics as well as alcoholics, is the diminished physical reserve occurring with advancing age (Schuckit, 1978c). For example, the brain's total weight at age 75 is only one-half to three-fourths that of its young adult years (Verwoerdt, 1976). As body systems lose resiliency, vital organs have less reserve, illnesses and injuries take longer to heal, and stressors, such as environmental change, infection, or an electrolyte imbalance caused by vomiting, can cause failure of these organs. This vulnerability includes reactions to alcohol, which can cause temporary failure of the cardiovascular, hepatic, or central nervous systems (CNS) in older people at levels easily tolerated in a 35- or 40-year-old.

The effects of diminished physical reserve are exacerbated by the accompanying changes in the metabolism of medications and toxins (Raskind, 1976). The tissue composition of older people changes from lean muscle mass to a greater proportion of adipose, leading to accumulation and a longer "wash out" period of certain drugs, as well as a protracted effect of others. Furthermore, changes in receptor site or end organ sensitivity may occur with aging. In addition, with increasing age there is probably less liver tissue available and there is some evidence that hepatic mitochondria are less efficient in their metabolic role (Lamy, 1974; Lenhart, 1976; and Vestal, et al., 1977). The result is that, at least theoretically, older individuals might be expected to obtain a higher or more persistent blood alcohol level when given the same amount of alcohol per body weight as a younger person.

There are many psychologic stresses involved in growing old in a youth-oriented culture. Most can be summarized as feelings of loss of stability and self-worth. Unemployment, inadequate income, immobility, absence of daily necessities and recreation, and fewer responsibilities all proclaim that the elderly person is no longer recognized nor valued. While these stresses may have nothing to do with the development of alcoholism per se (a direct cause and effect relationship is difficult to prove since many individuals with these factors do not develop serious alcohol misuse), they are important aspects of a patient's life to be considered when treating any disorder (Schuckit, 1977b; Schuckit and Pastor, 1978).

### Summary

The elderly now represent a significant and complex proportion of medical practice, and population studies indicate that they will become more and more prevalent. The risk factors for illness and disability steadily increase with age, and these risks abound in the "old" old (those past age 75), who are especially vulnerable to biologic insults, psychologic stress, and environmental change. When "normal" stress is imposed upon a vulnerable system, decompensation may ensue. Physical and psychologic treatment of the elderly must consider their diminished physical reserve, cumulative disease history, age-related alterations in drug response, biographical assets, and environmental supports.

## ALCOHOL

### The Dangers of Alcohol in the Non-alcoholic Older Individual

Alcohol-related problems in older people are not limited to those people who could be clinically regarded as alcoholics. Illness and the need for medication increase vulnerability to alcohol. Many elderly take prescription medications which can react adversely with alcohol, yet deliberately or unknowingly continue to drink (Schuckit, 1977b). Similarly, difficulties can arise from the interaction of alcohol and over-the-counter medications. The combination of alcohol and sleeping pills, for example, could decrease intellectual functioning and produce a state of confusion (an organic brain syndrome).

Despite the fact that cardiac disorders are very common in older individuals, few of those who suffer from these problems modify their drinking patterns. This may be dangerous since as little as one cocktail can significantly adversely affect cardiac efficiency in the presence of heart disease (Gould et al., 1971).

Similarly, those suffering from cardiac pain on exertion (angina) run the risk that alcohol can mask pain which might otherwise serve as a valuable warning signal (Horowitz, 1975). Alcohol can also exacerbate the problems of those with hepatic or pancreatic disease, diverticuli, anemia, neurologic disorders, and, in short, problems in almost all body systems in this highly vulnerable population (Schuckit, 1979).

As illustrated in Table 9–1, alcohol has important interactions with many classes of medical and psychotropic drugs, particularly those often prescribed to elderly patients. In acute intoxication or chronic abuse, alcohol augments the dangerous side effects of such common agents as aspirin, oral antidiabetic agents, nitroglycerin, digoxin, and many sedative-hypnotics. Alcohol also decreases the efficacy or produces unusual reactions when combined with anticonvulsants and some antibiotics. It is difficult to imagine another single agent with such widespread effects as alcohol on health and on our therapeutic armamentaria.

In short, as one grows older the number of prescribed and over-the-counter medications imbibed increases (Schuckit, 1977b). Alcohol interacts adversely with many of these drugs, a problem especially significant for other central nervous system depressants, whose actions are potentiated by ethanol (Raskind and Eisdorfer, 1976; Schuckit, 1977b). Through its effect on the liver, alcohol may also increase the rate of metabolism of *some* drugs but interfere with the degradation of others. Alcohol itself affects many organ systems and diseases. It is, thus, apparent that one cannot discuss alcohol problems in the elderly by limiting the notation to older alcoholics alone. Elderly individuals with diabetes, heart disease, liver disease, CNS degeneration, and other medical problems do not tolerate alcohol well. It is also wise to advise older individuals on certain medications to avoid alcohol or drink only with caution. While an adverse drug–alcohol or other interaction might be well tolerated in a 35-year-old, the decrease in reserves in vital organ systems can make such stress potentially life-threatening in the elderly person.

## Alcoholism

Drinking problems in older people receive much less attention than is deserved, a discrepancy partly explained by two factors. First, analysis of general population drinking patterns (Cahalan and Cisin, 1968; Rathbone-McCuan and Bland, 1974; U.S. Department of Health, Education,

Table 9–1
Interactions of Various Drugs and Alcohol

| *Drug* | *Adverse effect with alcohol* |
|---|---|
| Antibiotics | |
| Chloramphenicol | Disulfiram-like reaction |
| Griseofulvin | Disulfiram-like reaction |
| Isoniazid | Chronic abuse produces ↓ effect of isoniazid |
| Antidiabetics | |
| Oral Hypoglycemics | Minor disulfiram-like symptoms (tolbutamide, chlorpropamide)<br>↑ hypoglycemic effect<br>↓ hypoglycemic effect with chronic alcohol abuse with tolbutamide (Orinase®)<br>Lactic acidosis with phenformin (DBI®, Meltrol®) |
| Cardiovascular | |
| Digoxin | ↑ sensitivity to digitalis toxicity |
| Nitroglycerin | ↑ hypotension |
| Oral anticoagulants | ↓ anticoagulation effect with chronic alcohol abuse<br>↑ anticoagulation effect with acute intoxication |
| Sedative-hypnotics | |
| Barbiturate | ↑ CNS depression with acute intoxication<br>↓ overall effect with chronic alcoholism |
| Chloral Hydrate | Enhanced CNS depression |
| Diazepam | Enhanced CNS depression |
| Others | |
| Diphenylhydantoin | Decreased anticonvulsant effects with chronic alcohol abuse |
| Salicylates | ↑ GI bleeding |

and Welfare, 1971) reveals that the percentage of drinkers, especially heavy drinkers, decreases with advancing age, so that only 45 percent of people aged 65 and over are drinkers, as compared to 71 percent of those aged 30–49 years. There is a parallel decrease in the prevalence of alcohol problems after age 65 (Stotsky, 1972).

Second, the natural history of alcoholism causes a steady attrition of the young alcoholic. Many alcoholics die at a young age from cancer, cardiovascular disease, accidents, and suicide (Schmidt and DeLint, 1972; Schuckit and Gunderson, 1974; Sunby, 1967). At the same time, there is a high rate of spontaneous remission for alcoholism. It has been estimated that more than one-third of a group of alcoholics will permanently stop their problem drinking at some time during their career (Ludwig, 1971; McCance and McCance 1969; Schuckit and Cahalan, 1974). Both early death and spontaneous remission insure that a high percentage of alcoholics will not be found in the ranks of the 60–90-year-old problem drinkers.

In addition, most surveys of the prevalence of alcoholism miss or ignore the individual over the age of 60 (Rathbone-McGuan and Bland, 1974). Geriatric patients tend to receive care from several different agencies that communicate poorly with one another; thus, several different people may have picked up hints of alcoholism, but no one put the entire picture together and made a diagnosis (Rathbone-McCuan and Bland, 1974).

Yet a core of information on alcoholism is available. In this section we will begin by reviewing some problems in the definition of the disorder, then examine the epidemiology and clinical course of alcoholism in the elderly.

*Definition and Diagnostic Criteria.* Some of the difficulty in identifying, treating, and developing sound research into the causes and courses of alcoholism lies in the confusion over objective definitions and diagnostic criteria for the disorder. In recent years three major definitional approaches have dominated the field: the addiction approach, the socionormative approach (which includes a "quantity-frequency" definition), and the social-problem approach. Each of these displays distinct weaknesses when applied to elderly populations.

*Definitions of addiction.* The addiction definitions, which include psychological and physical addiction approaches, display limitations in both elderly and general populations. Psychological addiction means a compulsion to drink or a feeling of psychological discomfort when alcohol is not available. Such phenomena are very subjective and difficult to quantify. Nor is it easy to distinguish compulsion from free choice.

The physical-addiction definition is more objective. It employs the presence of definite behavioral-physiological signs (a withdrawal syndrome) arising from acute alcohol deprivation. The problem with this approach is that it portrays alcohol withdrawal as a dichotomous, either/or phenomenon. It is actually a syndrome of varying intensities, ranging from reactions associated with a mild hangover and tremor to those associated with severe delirium tremens (Becker et al., 1974). The physical-addiction approach defines addiction only in terms of the most severe withdrawal reactions; but reactions are common only among those who maintain consistently high blood alcohol levels (Sellers and Kalant, 1976). Even those who are in advanced stages of alcoholic cirrhosis may not show withdrawal reactions of sufficient severity to qualify as "addicted" (Feinman and Lieber, 1974). In short, using severe withdrawal reactions as a diagnostic criterion excludes many cases in which other objective evidence would clearly point to a diagnosis of alcoholism.

The physical-addiction approach is even less satisfactory when applied to the elderly, since their reactions to alcohol consumption and withdrawal are even more variable than those of younger persons. The identification of such reactions is further complicated in elder individuals by the fact that many of them may be taking medications which, when combined with even small amounts of alcohol, produce misleading signs.

*Socionormative definitions.* Socionormative definitions, especially those using quantity and frequency, also have several general limitations. Foremost among these is the complex nature of norms regarding drinking, norms which vary greatly with sex, race, culture, and socioeconomic category (Cahalan, 1970; Knupfer and Room, 1964). This variation frustrates attempts to distinguish the deviant drinker from the normal drinker.

Formulating criteria for deviant drinking is even more difficult for elderly people because so little is known about drinking practices in this group. Norms regarding quantity and frequency appear to change with age (Cahalan and Cisin, 1968), yet even minimal drinking may have important implications for the health of physically debilitated elderly individuals. An additional problem inherent in the quantity-frequency normative approach is its reliance on self-report information that may be inaccurate and intentionally distorted. Heavy drinkers may lose track of the amount consumed, and in some cases, the phenomenon of "blacking out" renders one completely unable to recall the details of recent drinking episodes.

*Social-problems definition.* The third definition, which portrays alcoholism as a disease characterized by the presence of significant alcohol-related life problems, was used in many of the studies cited here. The diagnostic criteria employed under this approach (the presence of marital, vocational, or legal problems related to alcohol or evidence that alcohol consumption had directly harmed health) have the advantage of being relatively specific and nonarbitrary. However, even these criteria have specific limitations with elderly populations. Although the elderly have important alcohol-related life problems, it is more difficult for an elderly person, as compared to a younger one, to be recognized as a case.

Using social-problems diagnostic criteria with the elderly is difficult because three of the four criteria have limited applicability. The elderly are less likely to be presently married and less likely to be employed than younger persons (U.S. Bureau of Census, 1975) and are also less likely to have police arrests than are other age groups. The fourth diagnostic criterion in the social-problem approach is alcohol-related health impairment. Here one must proceed cautiously, since differentiating between direct and indirect effects of alcohol consumption can be difficult in the elderly, with their higher levels of chronic illness and use of medication that may interact with alcohol.

Applying the social-problems diagnostic criteria to elderly populations presents difficulties even if the individual in question is married, employed, under medical care, and subject to legal processing. Marital problems are one example. In the elderly, such problems may arise from several sources including ill health and reduced income. If late-onset alcohol abuse occurs in conjunction with such circumstances, to what extent can the marital problems be regarded as alcohol-related? Relying on one of the involved parties to answer this question introduces a strong subjective element into diagnosis, and a report of no alcohol-related problems also may be biased.

Detecting vocational problems is equally complex. The employed elderly may face employers who encourage retirement despite continued ability to perform job tasks. Even a single episode of drinking may provide a convenient excuse to dismiss an elderly employee who is regarded as extraneous. On the other hand, elderly employees may be kept on the job for sentimental reasons, and heavy, debilitating drinking may be irrelevant to continued employment. Finally, firing or suspension may actually be due to drinking, but both employer and employee deny this and choose a less stigmatizing explanation for job loss.

The remaining two diagnostic criteria involve the actions of legal and medical officials, where errors of classification also may arise. In the area of legal problems, the discretion of police officers, prosecutors, and judges plays a major role. Arrest for public drunkenness is one example of an alcohol-related legal problem that elderly people may encounter. These arrests often occur in circumstances that maximize police discretion, and only a small proportion of police encounters with intoxicated elderly end in arrest (Bittner, 1967; Pastor, 1976).

Yet in some jurisdictions drunkenness is a charge employed for disorderly conduct that may or may not involve intoxication (Brittner, 1967; Stern, 1967). When an older person is arrested for drunkenness, it may arise either from the greater debilitating effect of intoxication in the elderly; an officer's attempt to assist a sober but "helpless old-timer" with temporary lodging; or the paternalistic practice of charging elderly petty offenders (shoplifter, morals violators) with the more convenient and less serious charge of drunkenness. In short, an official legal response may not accurately reflect the behavior of an individual who becomes a police case.

The manner in which the elderly come to the attention of medical authorities is relevant to the diagnostic criteria of alcohol-related health impairment. Several authors have demonstrated that health-care seeking is a complex process (Chrisman, 1974; Robinson, 1971). While an elderly person may seek help directly for an alcohol problem, physicians probably most often recognize alcoholism in the context of other presenting complaints (Graux, 1969; McCusker et al., 1971). Thus, whatever factors influence an individual to seek or avoid medical care or, once under a physician's care, to report or withhold complaints, can influence the likelihood that alcohol-related health problems will be diagnosed. Availability of medical care, fear of being diagnosed as terminally ill, denial of symptoms, and loathing of alcoholism-associated stigma are all relevant to health-care seeking in the elderly.

Even when an individual seeks medical care, it is easy for his physician to overlook the role of alcohol in creating a health problem, since some of alcohol's adverse effects mimic various degenerative diseases and various types of psychopathology. The physician who erroneously believes that alcohol abuse generally is limited to younger persons or skid-row derelicts will overlook alcoholism in the elderly.

In clinical psychiatry and in medicine a useful diagnosis is a guide for future treatment (Woodruff, 1974). Several clinical studies show that the life-problem definition of alcoholism, when applied to younger individuals, outlines a group with a relatively homogeneous prognosis and response to treatment (Schuckit, 1977a). There are no longitudinal studies of alcoholism in the elderly. The life problem definition is probably our best clinical label, even though it may not be as relevant when applied to older populations.

If an individual fulfills a life-problem definition of alcoholism, one must further evaluate whether alcohol problems occurred independent of any major preexisting psychiatric disorder (Schuckit, 1973, 1977a). By definition an individual who demonstrates alcohol-related difficulties *only* in the midst of a severe depression is labeled as having primary affective disorder and secondary alcoholism, while another individual with serious alcohol problems who shows a basically normal mood state *except* while drinking would be labeled as having primary alcoholism with a secondary affective disorder. The primary affective disorder patient with secondary alcoholism tends to drink when ill and abstain when well, implying, but not proving, that treatment might best be aimed at the affective disorder and not at alcoholism itself. Most of the material related below will deal with the primary alcoholic, since this group probably makes up 70–80 percent of groups of alcoholics in treatment (Schuckit, 1973, 1977a).

In conclusion the recognition of alcoholism in a clinical setting is often difficult, and imperfections in diagnostic criteria make the task even harder. The elderly's unique physiology and social status add further complexity to the problem. Nevertheless, the social-problems definition, which uses as criteria alcohol-related marital, vocational, legal, and health problems, is our best guide for clinical practice and research. This approach coupled with a search for any psychiatric disorder antedating the patient's alcoholism can lead to an effective treatment plan.

*Epidemiology.* We do not know the actual rate of alcoholism in elderly people, partly because epidemiologic studies of alcoholism in older individuals are hampered by problems in definition. Numerous attempts have been made to answer this question, but the figures given must be interpreted in light of the definition of alcoholism used, the survey methods, and the population under study.

Surveys of general populations, which usually base their diagnosis on either alcohol problems or alcohol intake (Bailey et al., 1965; Siassi et al., 1973), estimate the rate of alcoholism to be from 2–10 percent of the general elderly population, with higher rates for widowers, people in legal difficulty, and those never married. Reviews of nursing home populations (Graux, 1969; Lugand, 1969) indicate rates of alcoholism of about 20 percent; studies of psychiatrically ill older patients show a rate of alcoholism of between 5 and 50 percent (Busse, 1973; Daniel, 1972; Epstein and Simon, 1967; Gaitz and Baer, 1971; Kramer, 1969; Pfeiffer and Busse, 1973; Simon et al., 1968; Whittier and Korenyi, 1961). Surveys of general medical wards indicate a 15 to 30 percent rate of alcoholism (Moore, 1971; Barchha et al., 1968) which is equal to rates seen in geriatric medical inpatients (Schuckit and Miller, 1976). Between 5 and 15 percent of older medical outpatients have been estimated to be alcoholic (Barchha et al., 1968; Daniel, 1972; Epstein and Simon, 1967; Gaitz and Baer, 1971; Kramer, 1969; McCusker et al., 1971; Moore, 1971; Pequignot et al., 1969; Pfeiffer and Busse, 1973; Simon et al., 1968; Zimberg, 1974a). Roughly 10 percent of alcoholics in treatment are age 60 or over (Glatt, 1961; Rosin and Glatt, 1971; Vidojkovic et al., 1970).

*Possible Alcoholic Subtypes: Early Onset and Late Onset.* Studies of geriatric alcoholics raise some important questions about the possibility of diagnostic subtypes. One group of investigators believes that the elderly alcoholic is probably the young alcoholic grown old (Epstein et al., 1968; Fillmore, 1974; Patterson et al., 1974; Rathbone-McCuan and Bland, 1974); whereas another group (Lugand, 1969; Pascarelli, 1974; Stotsky, 1972) argues that old-age alcoholism begins in the elderly as a response to medical problems and environmental burdens. In one study (Pascarelli, 1974; Zimberg, 1974b), at least one-third of a group of old-age alcoholics in San Francisco began abusing alcohol after age 60.

The importance of the age of onset of alcoholism was addressed in a study of a random sample of men admitted to the San Diego Veterans Administration Medical Center medical and surgical wards (Schuckit and Miller, 1976). Information was gathered by personal interview, medical records review, and interview with a spouse or additional resource person. Fifteen to 20 percent of these individuals had at some point in their life fulfilled the criteria for alcoholism, there being equal subgroups of those who had their first alcohol problem before age 40 and those who did not demonstrate alcoholism until after that age. These two groups, one demonstrating the more typical age of onset and another the later onset, were very different.

The early-onset alcoholic reported a high rate of social, marital, legal, and job problems, experienced serious alcohol-related life difficulties over a span of 10 to 15 years, and had been "dry" or almost "dry" for an average of about 10 years before the interview; they were alcoholics who were no longer drinking at the time of entering the study. Those with a later age of onset of alcohol-related experienced far fewer social problems, had higher rates of medical disorder, and tended to be actively drinking at the time of investigation (Eisdorfer and Schuckit, 1977; Schuckit and Miller, 1976).

It is important that both potential subtypes of older-age alcoholics be recognized as each can present with alcohol-related pathology, the former related to their earlier intake and the latter to their present active drinking.

*The Clinical Course of Alcoholism in Older Age Groups.* About one-half of all older alcoholics begin their alcohol abuse at a younger age and survive past the age of 65 years, usually by acquiring abstinence sometime in their late 50s or early 60s. In contrast to the abstinent elderly alcoholic, the actively drinking older alcoholic tends to have a later age of onset for alcohol misuse and demonstrates a lowered level of social pathology—but has more medical problems. Once alcohol problems begin, the average practicing older alcoholic usually drinks four to five days a week, consuming about four drinks per occasion, a rate lower than that expected for younger alcoholics. This last finding is not surprising in light of the differences in body composition, metabolism of drugs, and increased medical pathology seen with advancing age. He or she also reports a mean of two or three alcohol-related life problems, also slightly lower than that seen for most younger drinking populations. Drinking history is paralleled by smoking as alcoholics appear to be less likely to abstain from smoking while actively drinking but seem to be better able to give up tobacco when they become abstinent from ethanol (Eisdorfer and Schuckit, 1977; Schuckit and Miller, 1976).

Primary alcoholism manifests much of the same course and clinical phenomenon in both older and younger individuals. We know this from comparing matched groups of young and elderly drinkers and nondrinkers and by charting their respective social, medical, and psychiatric disorders. Older alcoholics compared to age-matched nonalcoholics report higher rates of suicide attempts and are more likely to show signs of mental deterioration (Schuckit and Miller, 1976). Alcoholics are also more likely to be living alone, less likely to be married, and less likely to be living at their present address for five or more years (Schuckit and Miller, 1976).

It is also possible to compare the older alcoholic to other elderly patient groups. As opposed to the old-age *psychiatric* patients, the alcoholic more frequently lives alone (Glatt, 1961), is younger (Daniel, 1972;

Simon et al., 1968), and more frequently reports multiple marriages (Simon et al., 1968). When compared to the geriatric *medical* patient, the elderly alcoholic is also younger, is more isolated, has been married more times (Harrington and Price, 1962a; Lucas, 1969), shows a better employment record (Harrington and Price, 1962b), has a twofold higher rate of organic brain disease (Gaitz and Baer, 1971; Harrington and Price, 1962d), and more often reports a history of drug addiction and less frequently a history of cardiac disease (Harrington and Price, 1962c). One study compared the primary medical diagnoses for alcoholic and nonalcoholic elderly patients (Schuckitt and Miller, 1976), showing that 25 percent of the alcoholics reported chronic obstructive lung diseases, as against only 15 percent of the remaining subjects. Also, while 15 percent of the alcoholics had a primary admitting diagnosis of heart disease, the same was true for 27 percent of the remaining subjects. Both study groups had similar rates of pneumonia and cancer.

Again, compared to the *younger alcoholic,* the geriatric alcohol abuser is much less likely to have an obvious personality disorder (Rosin and Glatt, 1971). Older alcoholics demonstrate more life stability: they exhibit histories of better school and job performance, lower rates of drug and alcohol-related difficulties in early life, and fewer interpersonal problems. It appears as if many older alcoholics have been more stable in early life and then, for unknown reasons, in later years develop alcohol problems (Eisdorfer and Schuckit, 1977; Schuckit and Miller, 1976).

Alcoholics can enter medical care because of an array of psychopathologic problems ranging from obvious alcoholism, to depression, to psychosis, and alcohol abuse must be considered as part of a differential diagnosis of any psychiatric picture in older populations. The psychiatric problems seen in older alcoholics are very similar to those manifest in younger alcoholic populations. Depression nearly as severe as in primary affective disorder may appear during active drinking bouts but tends to clear spontaneously within two to seven days with proper detoxification; such episodes probably do not warrant treatment with antidepressants or lithium (Schuckit, 1977a). Acute confusional states, another common problem in older alcoholics, may appear at low blood alcohol levels or after relatively short periods of heavy drinking and persist longer than would be seen in younger alcoholics. An organic brain syndrome (OBS) is common in alcoholics, perhaps occurring in more than one-third of those studied (Gaitz and Baer, 1971). Compared to alcoholics without OBS, the organically impaired alcoholic is younger (Gaitz and Baer, 1971; Simon et al., 1968), has a higher rate of nursing needs (Gaitz and Baer, 1971), and has an elevated two-year mortality rate (Daniel, 1972; Gaitz and Baer, 1971; Simon et al., 1968). Paranoia and hallucinosis may occur at a higher rate in older individuals (Schuckit and Pastor, 1977) or arise from acute or chronic alcohol intoxication. These data point out again how alcoholism must be considered as part of the differential diagnosis for almost any psychiatric syndrome in older individuals.

The rates of specific life problems and of psychopathology are, as would be expected, apparently higher for actively drinking alcoholics than for nondrinking alcoholics (Schuckit and Miller, 1976). Thus, one study of medically and surgically hospitalized elderly alcoholics showed that, overall, 70 percent had health problems related to alcohol; this included 89 percent for the active versus 55 percent for the inactive drinkers; 56 percent of the active and 36 percent of the inactive drinkers had marital problems; and 44 percent of the active versus 36 percent of the inactive drinkers had alcohol-related driving problems. The 60 percent rate of other problems including life adjustment were seen for two-thirds of the active versus one-half of the inactive alcoholics (Schuckit and Miller, 1976).

Only a few studies examine older alcoholic women (aged 55 years or older) and compare older and younger women on alcohol histories. As with older men, older women demonstrate more life stability, reporting fewer antisocial problems in younger years and lower rates of drug use. Older women also show fewer psychiatric hospitalizations and lower rates of suicide attempts despite their greater tendency to live alone (Schuckit and Morrissey, 1976).

The older woman alcoholic usually does not begin to have alcohol difficulties until after age 40 and has an average of two years of alcohol abuse from her first major problem until first hospitalization. The development of alcohol-related difficulties in one sample of older women progressed from job problems and drunkenness in public (at a mean age of 44 years) to health problems (at a mean age of 46 years), divorce (at a mean age of 51 years), and automobile accidents (at a mean age of 55 years) (Schuckit and Morrissey, 1976). Older women as compared to men more often use drugs, especially barbiturates, stimulants, and opiates. In the scant literature on alcohol problems in older women, there is no evidence of any large differences in course and prognosis between alcoholic men and women, especially when one controls for socioeconomic status and primary diagnosis (Schuckit and Morrissey, 1976).

To summarize, current research indicates that a surprising percentage of alcoholics first develop drinking problems in later life. There is evidence for two subgroups of older alcoholics. The early-onset alcoholic has serious drinking problems before age 40 and lives into older age perhaps by becoming abstinent. The late-onset alcoholic has a better early history for social and personal adjustment, but develops alcohol-related problems after age 40 and continues drinking in his or her old age. The clinician should recognize that in the elderly alcoholic the amount of drinking and the number of alcohol-related problems is lower than for young alcoholics. Nevertheless, the older alcoholic has higher rates of divorce, suicide, and organic brain disease than nonalcoholics.

*Treatment of Alcoholism in Older Populations.* Because the older abuser is likely to be left out of treatment reviews for both geriatric and alcoholic patients (Riccitelli, 1967; Schuckit, 1974b), there is rather limited literature on the treatment of the geriatric alcoholic. Without strong evidence, most authors believe that the social and medical problems of the geriatric alcoholic require special care (Busse, 1973; Rathbone-McCuan and Bland, 1974; Rosin and Glatt, 1971), and some authorities consider that many medical facilities are ill-equipped to handle the geriatric alcoholic (Rathbone-McCuan and Bland, 1974). Because of his age and lack of physical reserves, the geriatric alcoholic needs excellent medical care. Yet it would seem that any facility providing good medical care and social work help, along with occupational and/or recreational therapy, should be able to deal effectively with the geriatric alcoholic.

One investigation demonstrated some interesting findings about the older alcoholic in treatment (Schuckit et al., 1977). Probably reflecting his advanced age and impaired physical reserve, he was more likely to be treated in a hospital setting and less likely to receive disulfiram (Antabuse®). He also appeared to have a better response to initial treatment, since 73 percent of the older versus only 40 percent of the younger ones completed their time in care.

There are few data indicating what the optimal treatment is for the older alcoholic, and no controlled studies demonstrate that one type of therapy is better than any other. One might make some commonsense modifications in the usual alcohol treatment program until adequate data accrues (Schuckit, 1978a, 1978b). These can be adapted to all stages of treatment ranging from detoxification, to rehabilitation, to outpatient follow-up.

**1.** *Detoxification.* Some alcoholics enter treatment solely because of medical or psychological problems caused by continued heavy drinking and do not desire rehabilitation, while others want help in stopping to drink but enter treatment in an intoxicated state. In either instance the patient must be carefully withdrawn from alcohol using the basic approach outlined by Sellers and Kalant (Sellers and Kalant, 1976) with some modifications for older individuals.

First, the serious physical pathology associated with alcoholism and the relative debilitation of the elderly make mandatory a thorough physical examination including a good neurologic evaluation and adequate blood screens. Any abnormalities must be carefully followed up as they might complicate later treatment.

Once this is accomplished, the alcoholic must be offered rest, nutrition, and vitamin supplementation. While multiple vitamins will frequently suffice, the decrease in body reserves of thiamine and the role this important vitamin plays in adequate heart functioning (beri-beri heart disease) and neurologic functioning (Wernicke-Korsakoff's disease) make thiamine supplementation of at least 100 mg intramuscularly each day for one to three days advisable. Intramuscular injections of B-complex vitamins should be considered in view of the possibility of multiple deficiencies. Especially in the case of Wernicke-Korsakoff's disease, it is wise to have a high index of suspicion; if detected early and treated vigorously, catastrophic and irreversible damage can be avoided (Wernicke's Encephalopathy, 1979).

If the individual is physically addicted to alcohol, the smoothest withdrawal with the best chance of preventing the serious abstinence symptoms of organic brain syndrome, hallucinations, or convulsions rests with the careful administration of another central nervous system depressant. The benzodiazepines such as chlordiazepoxide (Librium®) are effective and decrease respirations and cardiac functioning less than most other CNS depressants (Greenblatt and Shader, 1974). Because older people usually metabolize drugs more slowly and have greater CNS sensitivity to depressant drugs, benzodiazepines must be administered very carefully with close attention given to vital signs and the level of alertness. Thus, while the average younger alcoholic going through withdrawal might require 150 mg of chlordiazepoxide on the first day (which is then decreased by 20 percent of the original day's dose each subsequent day), the older alcoholic might conceivably require only 25 or 50 mg the first day. While no convincing data can be given on this point, it is safest to carefully monitor all doses of chlordiazepoxide, withholding the medication if the patient develops a drop in systolic blood pressure (of more than 20 mm Hg) or a decreased level of alertness. Some short-acting benzodiazepines like oxazepam (Serax®) have no active metabolites, do not tend to accumulate over time, and may prove to be especially useful agents for use in the elderly.

2. *The usual rehabilitation program.* Rehabilitating the alcoholic involves taking advantage of the patient's initial level of motivation and maximizing his chances of achieving abstinence by close support (Schuckit, 1978a). This usually is carried out through a short inpatient stay (often two weeks or less) under a physician's supervision during which the patient is educated about alcohol, counseled by paraprofessionals regarding day-to-day life problems, and introduced to Alcoholics Anonymous. Some settings use various forms of aversive conditioning (Elkins, 1975; Schuckit, 1978a, 1978b). At present, neither the comparative effectiveness of behavioral methods versus traditional treatment is known, nor have we identified those patients best suited for either approach.

There is no reason to believe that the elderly should receive any radical departure from the usual program, but common sense dictates the possible benefit of creating group discussions and Alcoholics Anonymous meetings involving other older alcoholics. This follows the assumption that the day-to-day life stresses and needs for counseling differ in the older individual from those in the 40-year-old patient.

Similarly, in dealing with the older alcoholic one might have to address interactions with grown children as much as with the spouse. It is also important to recognize that while vocational rehabilitation could have less relevance to the older alcoholic, volunteer work and other activities in the community might be important to sustain morale. The older alcoholic also has greater potential need for social service help in guaranteeing an adequate income for food and shelter. Of course, the older alcoholics' high risk of physical disorders requires adequate attention by a physician who can also coordinate all medical care for the patient.

**3.** *The older alcoholic in a nursing home.* Alcoholics afflicted by disabling physical illness or a persistent organic brain syndrome are often placed in nursing homes. Most such facilities have limited experience with alcoholics, and often the staff hold the erroneous opinion that alcoholics are hopeless skid-row bums who cause trouble. As a result, the staff may try to avoid having alcoholics placed in their facilities and attempt to transfer them as soon as possible once they are admitted. It is extremely unfortunate that there are so few adequate long-term treatment facilities for alcoholics with mental or physical deterioration. The shortage removes a valuable resource for patients and undercuts the efforts of rehabilitation programs interested in the treatment of alcoholism.

There is no easy answer for this situation. Ideally, specific facilities for the older impaired alcoholic might be developed, but limitations in public funding make this unlikely. For now the most useful approach is to (1) educate nursing home staffs about geriatric problems, and about alcoholism and its treatment, (2) work with them to establish programs aimed at controlling the patient's access to alcohol while in the nursing home, and (3) offer nursing home staff a high level of back-up from alcoholic treatment facilities and Alcoholics Anonymous. This kind of combined effort, while not perfect, usually is the best one can offer in a clinical setting.

Despite difficulties, the elderly alcoholic can be surprisingly amenable to treatment. It is therefore essential that professionals working with the alcoholic maintain a therapeutic stance and avoid punitive or rejecting attitudes toward relapses in drinking. Relapses often occur, and controlled drinking may be a more realistic treatment goal for some than absolute sobriety. The rigid professional with unrealistic expectations may only doom his patient and his treatment recommendations.

*Some Thoughts on Etiology.* Neither the course nor the etiology of alcoholism is known for any age group. The best data indicate that several mechanisms are involved and that individuals can enter an alcoholic life-style in different ways. Three very interesting areas seen in younger populations involve genetic aspects of alcoholism, alcohol abuse amidst a life crisis, and the effect of medical or psychiatric illness.

The average person demonstrating alcohol problems in his late 20s to early 30s would appear to be suffering from a genetically influenced disorder, with a level of heritability probably equal to that of diabetes. Family and twin studies, animal investigations, and genetic-marker studies all support this hypothesis but cannot separate the relative importance of heredity and environment. Yet adoption-type separation studies, utilizing adoption records (Goodwin, 1976) and half-siblings (Schuckit et al., 1972), consistently demonstrate that children of alcoholics separated from their parents close to birth and raised separately have rates of alcoholism at least as high as children of alcoholics raised by biologic parents. This phenomenon cannot be explained by separation and adoption alone, as adopted controls without biologic alcoholic parents have low rates of alcoholism, even when raised by alcoholic adoptive parents. The role of genetics is not completely clear, however, since no studies have been able to control for factors involved in the prenatal environment.

But if alcoholism is genetically influenced, how is it possible for a person to avoid problems in his 20s (when consumption is usually heaviest) and 30s (the age of onset for alcoholism in most individuals), only to succumb to alcohol problems in late life?

There are many possible explanations. For example, it is possible that people enter adulthood with varying levels of predisposition toward alcoholism. Whether and when alcohol problems arise would depend on an interaction between the degree of genetic vulnerability, the stresses encountered, and the character of a person's existing defenses against alcohol abuse. The stresses of increasing isolation and failing health which accompany aging may make some individuals much more vulnerable than did the stresses of developing a life occupation and raising a family. The more rigid demands of job and family may prevent drinking from getting out of hand—but this defense disappears as children leave home or retirement ensues.

Alcoholism can also occur as a complication of psychiatric disorders in the elderly. The peak age of onset for unipolar depressive disease is in the 40s and 50s (Winokur, 1969), and some older individuals with alcohol problems may drink in response to recurrent depressive episodes (Schuckit 1974a; Schuckit and Winokur, 1972). In addition, some of the psychiatric disorders more common in the elderly than in younger groups may predispose an individual to drink. One such syndrome, late paraphrenia (Schuckit and Miller, 1976), involves enhanced suspiciousness and paranoid delusions beginning in the 50s and 60s. It is possible that affected individuals drink in the midst of such stresses in an attempt to diminish their high levels of anxiety and antagonism. Only prospective studies will be able to determine whether this is true.

At present we can only speculate on the possible causes of alcoholism: a comprehensive approach should consider an interaction among genetic predisposition, life stress and assets, physical or psychiatric illness, and characteristic coping styles.

## Summary

Discussions of alcohol problems in older people must include not only the alcoholic but the nonalcoholic drinker. Elderly individuals even in good health may not tolerate alcohol well because of inevitable deficits in drug metabolism and decrements in physical reserve accompanying aging. The ill elderly may take medications which adversely interact with alcohol; alcohol affects virtually every organ system, and individuals with underlying brain or cardiac disease are especially vulnerable to its adverse effects.

Diagnosing alcoholism is a difficult task in any age group, but it is particularly difficult in the elderly. Of the three major definitional-diagnostic approaches, the social-problems approach is the most useful, although it, too, displays certain limitations, and variables unique to the elderly encourage both false-positive and false-negative diagnostic errors. The clinician diagnosing alcoholism in the elderly should be aware of the limitations of the diagnostic criteria for this population and should regard these criteria merely as areas from which to begin a much more detailed inquiry into the role of alcohol in any problems the patient may report.

Geriatric alcoholism's epidemiology and natural history is unknown, yet we have partial conclusions. The elderly alcoholic probably is not simply the young alcoholic grown old. Evidence indicates that there may be two equal subgroups of older alcoholics: those who exhibit their first alcohol problems before age 40 (early-onset alcoholics) and those who avoid alcoholism until after that age (late-onset alcoholics). Early-onset alcoholics have a high rate of personality disorders and of alcohol-related social, marital, legal, and job problems. They often become abstinent in their late 50s or early 60s. Late-onset alcohol abusers have a surprisingly placid early life, without psychiatric history, but have higher rates of medical disorders and are likely to be active drinkers. Psychiatric problems like depression, suicide, acute confusional states, and organic brain syndrome are common and occur at higher rates than in nonalcoholic populations. The actively drinking elderly have more social, interpersonal, and health problems than the nondrinking older alcoholic. Although the data are incomplete, the frequency and course of alcohol problems in older women is similar to those of older men.

No evidence indicates that the detoxification, rehabilitation, and outpatient follow-up of elderly alcoholics should differ substantially from that offered younger alcoholics. Nevertheless, more careful research needs to be addressed to this question. Meticulous medical care is the foundation of alcohol treatment. Awareness of common geriatric psychiatric disorders and of alcohol's ability to mimic psychopathologic states is essential. Treatment facilities should provide access to the extra social supports needed by elderly alcoholics. Education may help diminish staff prejudices against the elderly—especially elderly alcoholics. A therapeutic attitude and sound training based on current knowledge can go far in rehabilitation efforts.

Why so many older alcoholics have a stable early life and in later years develop alcohol problems is an important and unanswered question. Some possible etiologic factors may be an interaction of genetic vulnerability, life stress, coping mechanisms, and cultural and personal learned behavior patterns. We have no satisfactory etiologic explanation at this time.

## MISUSE OF MEDICATIONS BY THE ELDERLY

### Introduction

Illegal, recreational drug abuse among adolescents and young adults captures newspaper headlines—and the efforts of most health professionals interested in drug-related problems. As a counterpoint it is well to review the important information about over-the-counter and prescription medication use in the elderly and to become aware of the complexity of this problem.

### The Elderly Use Many Medications and Are at High Risk

There are four important facts about medication use by the elderly. The first two reveal the scope of the problem and the latter two the vulnerability of the older patient.

1. Persons age 55 years or older are the largest national consumers of legal drugs, receiving annually over 225 million prescriptions, in-

cluding almost 180 million for mood-altering drugs (Parry et al., 1973; Pascarelli and Fischer, 1974; Swanson et al., 1973), and accounting for 25–30 percent of all prescription drug costs. This is not a simple matter of reckless overprescribing, because the great majority of these scripts are warranted (Geriscope, 1972).

2. Elderly individuals mix prescribed medications with over-the-counter drugs and/or alcohol, a problem which will require both public education and prompting by physicians to warn older patients of adverse effects.
3. Adverse reactions to medication increase with the number of drugs taken (Gibson and O'Hare, 1968; Hemminki and Heikkila, 1975; Plutchnik et al., 1973) and with the complexity of the prescription's directions (Gibson and O'Hare, 1968; Petersen and Thomas, 1975).
4. The elderly have many symptoms, and "symptomatic" drugs are given for relief, especially the psychotropics, analgesics, vasodilators, antihistamines, and others (Hemminki and Heikkila, 1975). Since older persons are likely to use multiple drugs oriented to simultaneous disorders of sleep, appetite, mood, elimination, pain, and the like, the risk for misuse is high, especially if drugs are given on difficult or complicated schedules. Indeed, in a Helsinki study more than 50 percent of the symptomatic and psychotropic drugs were misused by aged patients, and this finding was considered to be underestimated (Hemminki and Heikkila, 1975).

Other issues believed to lead to abuse/misuse of prescribed medications include (1) the use of multiple physicians leading to polypharmacy and to duplication of essentially the same drugs; (2) borrowing of drugs from others in an effort to save money, or because that drug helped a neighbor in the past; (3) automatic refills, which may lead to storage of drugs; and (4) self-medication with over-the-counter drugs which complicate the polypharmacy. Drug interactions resulting from the patient's failure to report drugs given by other physicians and the lack of coordination of medical care occur regularly. The complications of adding over-the-counter medication, particularly bromides, antihistamines, or sleep preparations, to a frail individual, already on some drugs, certainly has the capacity to cause serious drug interaction. Furthermore, many physicians do not feel comfortable with psychiatric symptoms, and families and patients alike may not permit psychiatric evaluations. The result may be an over-reliance on psychotropic medications by physicians not experienced with such drugs. The data on this issues are more intuitive than empirical, however.

It is also wise to remember that when drugs are clinically investigated and approved, their dosage is often established using young, healthy individuals who are free from other disorders. When prescribed for the aged, the pharmacokinetics and results may be unpredictable (Bender, 1964; Hillestad et al., 1974) and include exacerbated side effects, inadvertent overdose, or other complications. Undesirable side effects to medical drugs occur in over 21 percent of hospitalized patients aged 70–79 years, compared to only 7.5 percent for those in their 40s, and 3 percent for those in their 20s (Friedel, 1978; Hurwitz, 1969). Adverse drug reactions occur in almost 25 percent of medical patients over age 80 and in only about 10–12 percent of patients below age 50 (Smith et al., 1966). We need much more investigation of drug interaction among the aged.

There are other serious problems to be considered, such as the problem of memory deficits in the elderly. Drugs may be taken improperly because they are forgotten or misplaced. Furthermore, even apparently simple directions may be complex or confusing to an impaired individual. As one suggestion, perhaps devices ought to be developed very much like postage meters and taken to registered pharmacists who will organize drug dispensing routines for the home: the machine could be filled with the needed drugs at the pharmacy and then appropriate medication would be dispensed to patients in single unit dosage at appropriate times (Eisdorfer and Schuckit, 1977).

The institutionalized older patient carries an extra burden of risk for medication misuse. Several serious problems in prescription drug use recently were reported by the Long-Term Care Subcommittee of the U.S. Senate Select Committee on the Aging (1974). At least 75 percent of nursing home patients were found to receive one or more psychotropic medications. Untrained nursing home attendants under virtually no supervision administered drugs to patients, often transferring drugs from one patient to another inappropriately. Drugs were overused because of economic incentives which allow the facility to buy the drug at wholesale and charge retail prices to the patient; they were prescribed by physicians only on the basis of telephone contact with nurses and without the benefit of careful examination or follow-up; and the use of sedatives as a substitute for trained personnel and individual care was common. Other surveys note ironically that the institutionalized patient who has the greatest total number of drug prescriptions may be the most active and least cognitively impaired (Ingman et al., 1975).

Drug misuse and abuse in the elderly is a complex biopsychosocial problem. Because the elderly are symptomatic, and often ill, they are prescribed numerous drugs, both by those who wish to provide relief and those who want to sedate them. Physician-shopping, polypharmacy, complicated prescriptions, borrowing drugs from others, use of other over-the-counter agents, and cognitive impairment contribute to the dilemma. To this one must add the elderly's special vulnerability and altered metabolic response to all medications.

## Intentional Drug Misuse

Some older individuals seek out drugs to abuse, getting their medications from several sources (Pascarelli and Fischer, 1974; Plutchnik et al., 1973; Swanson et al., 1973). The most frequently abused drugs in older patients are sleeping pills, like barbiturates (Subby, 1975; Swanson et al., 1973), and those we usually do not associate with abuse in younger populations, such as laxatives (Cummings et al., 1974) and aspirin compounds (Morrant, 1975). Surveys in both Australia and the United States have shown that the chance of abusing prescribed sedatives or analgesics increases with age in both men and women (Abrahams et al., 1970; George, 1972; Swanson, et al., 1973).

Substance-abuse problems are seen for a variety of over-the-counter medications. Bromide has long been abused and until recently existed in some medications including Sominex® and Bromo Seltzer®, among others. The symptoms of bromide intoxication (Carneh, 1971; Stewart, 1973) can mimic many psychiatric problems including an organic brain syndrome (confusion and disorientation) (Morrant, 1975). Antihistamines including Benadryl®, Dramamine®, and most cold medications and anticholinergics like scopolamine, found in almost all over-the-counter nerve medications, can also create confusion in the elderly, while heavy consumption of aspirin compounds is associated with a variety of physical as well as psychological symptoms (Bengtsson et al., 1975; Gault et al., 1968; George, 1972; Gillies and Skyring, 1972; Murray et al., 1971).

Barbiturates and other sedative drugs, which are among the most troublesome in terms of misuses and addictive properties, are still commonly used among the aged. Approximately one-third of all orders for phenobarbitol, and for related agents like glutethimide (Doriden®), ethchlorvynol (Placidyl®), and amobarbital (Amytal®) are issued to people aged 65 years or over (U.S. Department of Health, Education, and Welfare, 1979).

## Theories of Causation

Many authors have hypotheses relating problems of being old to the propensity to abuse medications. Psychologically, feelings of uselessness and being forgotten (Bergman and Amir, 1973), feelings of dependence

(Bergman and Amir, 1973), reactions to alienation (Garetz, 1974; Pascarelli and Fischer, 1974), poverty (Pascarelli and Fischer, 1974), and feelings of low status in society (Pascarelli and Fischer, 1974) have all been stated as contributing to substance abuse by the elderly.

Another variable involves acceptance of the sick role on the part of older persons who perceive their "illness" as an important explanation (unconsciously or otherwise) for their rolelessness in society. Loneliness itself can promote substance abuse, and people who are isolated are at heightened risk for physical and psychological problems. One area of stress deserves special mention. There is a general feeling that the loss of life structure and feelings of uselessness that accompany retirement or children's leaving home may play a role in the development of medication abuse in middle and old age. All of these commonsense theories deserve more thorough evaluations.

In addition, the available data indicate that the elderly may be at increasingly higher risk for the addiction to illicit drugs. This latter category may be primarily a function of the aging of young addicts rather than the late onset of compulsive abuse and addiction to illicit drugs (Eisdorfer and Schuckit, 1977).

However, many elderly people experience the stresses discussed without becoming substance abusers, and there are probably many geriatric drug abusers who never overtly experience these difficulties. Thus, while there is an association between many of these factors and growing old, there is no evidence that these factors cause substance abuse.

### Treatment of Drug Misuse in the Elderly

Treatment of inadvertent over-the-counter and prescription drug misuse begins with prevention. A reasonable approach toward prevention might emphasize the following points:

1. More research is needed to describe the characteristics of groups of greatest risk and to determine the course of drug misuse disorders.
2. Education of professionals and patients may help reduce inadvertent medication misuse: health professionals can be alerted to the extent of this problem and can emphasize patient education about drug interactions as a routine part of treatment planning.
3. Polypharmacy can be discouraged and drug regimens simplified. In some instances visiting nurses or home health aides can assist in drug compliance.

4. Detection of cognitive impairment and alcoholism will identify patients at especially high risk for adverse drug reactions.

The causes of *deliberate* drug abuse in the elderly are not known, and we can only speculate about determinants like ill health, loneliness, loss, and other stresses of growing old. Given the circumstances a preventive approach is difficult to adopt.

The treatment model developed for alcoholism probably provides our best guide to the treatment of both types of drug misusers and can be modified to fit the severity of the problem. Patients should be *detoxified* in settings that assure meticulous medical care, rest, and adequate nutrition. *Rehabilitation* beginning in an inpatient facility should provide social support, counseling, evaluation for predisposing psychiatric disorders, and connection to a network of social services. If necessary for medical or psychiatric reasons, *placement* in extended care facilities with adequately trained staff may be useful, and outpatient follow-up is essential.

Overall, well-designed pilot intervention programs to gather data on the nature and the treatment of unintended as well as deliberate drug misuse is the best way to proceed in this difficult area (Schuckit, 1977b). Until such programs are available we should try to control the patient's access to drugs, if possible, and to provide adequate medical and social service follow-up.

### Summary

Good research and new knowledge about geriatric medication problems is scarce. A better understanding of the aging body in relation to ingested substances is needed. We also need to have more knowledge of the extent of substance misuse and abuse, both legal and illicit, among the aged. We have slight understanding of the effects of the long-term use of psychotropic agents (major and minor tranquilizers and antidepressants), sleeping medication, over-the-counter concoctions, pain pills, laxatives, bromides, and the admixtures of all of these with alcohol.

Alternative explanations for causation have been reviewed (Haglund and Schuckit, 1977), but it must be pointed out that in alcohol as well as drug abuse it is hard to understand what influences a vulnerable group to misuse/abuse these substances while populations much larger in size are not influenced in the same way by similar stressors. Programs of intervention should involve heavy emphasis on the education of health professionals and the public, far better use of medication in long-term care, establishment of a centralized prescription memory bank to alert physicians and pharmacists to simultaneous prescription, control of over-the-counter drugs, better knowledge of drug effects, and more involvement of the aging in society at large. Perhap one way to deal with these issues is to make health care systems much more sensitive to drug and alcohol effects and to enable them to set up intervention programs and *simultaneously* to gather data on vulnerability, therapy, and long-term consequences.

Alcohol and prescription drug problems in older populations are an important area for future research. Both pose a potential difficulty for all older individuals, especially those with medical problems, whether or not they may be considered alcoholics or substance abusers. It is hoped that this review helps clinicians increase their awareness of these problems and provides a starting point for future readings and discussions in this area. It is also hoped that the National Institutes of Mental Health, Alcohol Abuse and Alcoholism, Drug Abuse, and Aging will devote more resources toward substance-abuse problems in older individuals.

## REFERENCES


Abrahams, M.J., Armstrong, J., and Whitlock, F.A. Drug dependence in Brisbane. *Medical Journal of Australia,* 1970, *2,* 397–404.

Bailey, M.D., Haberman, P.W., and Alksne, H. The epidemiology of alcoholism in an urban residential area. *Quarterly Journal of Studies on Alcohol,* 1965, *26,* 20–40.

Barchha, R., Stewart, M.A., and Guze, S. The prevalence of alcoholism among general hospital ward patients. *American Journal of Psychiatry,* 1968, *125,* 681–684.

Becker, C.E., Roe, R.L., and Scott, R.A. *Alcohol as a Drug: A Curriculum on Pharmacology, Neurology and Toxicology.* New York: Medcom, 1974.

Bender, A.D. Pharmacologic aspects of aging: a survey of the effect of increasing age on drug activity in adults. *Journal of American Geriatric Society,* 1964, *12,* 114–134.

Bengtsson, U., Angerval, L., and Johansson, L. Phenacetin abuse and renal pelvic carcinoma. *International Journal of Clinical Pharmacology,* 1976, *12,* 290–294.

Bergman, S., and Amir, M. Crime and delinquency among the aged in Israel. *Geriatrics,* 1973, *28,* 149–157.

Bittner, E. The police on skid row: a study in peace keeping. *American Sociology Review,* 1967, *32,* 699–715.

Butler, R.N. *Why Survive? Being Old in America.* New York: Harper & Row, 1976.

Busse, E.W. Mental disorders in later life—organic brain syndromes. In E.W. Busse and E. Pfeiffer (Eds.), *Mental Illness in Later Life.* Baltimore, Maryland: Garamond/Pridemark Press, 1973.

Cahalan, D. *Problem Drinkers.* San Francisco: Jossey-Bass, 1970.

Cahalan, D., and Cisin, I.H. American drinking practices: summary of findings from a national probability sample. I. Extent of drinking by population subgroups. *Quarterly Journal of Studies on Alcohol,* 1968, *28,* 130–151.

Carneh, M.W.P. Five cases of bromism. *Lancet,* 1971, *2,* 523–524.

Chrisman, N.J. American patterns of health care seeking behavior. Paper presented at Annual Meeting of American Anthropological Association, Mexico City, 1974.

Cummings, J.H., Sladen, G.E., James, O.F.W., Sarner, M., and Misciewiz, J.J. Laxative-induced diarrhea: a continuing clinical problem. *British Medical Journal,* 1974, *1,* 537–541.

Daniel, R. A five-year study of 693 psychogeriatric admissions in Queensland. *Geriatrics,* 1972, *27,* 132–155.

Eisdorfer, C., and Schuckit, M.A. Drug and alcohol misuse in the elderly. Drug use patterns, consequences and the federal response: a positive review. Washington, D.C.: Office of Drug Abuse Policy, March, 1978.

Elkins, R.L. A note on aversion therapy for alcoholism. *Behavioral Research and Therapy,* 1976, *4*(2), 159–160.

Epstein, L.J., and Simon, A. Organic brain syndrome in the elderly. *Geriatrics,* 1967, *22,* 145–150.

Feinman, L., and Lieber, C.S. Liver disease in alcoholism. In B. Kissin and H. Begleiter (Eds.), *The Biology of Alcoholism,* vol. 3, *Clincal Pathology.* New York: Plenum, 1974, p. 304.

Fillmore, L.M. Drinking and problem drinking in early adulthood and middle age. An exploratory 20-year follow-up study. *Quarterly Journal of Studies on Alcohol,* 1974, *35,* 819–840.

Friedel, R.O. Pharmacokinetics in the geropsychiatric patient in psychopharmacology. In M.A. Lipton, A. Dimascio, and K.F. Kollam (Eds.), *Psychopharmacology: A Generation of Progress.* New York: Raven Press, 1978, pp. 1499–1505.

Gaitz, C.M., and Baer, P.E. Characteristics of elderly patients with alcoholism. *Archives of General Psychiatry,* 1971, *24,* 372–378.

Garetz, F.K. Common psychiatric syndromes of the aged. *Minnesota Medicine,* 1974, *57,* 618–620.

Gault, M.H., Rudwal, A., and Redmond, N.I. Analgesic habits of 500 veterans: incidence and complications of abuse. *Canadian Medical Association Journal,* 1968, *98,* 619–626.

George, A. Survey of drug use in a Sydney suburb. *Medical Journal of Australia,* 1972, *2,* 233–237.

Geriscope. *Geriatrics,* 1972, *27,* 120–125.

Gibson, I., and O'Hare M.M. Prescription of drugs for old people at home. *Gerontologica Clinica,* 1968, *10,* 271–280.

Gilles, M.A., and Skyring, A.P. The pattern and prevalence of aspirin ingestion as determined by interview of 2,921 inhabitants of Sydney. *Medical Journal of Australia,* 1972, *1,* 974–979.

Glatt, M.M. Drinking habits of English alcoholics. *Acta Psychiatrica Scandinavica,* 1961, *37,* 88–113.

Graux, P. Alcoholism of the elderly. *Review on Alcohol,* 1969, *15,* 61–63.

Goodwin, D. *Is Alcoholism Hereditary?* New York: Oxford University Press, 1976.

Gould, L., Zahir, M., and Demartino, A. Cardiac effects of a cocktail. *Journal of the American Medical Association,* 1971, *218,* 1799–1802.

Greenblatt, D.J., and Schader, R.I. *Benzodiazepines in Clinical Practice.* New York: Raven Press, 1974.

Haglund, R.M.J., and Schuckit, M.A. The epidemiology of alcoholism. In N.

Estes & E. Heinemann (Eds.), *Alcoholism: Development, Consequences and Interventions*. St. Louis: C.V. Mosby Co., 1977, pp. 28–43.

Harrington, L.G., and Price, A.C. Alcoholism in a geriatric setting. I. Disciplinary problems, marital status and income level. *Journal of the American Geriatric Society*, 1962a, *10*, 197–200.

Harrington, L.G., and Price, A.C. Alcoholism in a geriatric setting. II. Education, milltary service and employment records. *Journal of the American Geriatric Society*, 1962b, *10*, 201–203.

Harrington, L.G., and Price, A.C. Alcoholism in a geriatric setting. IV. Incidence of drug addiction and disease. *Journal of the American Geriatric Society*, 1962c, *10*, 207–208.

Harrington, L.G., and Price, A.C. Alcoholism in a geriatric setting. V. Incidence of mental disorders. *Journal of the American Geriatric Society*, 1962d, *10*, 209–211.

Hemminki, E., and Heikkila, J. Elderly's people's compliance with prescriptions, and quality of medication. *Scandanavian Journal of Social Medicine*, 1975, *3*, 87–92.

Hillestad, L., Hansen, I., Melsom, H., and Privenes, A. Diazepam metabolism in normal man: I. Serum concentrations and clinical effects after intravenous, intramuscular and oral administration. *Clinical Pharmacology and Therapeutics*, 1974, *16*, 479–498.

Horowitz, L.A. Alcohol and heart disease. *Journal of the American Medical Association*, 1975, *239*, 959–960.

Hurwitz, N. Predisposing factors in adverse reactions to drugs. *British Medical Journal*, 1969, *1*, 536–539.

Ingman, S.R., Lawson, I.R., Pierpaoli, P.G., and Blake, P. A survey of the prescribing and administration of drugs in a long term care institution for the elderly. *Journal of the American Getriatric Society*, 1975, *23*, 309–316.

Knupfer, G., and Room, R. Age, sex and social class factors in amount of drinking in a metropolitan community. *Social Problems*, 1964, *12*, 224–240.

Kovar, M.G. Health of the elderly and use of health services. *Public Health Report*, Jan.-Feb., 1977, *92*(1), 9–19.

Kramer, M. *Patients in State and County Mental Hospitals*. Chevey Chase, Maryland: Public Health Service Publication No. 1921, 1969.

Lamy, P.P. Geriatric drug therapy. *Clinical Medicine*, 1974, *81*, 52–57.

Lenhart, D.G. The use of medications in the elderly population. *Nursing Clinics of North America*, 1976, *11*, 135–143.

Long-Term Care Subcommittee of the U.S. Senate Select Committee on the Aging. Special Committee on Aging. Washington, D.C.: U.S. Government Printing Office, 1974.

Lucas, M. Alcoholism in homes for the aged in the Paris region. *Review on Alcoholism*, 1969, *14*, 268–284.

Ludwig, A.M. The design of clinical studies in treatment efficacy. Presented at the First Annual Alcoholism Conference of the National Institute of Alcohol Abuse and Alcoholism. Washington, D.C., 1971.

Lugand, A. The situation in a hospital in Isere. *Review on Alcoholism*, 1969, *15*, 61–63.

McCusker, J., Cherubin, C.F., and Zimberg, S. The prevalence of alcoholism in general municipal hospital population. *New York State Journal of Medicine*, 1971, *71*, 751–754.

McCance, C., and McCance, P.F. Alcoholism in northeast Scotland: Its treatment and outcome. *British Journal of Psychiatry,* 1969, *115,* 189–198.

Moore, R.A. The prevalence of alcoholism in a community general hospital. *American Journal of Psychiatry,* 1971, *128,* 638–639.

Morrant, J.C.A. Medicines and mental illness in old age. *Canadian Psychiatric Association Journal,* 1975, *20,* 309–312.

Murray, R.M., Adams, J.H., and Greene, J.G. Analgesic abuse and dementia. *Lancet,* 1971, *2,* 242–245.

Parry, H.J., Balter, M.B., Mellinger, D.G., Cisin, I.H., and Manheimer, D.I. National patterns of psychotherapeutic drug use. *Archives of General Psychiatry,* 1973, *28,* 769–783.

Pascarelli, E.F. Drug dependence: an age-old problem compounded by old age. *Geriatrics,* 1974, *29,* 109–115.

Pascarelli, E.F., and Fischer, W. Drug dependence in the elderly. *International Journal of Aging and Human Development,* 1974, *5,* 347–356.

Pastor, P.A., Jr. The control of public drunkenness: a comparison of the legal and medical models. Unpublished doctoral dissertation, Department of Sociology, Yale University, New Haven, Connecticut, 1976.

Patterson, R.D., Abrahams, R., and Baker, F. Preventing self-destructive behavior. *Geriatrics,* 1974, *29,* 115–121.

Pequignot, H., Voisin, P., Guerre, J., Christoforov, B., and Portos, J.L. Aspects of alcoholism in the aged, hospitalized on a general medical ward. *Review on Alcoholism,* 1969, *15,* 33–45.

Petersen, D.M., and Thomas, C.W. Acute drug reactions among the elderly. *Journal of Gerontology,* 1975, *30,* 555–556.

Pfeiffer, E., and Busse, E.W. Mental disorders in later life—affective disorders; paranoid, neurotic, and situational reactions. In E.W. Busse and E. Pfeiffer (Eds.), *Mental Illness in Later Life.* Baltimore, Maryland: Garamond/Pridemark Press, 1973.

Plutchnik, R., McCartley, M., and Hall, B.H. Evaluation of a comprehensive psychiatric and health care program for elderly welfare tenants in a single room occupancy hotel. *Journal of the American Geriatrics Association,* 1973, *21,* 452–457.

Raskind, M., and Eisdorfer, C. Psychopharmacology of the aged. In L.L. Simpson (Ed.), *Drug Treatment of Mental Disorders.* New York: Raven Press, 1976, pp. 237–266.

Rathbone-McCuan, E., and Bland, J. Diagnostic and referral considerations for the geriatric alcoholic and aging problem drinker. Presented at the Gerontological Society's 27th Annual Meeting, Portland, Oregon, 1974.

Riccitelli, M.L. Treatment of alcoholism—modern concepts. *Journal of the American Geriatric Society,* 1967, *15,* 523–534.

Robinson, D. *The Process of Becoming Ill.* London: Routledge & Kegan Paul, 1971.

Rosin, A.J., and Glatt, M.M. Alcohol excess in the elderly. *Quarterly Journal of Studies on Alcohol,* 1971, *32,* 53–59.

Schmidt, W., and DeLint, J. Causes of death of alcoholics. *Quarterly Journal of Studies on Alcohol,* 1972, *33,* 171–185.

Schuckit, M.A. Alcoholism and sociopathy—diagnostic confusion. *Journal of Studies on Alcohol,* 1973, *34,* 157–164.

Schuckit, M.A. *Depression and Alcoholism in Women.* U.S. Department of

Health, Education and Welfare, Alcohol, Drug Abuse and Mental Health Administration. Reprinted. Washington, D.C., 1974a.

Schuckit, M.A. Unrecognized psychiatric illness in elderly medical-surgical patients. Presented at the 27th Annual Scientific Meeting of the Gerontological Society, Portland, Oregon, 1974b.

Schuckit, M.A. Alcoholism and affective disorder: diagnostic confusion. Presented at NIAAA Workshop on Alcoholism and Affective Disorder. Hilton Head Inn, Hilton Head, South Carolina, March, 1977a.

Schuckit, M.A. Geriatric alcoholism and drug abuse. *The Gerontologist,* 1977b, *17,* 168–174.

Schuckit, M.A. Inpatient and residential approaches to the treatment of alcoholism. In J.H. Mendelson and N.K. Mello (Eds.), *Diagnosis and Treatment of Alcoholism.* Springfield, Illinois: Charles C. Thomas, 1978a.

Schuckit, M.A. Treatment of alcoholism in office and outpatient settings. In J.H. Mendelson and N.K. Mello (Eds.), *Diagnosis and Treatment of Alcoholism.* Springfield, Illinois: Charles C. Thomas, 1978b.

Schuckit, M.A. *Drug and Alcohol Abuse: A Clinical Guide to Diagnosis and Treatment.* New York: Plenum Publishing Company, 1979.

Schuckit, M.A., and Cahalan, D. Evaluation of alcohol treatment programs. In Filstead, W.J., Rossi, J.J., and Keller, M. (Eds.), *Alcohol and Alcohol Problems: New Thinking and New Directions.* Cambridge, Mass.: Ballinger Publishing Company, 1967, pp. 229–262.

Schuckit, M.A., and Gunderson, E.K.E. Deaths among young alcoholics in the U.S. naval service. *Quarterly Journal of Studies on Alcohol,* 1974, *35,* 856–862.

Schuckit, M.A., and Miller, P.L. Alcoholism in elderly men: a survey of a general medical ward. *Annals of the New York Academy of Sciences,* 1976, *273,* 558–571.

Schuckit, M.A., and Morrissey, E.R. Alcoholism in women: some clinical and social perspectives with an emphasis on possible subtypes. In M. Greenblatt and M.A. Schuckit (Eds.), *Alcoholism Problems in Women and Children.* New York: Grune & Stratton, 1976.

Schuckit, M.A., and Pastor, P.A. Alcohol-related psychopathology in the aged. In Kaplan, O.J. (Ed.), *Psychopathology of Aging.* New York: Academic Press, 1977, pp. 211–227.

Schuckit, M.A., and Pastor, P.A. The elderly as a unique population. *Alcoholism: Clinical and Experimental Research,* 1978, *2,* 31–38.

Schuckit, M.A., and Winokur, G. A short term follow-up of women alcoholics. *Diseases of the Nervous System,* 1972, *33,* 672–678.

Schuckit, M.A., Goodwin, D., and Winokur, G. A study of alcoholism in half siblings. *American Journal of Psychiatry,* 1972, *128,* 1132–1136.

Schuckit, M.A., Morrissey, E.R., and O'Leary, M.R. Alcohol problems in elderly men and women. *Addictive Diseases,* 1978, *3,* 405–416.

Sellers, E.M., and Kalant, H. Medical intelligence—alcohol intoxication and withdrawal. *The New England Journal of Medicine,* 1976, *2,* 757–762.

Siassi, I., Crocetti, G., and Spiro, H.R. Drinking patterns and alcoholism in a blue-collar population. *Quarterly Journal of Studies on Alcohol,* 1973, *34,* 917–926.

Simon, A., Epstein, L.J., and Reynolds, L. Alcoholism in the geriatric mentally ill. *Geriatrics,* 1968, *23,* 125–131.

Smith, J.W., Seidl, L.G., and Cluff, L.E. Studies of epidemiology of adverse drug reactions: V. Clinical factors influencing the susceptibility. *Annals of Internal Medicine,* 1966, *65,* 629–640.

Stern, G. Public drunkenness: crime or health problem? *Annual American Academy of Political Social Sciences,* 1967, *374,* 146–156.

Stewart, R.B. Bromide intoxication from a nonprescription medication. *American Journal of Hospital Pharmacy,* 1973, *30,* 85–86.

Stotsky, B.A. Social and clinical issues in geriatric psychiatry. *American Journal of Psychiatry,* 1972, *129,* 117–126.

Subby, P. A community based program for the chemically dependent elderly. Presented at North American Congress on Alcohol and Drug Problems, San Francisco, December, 1975.

Sunby, P. *Alcoholism and Mortality.* Oslo, Norway: Universitetsforlaget, 1967.

Swanson, D.W., Weddige, R.L., and Morse, R.M. Abuse of prescription drugs. *Mayo Clinic Proceedings,* 1973, *48,* 359–367.

U.S. Department of Health, Education and Welfare. *First Special Report to the U.S. Congress on Alcohol and Health (23,26).* Rockville, Maryland: National Institute of Alcohol Abuse and Alcoholism, 1971.

U.S. Department of Health, Education and Welfare. *The Aging Process and Psychoactive Drug Use.* Rockville, Maryland: National Institute on Drug Abuse, 1979.

U.S. Bureau of Census. *Statistical Abstracts of the United States of America.* Washington, D.C.: U.S. Government Printing Office, 1975.

Verwoerdt, A. *Clinical Geropsychiatry.* Baltimore: Williams & Wilkins, 1976.

Vestal, R.E., McGuire, E.A., Tobin, J.D., Andres, R., Norris, A.H., and Mezey, E. Aging and ethanol metabolism. *Clinical Pharmacology and Therapeutics,* 1977, *21,* 343–353.

Vidojkovic, P., Grbesa, B. Miljkovic, S., and Sreckovic, M. Alcoholism in the aged. *Alkoholizam,* 1970, *10,* 52–59.

Wernicke's Encephalopathy. *British Medical Journal,* August 4, 1979, *2,* 291.

Whittier, J.R., and Korenyi, C. Selected characteristics of aged patients: a study of mental hospital admissions. *Comprehensive Psychiatry,* 1961, *2,* 113–120.

Winokur, G., Clayton, P., and Reich, T. *Manic Depressive Illness.* St. Louis: C.V. Mosby, 1969.

Woodruff, R.A., Goodwin, D.W., and Guze, S.B. *Psychiatric Diagnosis.* New York: Oxford University Press, 1974.

Zimberg, S. The elderly alcoholic. *The Gerontologist,* 1974a, *14,* 221–224.

Zimberg, S. Two types of problem drinkers: both can be managed. *Geriatrics,* 1974b, *29,* 135–138.

CHAPTER 10

# Past and Future Directions in Gerontological Nursing Research

Sue B. Foster, R.N., M.S.N., F.A.A.N.
Nursing Education Programs
Beth Israel Hospital
Boston, Massachusetts

Patricia G. Archbold, R.N., M.S.
School of Nursing
University of California
San Francisco, California

Nurse educators and researchers have made substantial strides in developing a gerontological nursing knowledge base. Although gerontological nursing papers have increased from two in 1966 to 114 ten years later, the majority of these are not directly related to research (Brimmer, 1979). The sparse research reported has focused on the psychosocial characteristics of the elderly, the attitudes of caretakers to the psychosocial needs of the elderly, and interventions to meet these needs. The research setting has usually been the institution, that is, nursing and old-age homes.

Our review of selected nursing studies delineates trends and identifies deficiencies, thus targeting critical areas in which further research could improve practice. This review is organized into four areas: descriptive studies; nursing interventions; attitudinal research; and evaluative instruments.

## DESCRIPTIVE STUDIES

### General Studies

Several studies documenting the nursing needs of elderly persons are cited. Health nurses surveyed a 5 percent stratified random sample of noninstitutionalized elderly in DuPage County, Illinois (Managan et al.,

1974). The investigators gathered data on the subjects' health condition, physical functioning, access to medical care, social isolation, and service needs. Survey data identified major problems of functional impairment, lack of a family physician, and social isolation. At the time of the survey 4.2 percent of the subjects were followed by health department nurses, although the survey indicated that 15 percent actually needed service. This represents a large, hidden, underserved population of elderly.

Franck (1979) replicated the DuPage County study in rural Johnson County, Iowa. The findings for all parameters resembled those in the DuPage study. These studies demonstrate the importance of first identifying needs of community elderly so that carefully planned services can then be developed and funding generated.

In another survey study, Hain and Chen (1976) questioned elderly persons living in a high-rise apartment building to identify health needs. The area of most difficulty was in activities requiring ambulation. Those having the most difficulty managing in this type of congregate dwelling were females living alone, constituting a high-risk group within the elderly population.

To determine whether patients over 60 years of age who live at home take their medications as prescribed, Neely and Patrick (1968) replicated an earlier study by Schwartz (1960). The investigators interviewed a 25 percent random sample of persons 60 years of age and older attending a clinic during a particular month. Fifty-nine percent of the sample made errors; half of the errors were omission of a dose. Serious medication errors were related to the number of prescribed medications, the method of remembering to take medications, and the respondent's perceptions of his or her illness as a major problem.

In 1975 Cumming suggested that attention be given to the neurophysiologic findings indicative of disengagement. Edsall and Miller (1978) interviewed 122 residents aged 58–95 years in two high-rise dwellings to obtain measures of social life, perceived life space, and role count, and an index of total disengagement. Additionally, they tested the subjects' hearing and vision. No relationships were found among the variables or between the variables and age or sex.

Henthorn (1979) examined the relationship between disengagement and social reinforcement in 50 nursing home residents and 50 community-based registered voters. A disengagement index included role-set counts, role participation, role importance, and perceived life space. A Reinforcement Survey Schedule was used to identify positive reinforcers, level of reinforcement, and anticipated reinforcement. For both groups, disengagement and reinforcement were strongly related; the greater the degree of disengagement, the lower the reported reinforcement.

Such studies as these contribute to our knowledge of the elderly. Future productive research might include identifying (1) needs of institutionalized elderly from their own perspective, (2) characteristics of families engaged in successful caregiving for an elderly member, and (3) factors influencing health-promoting behavior in the elderly.

**Psychosocial Studies**

Most nursing studies of psychosocial aspects of aging and the aged individual concentrate on institutional residents.

Chang (1978, 1979) reported on generalized expectancy, situational perception, and morale among institutionalized elderly. Thirty residents of four skilled-nursing facilities were studied using scales measuring locus of control, self-reported trust, self-rated health and morale, and perceived situational control of daily activities. Findings of internal orientation and self-determined situational control of daily activities were associated with high morale; whereas, conversely, findings of external orientation and other-determined control over daily activities resulted in low morale. These findings underscore the need to incorporate opportunities for patients to control their own activities in care plans.

Francis and Odell (1979) measured secondary loneliness in a probability sample of 44 persons in a home for the aged. Secondary loneliness was defined as a reactive response to separation from persons and things in which one has invested energy. Subjects were found not to be lonely, as measured by objective measures and their subjective assessment. These data challenge assumptions held by many professionals concerning the emotional state of institutionalized elderly.

Muhlenkamp and co-workers (1975) administered the Holmes and Rahe (1967) Social Readjustment Rating Scale to 41 members of a senior citizens' club, aged 65–84 years. The investigators found significant agreement between elderly subjects and a normative sample with regard to rank ordering of life events; compared with the normative sample, the elderly assigned a greater value to most items.

Although these studies address key issues in gerontological nursing, many other important issues related to the psychosocial characteristics of the elderly need clarification. Some examples include identification of (1) strengths and specific coping strategies in older persons and their families; (2) major psychological factors enabling an old person to live independently; (3) the stresses produced by family caregiving; and (4) cultural variability in dependency expectations associated with illness and age.

### Physical Studies

Surprisingly few nursing investigations of important physical characteristics of the elderly population exist. This gap is especially disturbing when one considers the physical changes which occur with normal aging and the changes secondary to chronic illnesses common in the older population.

Schank and Conrad (1977), interviewing 125 well elderly regarding their podiatric health, reported a 75 percent prevalence of foot problems. Most commonly identified were corns, callouses, toenail abnormalities, bunions, edema, fungus, and poor circulation. A follow-up study delineated an educational program for the prevention and care of foot problems.

Falls were twice as frequent in the early weeks after admission to a small nursing home compared with falls in periods later on in a resident's stay (Feist, 1978). During a 24-hour period, the peak time for falls was 6–9 p.m., when persons were fatigued and preparing for bed. Twenty-six percent of the falls occurred in well-oriented residents, and 57 percent in confused residents; 3.8 percent of the falls led to "major " injuries. Accidents resulting from nighttime fatigue might be prevented by alert nursing staff.

## NURSING INTERVENTIONS

Well designed and controlled experimental studies are imperative. Small samples, inadequate evaluative instruments, and lack of controls for environmental variables plague most studies.

### General Studies

In ten years only two studies based on the nursing process, that is, assessing, planning, intervening, and evaluating care, were found.

Hefferin and Hunter (1975) investigated the effectiveness of a structured patient assessment tool in facilitating clinical judgments and in formulating care plans. Results indicated that use of the tool was positively associated with the number of documented nursing assessments and written plans in the patient record. Secondary analysis showed that planning occurred predominantly for physical rather than psychosocial needs.

Sullivan and Armignacco (1979) evaluated the effectiveness of three nursing approaches on care delivery to the elderly. Matched resident groups in three elderly housing units were assigned to groups differing in the degree of physical and psychosocial assessment and in the level of screening, counseling, and education. Health status measures were obtained before the interventions and after one year. Those residents who received the most extensive nursing program reported more positive health perceptions, utilized health screening programs more appropriately, and were more likely to utilize diagnostic and medical services.

### Psychosocial Outcomes

A number of studies investigated the relationship of nursing activities and psychosocial status. Williams and colleagues (1979) in a nonexperimental design examined postoperative confusion in 91 elderly patients following surgical correction for fractured hips. The most consistent predictor of postoperative confusion was the presence preoperatively of confusion. Less postoperative confusion was associated with mobility, freedom from urinary problems, and use of time pieces and television. The exact relationship of nursing activities to mental status was not discernible. For all parameters, cause and effect relationships were not demonstrated.

In another group of elderly patients undergoing surgery for fractured hips, Lamb (1979) investigated the effect of positioning on postoperative comfort. No significant relationship was found in turning patients away from the operative side and their level of comfort. In fact, half favored lying on the operative side. For this group of patients the need to individualize decisions on positioning based on sleep habits, position preferences, and surgical procedure is clear.

Dittmar and Dulski (1977), investigating the effect of administering early evening sleep medication to 21 elderly hospitalized patients, found, paradoxically, improved daily living activities and more "negative" social behavior. Negative behavior was described as depressed, aggressive, suspicious, rejecting, demanding, hostile, and indifferent. These findings are limited by the small sample size and by serious methodologic problems.

In chronically ill, hospitalized elderly, Brown and Brown (1976) studied the effect of nurse–patient interaction on physical fitness and psychosocial behavior. Patients who received skilled nursing care had longer and more frequent communication with others. The impact of skilled nursing was greatest in the most deprived settings.

Hogstell (1979) administered a three-week reality-orientation program to 20 elderly, confused patients residing in a nursing home. Although no statistically significant difference in the degree of confusion between the experimental group who participated in the program and a control group was found, the experimental group socialized more and their families were pleased with the program.

### Physical Function

Investigations of nursing interventions on physical function of the elderly include the reestablishment of self-feeding in a nursing home (Baltes and Zerbe, 1976), the effect of operant conditioning or modification of incontinence in neuropsychiatric geriatric patients (Grosicki, 1968), the effect of increased dietary fiber content on constipation in nursing home residents (Wichita, 1977), and the effect of timed hygienic measures on oral mucosa of the elderly (DeWalt, 1975). Another study (Pope et al., 1975) demonstrated that a biweekly oral hygiene program (1) successfully prevented extension of gingivitis and (2) increased food intake.

## ATTITUDINAL RESEARCH

Attitudes, knowledge, and expectations of providers and patients alike have been extensively studied.

Thirty randomly selected stroke patients were studied in their homes over a six-month period (Kratz, 1976). Using a grounded theory approach, patient care was shown to be influenced by the knowledge and values of nurses, professional and lay expectations, and organizational constraints. The patient's medical condition was merely one aspect determining the care of these old people with strokes.

Many attitudinal studies reported in the nursing literature have small samples and present conflicting findings (Campbell, 1971; Futrell and Jones, 1977; Gillis, 1973; Taylor, 1978). None assesses the relationship between attitude and quality of nursing care.

Few nursing studies have examined the influence of professional expectations on the care or the health status of older persons; however, Grier (1977) used decision-making theory to plan a study comparing visiting nurses', hospital nurses', and elderly subjects' choices of living arrangements for older patients. Visiting nurses intuitively chose the patient's own apartment, hospital nurses chose the nursing home, and the elderly were divided in their choice of the two living situations. When decision making involved applying numerical values to the expected and desired outcomes of each choice, the three groups had a high rate of agreement in their choices of living arrangements. Certainly, for making important decisions, such an approach is superior to one based upon intuition.

Wilson and Heinert (1977) examined perceptions held by elderly Mexican Americans in rural California about their sociomedical problems. The respondents identified the greatest problems as financial, housing, transportation, legal services, and nutrition. More nursing research is needed to determine the constraints placed by social policy on the availability and distribution of services. To illustrate, we know experientially that the delivery of nursing services in the home is related more to funding guidelines than to patient needs. Documenting unmet service needs is essential to favorably modify the health care delivery system for community elderly.

## EVALUATIVE INSTRUMENTS

The two volumes of *Instruments for Measuring Nursing Practice and Other Health Care Variables* (Ward and Lindemann, 1978) contain 19 instruments relevant to gerontological research. Ten instruments measure psychosocial coping, daily living functioning, or health needs. Others measure the functional competence of the old person, as well as the environmental, human, and social resources available as predictors of (1) institutional care need; (2) pressure sore potential; (3) state of the oral cavity; and finally, (4) perceived impact of sickness on behavior and activities of daily living dysfunction.

Four instruments measuring professional and environmental variables include: (1) attitudes of nursing personnel toward the elderly; (2) attitudes toward the dying; (3) the professional's perceptions of the health needs of the elderly and the degree to which they are met; and (4) nursing home climate.

The lack of instruments, let alone valid and reliable instruments, reflects the immaturity of a gerontological nursing science. Instrument development is a clear priority for future work in the field.

## DIRECTIONS FOR FUTURE RESEARCH IN GERONTOLOGICAL NURSING

Based upon this review of the gerontological nursing literature, the following guidelines and priorities for future research emerge. Descriptive studies of the lives of older persons and their families, specifically focusing on the process of change in their lives and the presence and psychosocial impact of functional impairment, are needed. Other priorities include experimental research testing nursing interventions, research applying theory and findings from other discplines, instrument development, and policy and ethics research.

### Descriptive Studies

Currently, gerontological nursing needs theory-generating (inductive) studies. Much crucial information needs to be collected about the lives of older people and their families, their perceptions of health, functional abilities, and meaning of loss. Little is known about the factors associated with a family's decision to provide care or to institutionalize an older member, or of the capacity of families to cope with an impaired elderly member. To ensure comparability of studies, standardized operational definitions of old age and sampling frames should be used.

### Nursing Interventions

There is a clear need to study the effectiveness of (1) graduated dependence and independence, (2) variation in degrees of sensory stimulation, (3) variation in degrees and kinds of energy expenditure, (4) stress reduction, and (5) disengagement prevention. Better designed studies with larger samples and clear outcome measures are vital.

### Application of Theory from Other Disciplines

Existing data from other disciplines are often not used. To illustrate, available knowledge on the use of color, space, and lighting on preventing and reducing sensory impairment has not yet been adequately tested in the elderly. Furthermore, effects of color and space in different clinical disorders, such as depression and senile brain disease, could be another area investigated. More collaborative research with other disciplines is indicated.

### Instrument Development

The lack of outcome measures for evaluating the effectiveness of interventions is a major obstacle to valid research. The gerontological nurse researcher must develop valid and reliable measures to evaluate the old person's physical and psychological well-being, patient and family coping abilities in the face of declining functional capacity, and the social, psychological, and economic costs of family caregiving.

### Policy Research

Social policy has major impact on health in old age. Researchers must examine to what extent the health care delivery system is meeting the unique needs of the aged population. Specific services, for example, respite services for families caring for old persons with senile brain disease, are needed for certain subgroups of the aged. In the United States funding is a major determinant of services. Hence, research into social policies per se and their impact on the lives of the elderly must be a major thrust of gerontological nursing research.

### Ethical Research

Several crucial ethical issues confronting nurses working with the elderly are (1) respect for persons and the related issue of autonomy; (2) distributive justice; and (3) the quality of life. These issues permeate all decisions about practice and research with the elderly. Identification of the ethical dilemmas in gerontological nursing, and investigation of the decision-making process which occurs when nurses are confronted with specific situations involving ethical dilemmas, are necessary.

## CONCLUSION

To date few well-designed studies have been produced in gerontological nursing. Improved gerontological nurse specialist programs promise a bright future. Well defined nursing interventions need to be tested with reliable and valid measures, taking the various determinants of care into account. From these studies nursing theories will develop which will then trigger research geared toward answering more difficult and complex problems in care of the elderly.

## REFERENCES

Baltes, M., and Zerbe, M. B. Reestablishing self-feeding in a nursing home resident. *Nursing Research*, 1976, *25*, 24–26.

Brimmer, P. F. Past, present and future in gerontological nursing research. *Journal of Gerontological Nursing*, 1979, *5*, 27–34.

Brown, M. M., and Brown, P. R. Nurse-patient interchange in the arrestment of psycho-social atrophy of aged institutionalized patients. *Nursing Research Conference,* 1976, *6,* 1–32.

Campbell, M. E. Study of the attitudes of nursing personnel toward the geriatric patient. *Nursing Research,* 1971, *20,* 147–151.

Chang, B. L. Generalized expectancy, situational perception and morale among institutionalized aged. *Nursing Research,* 1978, *27,* 316–324.

Chang, B. L. Locus of control, trust, situational control and morale of the elderly. *International Journal of Nursing Studies,* 1979, *16,* 169–182.

DeWalt, E. M. Effect of timed hygienic measures on oral mucosa in a group of elderly subjects. *Nursing Research,* 1975, *24,* 104–108.

Dittmar, S. S., and Dulski, T. Early evening administration of sleep medication to the hospitalized aged: a consideration for rehabilitation. *Nursing Research,* 1977, *26,* 299–303.

Edsall, J. O., and Miller, L. A. Relationship between loss of auditory and visual acuity and social disengagement. *Nursing Research,* 1978, *27,* 296–298.

Feist, R. R. A Survey of accidental falls in a small home for the aged. *Journal of Gerontological Nursing,* 1978, *4,* 15–17.

Francis, G., and Odell, S. H. Long-term residence and loneliness: myth or reality. *Journal of Gerontological Nursing,* 1979, *5,* 9–11.

Franck, P. A survey of health needs of older adults in Northwest Johnson County, Iowa. *Nursing Research,* 1979, *28,* 360–364.

Futrell, M., and Jones, W. Attitudes of physicians, nurses and social workers toward the elderly and health maintenance services for the aged: implications for health manpower. *Journal of Gerontological Nursing,* 1977, *3,* 41–46.

Gillis, S. M. Attitudes of nursing personnel toward the aged. *Nursing Research,* 1973, *22,* 517–520.

Grier, M. R. Living arrangements for the elderly. *Journal of Gerontological Nursing,* 1977, *3,* 19–22.

Grosicki, J. P. Effect of operant conditioning on modification of incontinence in neuropsychiatric geriatric patients. *Nursing Research,* 1968, *17,* 304–311.

Hain, M. J., and Chen, S. P. Health needs of the elderly. *Nursing Research,* 1976, *25,* 433–439.

Hefferin, E. A., and Hunter, R. E. Nursing observation and care planning for the hospitalized aged. *Gerontologist,* 1975, *15,* 57–60.

Henthorn, B. S. Disengagement and reinforcement in the elderly. *Research in Nursing and Health,* 1979, 2, 1–8.

Hogstell, M. O. Use of reality orientation with aging confused patients. *Nursing Research,* 1979, *28,* 161–165.

Kratz, C. R. Some determinants of care of patients with stroke who were nursed in their own homes. *Journal of Advanced Nursing,* 1976, *1,* 89–96.

Lamb, K. Effect of positioning of postoperative fractured-hip patients as related to comfort. *Nursing Research,* 1979, *28,* 291–294.

Managan, D. et al. Older adults: a community survey of health needs. *Nursing Research,* 1974, *23,* 426–432.

Muhlenkamp, A. F., Gress, L. D., and Flood, M. A. Perception of life change events by the elderly. *Nursing Research,* 1975, *24,* 109–113.

Neely, E., and Patrick, M. L. Problems of aged persons taking medications at home. *Nursing Research,* 1968, *17,* 52–55.

Pope, W., Reitz, M., and Patrick, M. A study of oral hygiene in the geriatric patient. *International Journal of Nursing Studies,* 1975, *12,* 65–92.

Schank, M. J., and Conrad, D. A survey of the well elderly: their foot problems, practices and needs. *Journal of Gerontological Nursing,* 1977, *3,* 10, 12–14.

Schwartz, D. Nursing needs of chronically ill ambulatory patients. *Nursing Research,* 1960, *9,* 185–188.

Sullivan, J. A., and Armignacco, F. Effectiveness of a comprehensive health program for the well-elderly by community health nurses. *Nursing Research,* 1979, *28,* 70–75.

Taylor, K. H., and Harned, T. L. Attitudes toward old people: a study of nurses who care for the elderly. *Journal of Gerontological Nursing,* 1978, *4,* 43–47.

Ward, M. J., and Lindemann, C. A. (Eds.). Instruments for measuring nursing practice and other health care variables. Hyattsville, Maryland: U.S. Department of Health, Education and Welfare, Health Manpower References, DHEW Publication No. HRA 78-53, 1978.

Wichita, C. Treating and preventing constipation in nursing home residents. *Journal of Gerontological Nursing,* 1977, *3,* 35–39.

Williams, M. A., Holloway, J. R., Winn, M. C., Wolanin, M. O., Lawler, M. L., Westwick, C. R., and Chin, M. H. Nursing activities and acute confusional states in elderly hip-fractured patients. *Nursing Research,* 1979, *28,* 25–35.

Wilson, . S., and Heinert, J. Los viejitos: the old ones. *Journal of Gerontological Nursing,* 1977, *3,* 19–25.

## SELECTED READINGS

Ankenbrandt, M. D., and Tanner, L. K. Role-delineated and informal nurse-teaching and food selection behavior of geriatric patients. *Nursing Research,* 1971, *20,* 61–64.

Baltes, M. M., and Lascomb, S. L. Creating a healthy institutional environment for the elderly via behavior management: the nurse as a change agent. *International Journal of Nursing Studies,* 1975, *12,* 5–12.

Bartol, M. A. Dialogue with dementia. Nonverbal communication in patients with Alzheimer's Disease. *Journal of Gerontological Nursing,* 1979, *5,* 21–31.

Basson, P. H. The gerontological nursing research literature. *Nursing Research,* 1967, *16,* 267–272.

Brimmer, P. F. Past, present and future in gerontological nursing research. *Journal of Gerontological Nursing,* 1979, *5,* 27–34.

Brower, H. T. A study of graduate programs in gerontological nursing. *Journal of Gerontological Nursing,* 1977, *3,* 40–46.

Brown, M. I. Social theory in geriatric nursing research. *Nursing Research,* 1968, *17,* 213–217.

Cumming, E. Engagement with an old theory. *International Journal of Aging,* 1975, *6,* 187–191.

Dufalt, S. K. Recognition of a classic in gerontological nursing. *Journal of Gerontological Nursing,* 1979, *5,* 56–58.

Gioiella, E. C. The relationship between slowness of response, state anxiety, social isolation and self-esteem, and preferred personal space in the elderly. *Journal of Gerontological Nursing,* 1978, *4,* 40–43.

Glaser, B. G., and Strauss, A. L. *The Discovery of Grounded Theory: Strategies for Qualitative Research.* Chicago: Aldine, 1967.

Grier, M. R. Choosing living arrangements for the elderly. *International Journal of Nursing Studies,* 1977, *14,* 69–76.

Gunter, L. M., and Estes, C. A. *Education for Gerontic Nursing.* New York: Springer Publishing Co., 1979.

Gunter, L., and Miller, J.C. Toward a nursing gerontology. *Nursing Research,* 1977, *26,* 208–220.

Hatton, J. Nurse's attitudes toward the aged: relationship to nursing care. *Journal of Gerontological Nursing,* 1977, *3,* 21–26.

Kiesel, M., Sr., and Bininger, C. An application of psycho-social role theory to the aging. *Nursing Forum,* 1979, *18,* 80–91.

Lester, P. B., and Baltes, M. M. Functional interdependence of the social environment and the behavior of the institutionalized aged. *Journal of Gerontological Nursing,* 1978, *4,* 23–27.

Luker, K. A. Measuring life satisfaction in an elderly female population. *Journal of Advanced Nursing,* 1979, *4,* 503–511.

Miller, C., Meier, R., and Feldhusen, J. Measurement of stroke care nursing proficiency. *International Journal of Nursing Studies,* 1974, *11,* 211–222.

Nichols, L. W. A study of sociopsychological needs of institutionalized chronically ill and aging patients. ANA Clinical Sessions, 1970, 82–92.

Nursing Clinics of North America. *Gerontological Nursing,* March 1976, *11,* and December 1979, *14.*

Piotrowski, M. M. Aphasia: providing better nursing care. *Nursing Clinics of North America,* 1978, *13,* 543–554.

Strow, C., and Mackreth, R. Family group meetings—strengthening a partnership. *Journal of Gerontological Nursing,* 1977, *3,* 30–35.

Voelkel, D. A study of reality orientation and resocialization groups with confused elderly. *Journal of Gerontological Nursing,* 1978, *4,* 13–18.

SECTION IV

# Policy and Planning

## CHAPTER 11

# Aging, Retirement, and the Economic Security of the Elderly: An Economic Review

ROBERT L. CLARK, PH.D.
DEPARTMENT OF ECONOMICS
NORTH CAROLINA STATE UNIVERSITY
RALEIGH, NORTH CAROLINA

Changes in mortality and fertility during the past decade have lengthened life expectancy and generated an aging of the population. Past fertility decisions and the anticipation of future relatively low rates of fertility along with mortality improvements have given rise to projections of a continuation of the aging of the population. These events stimulated considerable new research into individual life-cycle decisions as they pertain to the retirement process, the economic responses to the changing population age structure, and ability of the nation to provide for economic security of the elderly. This chapter examines the emerging literature on these interrelated topics from an economic perspective and seeks to identify the principal research questions that comprise the economics of aging.

The aging of the population is reflected in shifts in the relative size of cohorts, which gives rise to a changing age distribution. Increases in the size of the population in the older age groups results in economic responses that influence the welfare of the nation. In addition, there are specific inferences for the income security of the elderly. The cost of public transfers to elderly incidence on the working population rises as the ratio of workers to retirees falls. This review outlines the relationship between the demographic changes and the prospective welfare of older persons.

The demographic pressures threaten the adequacy of income transfers to the elderly. However, the rising costs associated with population aging can be moderated with delayed retirement. The recent trend in labor force participation of the aged is not encouraging on this point. There has been an increasing tendency toward early retirement over the past two decades. The labor force participation rate of males aged 55–64 years has declined from 87 percent in 1960 to less than 74 percent in 1978. Over the same period, the participation rate of men aged 45–54 years declined from 96 to 91 percent. This pattern of early retirement will necessitate even greater taxes to support a given level of income transfers.

One of the principal factors causing this trend toward early retirement has been the increasing generosity of public and private pension benefits. The provision of more adequate retirement benefits, of course, directly raises the total cost of providing these benefits. Costs are increased further as more people choose to withdraw from the labor force and accept pension benefits. Thus, there is a close link between the level of income transfers and the decision to retire, and this relationship becomes increasingly important in an aging population. The research examined in this review identifies these relationships and estimates their importance. One of the most important issues in the economics of aging is whether the trend toward early retirement will continue. Within the projected demographic framework, the answer to this question will determine, in part, the future income security of the older population.

## ECONOMIC RESPONSES TO POPULATION AGING

The aging of the population is illustrated by the increase in the proportion of the population in the older age groups. During this century, the percentage of the population aged 65 years and over has risen from 4 percent in 1900 to 11 percent in 1980. Table 11–1 indicates the current population projections under the assumption that the fertility rate will gradually rise to the replacement level of 2.1 births per woman. These projections indicate that the older population will double by 2020 and rise to over 16 percent of the total population. The fraction of the population aged 65 years and older will further increase to 19 percent in 2055. The projected age structure changes will influence aggregate economic activity to the extent that there are age-specific differences in economic responses and to the degree to which the change in cohort size affects the decisions of individuals at a particular age. A cohort is composed of individuals who were born at approximately the same time, the initial size of which is determined at birth. Thus, the age distribution of the population reflects patterns of annual births and the differential cohort mortality experience. In a country experiencing the aging of its population, successive cohorts at birth would be declining in number. The remainder of this section is devoted to examining the economic responses to population aging.

### The Labor Force and the Dependency Ratio

Low fertility and its concomitant population aging result in a relatively high proportion of the population in the primary working ages. Table 11–1 illustrates the projected trend in the total dependency ratio (population aged 0–20 years plus those age 65 and over divided by the population aged 20–64 years). This ratio is projected to decline until 2010 and by itself would appear to indicate an increase in the productive potential of the population as the size of the working population relative to the total increases during this period. In the demographic literature, the dependency ratio is used to compare the potential well-being of different populations with reductions in this rate being associated with increases in per capita output or income. A series of factors may tend to offset or even reverse this seemingly favorable effect.

*Labor Force Participation.* Clark and Spengler (1980a) indicate that the favorable relationship between population aging and the dependency ratio depends on the ages used to approximate the age of entry into the labor force and retirement. A lower retirement age tends to reduce the advantage ascribed to a lower rate of population growth. The difference between the higher dependency rate with an increasing population and lower rate with a stationary population is reduced as the age of retirement is lowered. Thus, the downward trend in the labor force participation of older workers (U.S. Department of Labor, 1979) during the post–World War II period and its projected continuation (Flaim and Fullerton, 1978) produce a higher dependency ratio than is indicated by the population trends. Obviously, such changes in participation should make one cautious concerning the use and interpretation of the dependency ratio. The determination of a dependency ratio requires the arbitrary selection of ages of entry into and retirement from the labor force. Shifts in these ages are endogeneous in an economic system and can significantly alter the magnitude of the dependency ratio.

*Age Structure Change Within the Labor Force.* The same forces that alter the dependency ratio influence the age composition of the labor force. Slowing population growth reduces the relative number of new entrants into the labor force and increases the number of older workers. This shift will alter the rate of introduction of new human capital, decrease the average physical ability of the labor force, but increase the degree of experience of workers. Studies by Serow (1976), Sweezy and

Table 11–1.
U.S. Population as of July 1 and Dependency Ratios by Broad Age Group, Calendar Years 1975–2055[a]

| | *Population (in thousands)* | | | | *Dependency ratios* | |
|---|---|---|---|---|---|---|
| *Year* | UNDER 20 | 20–64 | 65 AND OVER | TOTAL | AGED[b] | TOTAL[c] |
| 1975 | 77,667 | 121,849 | 23,132 | 222,648 | 0.190 | 0.827 |
| 1976 | 76,860 | 123,861 | 23,630 | 224,351 | 0.191 | 0.811 |
| 1977 | 76,024 | 126,037 | 24,105 | 226,166 | 0.191 | 0.794 |
| 1978 | 75,133 | 128,217 | 24,645 | 227,995 | 0.192 | 0.778 |
| *Projections* | | | | | | |
| 1979 | 74,345 | 130,383 | 25,187 | 229,915 | 0.193 | 0.763 |
| 1980 | 73,660 | 132,506 | 25,756 | 231,922 | 0.194 | 0.750 |
| 1985 | 71,700 | 142,345 | 28,629 | 242,674 | 0.201 | 0.705 |
| 1990 | 73,183 | 148,687 | 31,577 | 253,447 | 0.212 | 0.705 |
| 1995 | 75,811 | 153,914 | 33,611 | 263,336 | 0.218 | 0.711 |
| 2000 | 77,667 | 159,764 | 34,448 | 271,919 | 0.216 | 0.702 |
| 2005 | 77,781 | 166,661 | 35,441 | 279,882 | 0.213 | 0.679 |
| 2010 | 77,950 | 171,929 | 38,160 | 288,039 | 0.222 | 0.675 |
| 2015 | 78,987 | 174,016 | 43,257 | 296,260 | 0.249 | 0.702 |
| 2020 | 80,760 | 173,673 | 49,452 | 303,885 | 0.285 | 0.750 |
| 2025 | 82,338 | 171,999 | 56,118 | 310,456 | 0.326 | 0.805 |
| 2030 | 83,194 | 171,630 | 61,215 | 316,038 | 0.357 | 0.841 |
| 2035 | 83,828 | 174,234 | 62,896 | 320,958 | 0.361 | 0.842 |
| 2040 | 84,855 | 178,039 | 62,548 | 325,443 | 0.351 | 0.828 |
| 2045 | 86,303 | 181,437 | 61,881 | 329,621 | 0.341 | 0.817 |
| 2050 | 87,739 | 183,360 | 62,639 | 333,738 | 0.342 | 0.820 |
| 2055 | 88,857 | 185,102 | 64,232 | 338,191 | 0.347 | 0.827 |

[a]These projections are based on an assumed total fertility rate that rises from 1,793 in 1979 to 2,100 in 2000 and then remains at that level. The fertility rate indicates the number of children ever born to a cohort of 1,000 women. Mortality rates are assumed to decline throughout the period. These projections are the intermediate alternative constructed by the actuaries of the Social Security Administration.

[b]Population aged 65 years and over as ratio to population aged 20–64 years.

[c]Population aged 65 years and over plus population under age 20 as ratio to population aged 20–64 years.

Source: *1979 Annual Report of the Board of Trustees of the Federal Old-Age and Survivors Insurance and Disability Insurance Trust Funds*, p. 98.

Owens (1974), and Ryder (1975) find little relationship between the level of labor force growth and productivity. Other potential effects of these age structure changes include inventiveness, political power, and responsiveness to changing economic conditions (see Clark and Spengler, 1980a).

*Unemployment.* The age-structure changes of the labor force will also influence the unemployment rate. The reduced number of young workers with relatively unstable employment patterns should reduce the level of unemployment associated with full employment. Wachter and Wachter (1978) estimate the increase in the number of youths in the labor force played a major role in the rise in the unemployment rate during the past decade; however, the smaller cohorts entering into the labor foce in the 1980s will tend to lower the rate of unemployment.

*Cost of Young and Old Dependents.* The discussion of the total dependency rate overlooks changes that occur within the dependent groups. Table 11–1 notes that while the total dependency rate is falling, the old-age ratio is steadily increasing. Population aging reduces the nnmber of youths relative to older dependents. These shifts are important because expenditures on youths differ in magnitude and concept from public transfers to the elderly. Clark and Spengler (1978, 1980a) estimate that public expenditures per elderly persons exceed those per youth (perhaps by as much as three-fold). Thus, a declining total dependency ratio does not necessarily imply lower total dependency costs and the related advantages to society. In addition, much of the expenditures on youth that would be reduced are investments in the productive potential of the economy. A reduction in these expenditures would tend to lower the rate of accumulation of human capital in the country.

### Labor Mobility

The mobility and flexibility of the labor force is in part a function of its age structure and rate of growth. Keyfitz (1973) demonstrated that upward mobility or promotional prospects were retarted by population aging, which is caused by a reduction in fertility. A lower rate of fertility increases the number of older workers compared to young employees. This age structure change reduces the opportunity for job advancement. Cantrell and Clark (1979) have shown that declines in labor force participation of older workers partially offset this effect. They also indicate that increasing the age of mandatory retirement will produce only minor delays in promotions (Cantrell and Clark, 1980).

Considerable research indicates that job changes and migration decline with age. For those elderly who do relocate, Serow (1978) finds a higher proportion are returning to the state of their birth than is true for younger migrants. [Also see Yee and van Arsdol (1977) for residential changes.]

### Consumption and Savings

Consumption and savings decisions vary over the life cycle of an individual. However, the extent to which an aging of the population and the slowing of population growth will influence per capita consumption and patterns of expenditures is subject to considerable debate. Ridker (1978) and Espenshade (1978b) conclude on the basis of current research that movement toward a stationary population will not produce a significant change in per capita consumption. Age-structure changes can be expected to alter the demand for specific commodities; however, evidence tends to indicate that the consumption across broad commodity groups will be little affected (Ridker, 1978; Espenshade, 1978a). Of course, firms may attempt to alter the demand for their product by appealing to different segments of the population and by modifying their products.

While there are clear life-cycle patterns of savings, research studies are not uniform in their assessment of the effect of population growth and aging on the rate of savings (Serow and Espenshade, 1978). A related debate concerning the effect of social security financing on savings has recently emerged. Munnell (1974) and Feldstein (1974) first identified that the pay-as-you-go method of financing social secrurity curtailed private saving. Their estimates showed that aggregate savings in the economy fell because individuals reduced their savings and there was no corresponding accumulating of savings in a social security fund. Numerous recent studies have attempted to verify this effect (Barro, 1978; Hemming, 1978; Munnell, 1977; Pogue and Sgontz, 1977); however, most indicate that this effect is statistically insignificant and not robust to alternative econometric specifications (Esposito, 1978).

### Income Transfers to the Elderly

The tax burden on the working population necessary to provide any given level of benefits is a function of the ratio of older beneficiaries to the working population. Concern was expressed in the 1970s for the growth in the proportion of government expenditures on old-age benefit programs (Califano, 1978; Hudson, 1978). Official projections of the future cost increases of social security following the 1972 Amendments (see Board of Trustees Report, various years) gave impetus to the debate over the bankruptcy of this system. The projected cost increases were due to overindexing of future benefits for inflation (Campbell, 1976; Munnell, 1977, pp. 32–38) and the changing worker–beneficiary ratio (Clark, 1977; Rejda and Shepler, 1973). The indexing problem was corrected by legislation in 1977; however, the demographic factors are still expected to force substantial increases in future taxes (Robertson, 1978).

Population aging raises the cost of providing benefits to the elderly and as a result can be expected to increase opposition to higher benefits (Hudson, 1978). Thus, the future age-structure changes make the maintenance of an adequate level of income for the elderly more tenuous (Clark and Spengler, 1980a, pp. 33–40, 157–63; Spengler, 1978). This effect increases the importance of the age of transition from work to retirement. Population aging is conducive to delayed retirement and the deferment of beneficiary status to a later age would significantly lower the cost of retirement benefits (Clark and Spengler, 1980b; Kreps, 1977; Munnell, 1977, pp. 76–77).

## ECONOMIC SECURITY OF THE ELDERLY

Over the past two decades, the economic position of the elderly has substantially improved. The number of individuals aged 65 years and over below the poverty level set by the Social Security Administration has declined from 5.5 million in 1959 to 3.2 million in 1977. As a result, the proportion of older persons in poverty dropped from 35.3 to 14.1 percent during this period (U.S. Bureau of Census, 1978). The income status of the elderly has also improved relative to the rest of the population. The median income of families whose head is 65 years old or over increased from 49.3 percent of the income of all families in 1965 to 58.3 percent in 1976 (U.S. Bureau of Census, 1977; also see Torda, 1972). This improvement is due in part to the growth and development of public and private pensions and to the introduction of new government transfer programs. The effect of these programs on the consumable income of the elderly is clearly shown in Table 11–2, as public tax and transfer programs lower the poverty rate from 59.9 percent to 6.1 percent in 1976.

The level of income and sources of income are a function of age with average incomes falling with age (Grad, 1977; Schulz, 1980, pp. 14–27). Table 11–3 shows Moon's (1977) calculation of income by source for various age groups. Earnings decline in relative importance while social security, other transfers, and property income increase in significance. The importance of social security is shown by the fact that over 90 percent of the persons over 65 years of age receive benefits and that these benefits represented more than half of the annual income of 44 percent of married couples and 65 percent of nonmarried persons who received these payments in 1971 (Grad, 1977). For married couples, 28 percent received income from private pensions and another 16 percent received benefits from other public pensions in 1976. Earnings remain an impor-

Table 11–2.
Families Aged 65 Years and Over Below the Poverty Level Under Alternative Definitions; Fiscal Year 1976

| | Families below poverty level | |
|---|---|---|
| | NUMBER (000) | PERCENTAGE |
| Pretax/pretransfer income | 9,647 | 59.9 |
| Pretax/post-social insurance income | 3,459 | 21.5 |
| Pretax/post-money transfer income | 2,686 | 16.7 |
| Pretax/post money and in-kind transfer income | 977 | 6.1 |
| Post tax/post total transfer income | 982 | 6.1 |

Source: U.S. Congressional Budget Office, *Poverty Status of Families Under Alternative Definitions,* Background paper No. 17 (revised). Washington, D.C.: U.S. Government Printing Office, 1977, p. 12.

tant source of income for many older families with over 40 percent of couples having income from earnings in 1976 (Grad and Foster, 1979). The remainder of this section concentrates on recent research on the nonwage sources of income while the concluding section examines work decisions.

### Social Security

The liberalization and extension of social security benefits have played a major role in improving the economic status of the elderly. Some researchers have argued that many low- and middle-income workers with eligible spouses can achieve a retirement income approximately equal to their preretirement income solely through social security benefits (Feldstein, 1977; Munnell, 1977, p. 26). These estimates of replacement ratios (pension benefits/preretirement earnings) are based on hypothetical earnings histories constructed by the Social Security Administration. Schulz (1978a) argues that these hypothetical replacement ratios do not accurately reflect the actual experience of beneficiaries because they do not recognize life-cycle patterns of earnings and they exclude the wife's earnings from the income base (Fox, 1979). This point is central to the discussion of adequacy of the current social security benefit formula.

Research has been conducted on the economic implications of the characteristics of the social security systems which directly or indirectly affect the economic security of the aged. Some of these are briefly noted below.

Table 11–3
Components of Income by Age of Head, 1972

| *Age of Family head* | *Mean income* | *Sources of income (as percentage of total)* | | | | | |
|---|---|---|---|---|---|---|---|
| | | EARNINGS | PROPERTY INCOME | SOCIAL SECURITY | WELFARE PUBLIC ASSISTANCE | REMAINING TRANSFERS | OTHER INCOME |
| 41–55 | $14,155.19 | 92.26% | 2.99% | 1.39% | 0.55% | 2.18% | 0.91% |
| 56–61 | 12,087.97 | 87.57 | 5.44 | 2.41 | 0.62 | 2.86 | 1.44 |
| 62–64 | 9841.29 | 76.64 | 7.65 | 7.65 | 0.77 | 4.00 | 3.35 |
| 65–69 | 7432.93 | 49.95 | 12.78 | 24.01 | 1.11 | 4.91 | 7.54 |
| 70–74 | 5895.25 | 31.56 | 18.35 | 35.76 | 1.63 | 5.88 | 7.46 |
| 75–79 | 5237.44 | 26.30 | 17.65 | 40.03 | 1.83 | 7.17 | 7.14 |
| 80–99 | 4566.42 | 22.85 | 22.70 | 39.06 | 2.88 | 6.50 | 6.03 |

Source: Moon, M. *The Measurement of Economic Welfare: Its Application to the Aged Poor*. New York: Academic Press, 1977, p. 6.

*Inflation adjustment.* Prior to the 1977 legislation revising the adjustment mechanism, discussion centered on the most appropiate method of indexing past wages in order to prevent a continuous rise in the replacement rate with high rates of inflation (Campbell, 1976; Munnell, 1977). The enactment of the 1977 amendments created a framework that will produce a constant replacement ratio over time. Recently, attention has turned to the advantages of social security with automatic inflation adjustments in comparison to private pensions that generally do not rise with inflation (Munnell, 1980).

*Cost and Method of Financing.* The effect of projected demographic changes on the cost of the system and the projected future tax rates was noted above. Concern has been expressed over whether all of this forecasted tax increase should come from the payroll tax. The debate concerns the incidence of this and alternative taxes and how changes in the tax structure would affect future support for the program (see Friedman, 1977; Munnell, 1977; Okner, 1975; and Pechman, 1977).

*Rate of Return on Taxes.* Workers are required to pay taxes throughout their work life to support the social security system. In retirement they receive a continuing flow of benefits for the duration of their lives. By comparing the taxes paid to the anticipated benefits, implied rates of return can be calculated. Everyone retiring prior to the 1970s has received a very large return to their contributions as the system has matured. Questions have been raised whether future retirees will receive a fair return on their social security "investment." The answer depends on the assumptions used to estimate the returns and differs by the characteristics of the worker (Aaron, 1977; Leimer, 1978). The progressive benefit formula is used to calculate benefits under social security. Thus, lower earnings give rise to higher dollar return. Obviously, then, the longer one lives the more they will receive in benefits. In addition, couples in which only one spouse works receive a higher return than single individuals or dual career families.

*Earnings Test.* The earning test taxes the earnings of individuals who are currently eligible for social security. For individuals aged 62–65 years, the actuarial adjustment from delayed retirement is probably sufficient to offset the taxes on earnings. The bonus for working beyond age 65 is less generous and the tax is therefore more restrictive (Blinder et al., 1979). Thus, the tax lowers potential income for older workers and has produced proposals for its elimination. The tax has been steadily liberalized and the age of its removal lowered to 70 beginning in 1982.

The employment effects of the removal of this tax are examined below; however, it would seem that its elimination would increase the number of older workers. Objections to the abolition of the earnings test have been the cost in extra benefits and the distributional effects. Gordon and Schoeplein (1979) estimate that using the 1982 earnings ceiling adjusted to 1978, the cost of the removal of the earnings test for workers aged 65–69 years for 1978 would have been $2.1 billion. However, they argue that the increase in work effort would raise social security payroll tax revenues by 32 percent of this total while income taxes would be increased by $786 million. Thus, 79 percent of the costs would be offset by higher tax revenues. Schulz (1978b) illustrates that the complete elimination of the earnings test would primarily benefit the high income elderly, but indicates that significant liberalization could occur without this distributional effect.

## Pensions

Coverage by pensions increased from 10 million workers in 1950 to 30 million in 1975, while rising as a percent of wage and salary workers in private industry from 22.5 percent to 46.2 percent (Yohalem, 1977). Replacement rates from private pensions can be in the range of 20–30 percent of final salary (Schulz et al., 1974) and thus for long-tenured workers with a pension in addition to social security their income in retirement may approach their preretirement disposable income. (On adequacy of pension benefits, see Schulz et al., 1974; for a general discussion of pension issues, see Greenough and King, 1976.)

Recent public debate has centered on the impact of the Employee Retirement Income Security Act of 1974 (ERISA) and of inflation on the future of private pensions. Little direct evidence has been examined on the influence of ERISA on the future growth of pensions. This legislation raised the cost of providing pension benefits and therefore may tend to retard further expansion of coverage even while increasing the protection of those already covered (Pension Benefit Guaranty Corporation, 1977).

Inflation erodes the real value of pension benefits that are not adjusted for price increases and makes pension coverage less desirable (Clark and McDermed, 1979; see below). Therefore, continued high rates of inflation may lead to greater support for an expanded role for social security at the expense of private pensions (Munnell, 1980).

## Other Sources of Income

Pension income can be supplemented by the drawing down of accumulated wealth; however, most individuals do not accumulate a significant amount of private savings during their worklife. Grad and Foster (1979) find that 66 percent of older families had income from assets in 1976. The extent of this income has been rather small. Sherman (1973) reported that 19 percent of those in the Retirement History Study (RHS) had an estimated net worth reported to be negative or equal to zero and the net worth of another 30 percent was reported to be less than $10,000. Diamond (1977) argues that inadequate savings is a widespread phenomenon not limited to low-income families.

In-kind benefits have played an increasing role in the income security of the elderly. The largest programs are Medicare, Medicaid, food stamps, and public housing but a large number of other in-kind benefit programs are currently in place (U.S. Congress, House Committee on Aging, 1976). Moon estimates (1977) that in-kind transfers to the aged average more than 10 percent of the mean current money income for aged families. In a later article (Moon, 1979) she critically examines how these programs should be included in assessments of the economic security of the elderly. Her principal point is that in-kind benefits should not be valued at cost for determining the well-being of the recipient because if given cash the individual would not purchase this amount of that commodity.

### Distribution of Income

Grad and Foster (1979) compare the distribution of income for older families and individuals. Table 11–4 illustrates the substantial differences in these income distributions with increasing age (also see Brotman, 1978). Henson (1967) notes that the income of the elderly is more unequally distributed than that for the other age groups. Moon (1977) argues that measures of income levels and distributions should include in-kind benefits, annuitized flow of wealth, and earnings potential. She finds that this procedure reduces the measure of inequality, reorders the income ranking of families, and increases their estimated level of well-being.

### Inflation

Inflation erodes the real value of income streams that do not adjust to reflect the new higher price levels. At present, only limited conclusions can be drawn from previous research concerning the inflation effect on the income of the elderly. Schulz (1980, pp. 46–50) identifies the following five principal ways that the aged may be affected adversely by unanticipated increases in inflation:

1. Assets which do not adjust with inflation depreciate in value.
2. Transfer payment may adjust only with a lag.

Table 11–4
Distribution of Money Income, 1976 in Percent

| | Age and family status | | | | | |
|---|---|---|---|---|---|---|
| | MARRIED COUPLES | | | NON-MARRIED | | |
| Money income | 55–61 | 62–64 | 65 AND OLDER | 55–61 | 62–64 | 65 AND OLDER |
| Less than $3,000 | 4 | 4 | 5 | 31 | 34 | 43 |
| 3,000–4,999 | 5 | 8 | 17 | 18 | 20 | 30 |
| 5,000–6,999 | 6 | 10 | 21 | 11 | 13 | 15 |
| 7,000–9,999 | 11 | 13 | 20 | 14 | 12 | 8 |
| 10,000–14,999 | 20 | 23 | 19 | 14 | 12 | 5 |
| 15,000–19,999 | 22 | 18 | 9 | 6 | 5 | 2 |
| 20,000 or more | 35 | 23 | 10 | 5 | 3 | 1 |
| Median income | $16,490 | $12,750 | $7,890 | $5,260 | $4,450 | $3,360 |

Source: Grad, S., and Foster, K. "Income of the Population Aged 55 and Older, 1976." *Social Security Bulletin*, July 1979, pp. 22–23.

3. Earnings may lag behind prices.
4. Real tax burden may rise.
5. Elderly persons may allocate their budget differently from others. Thus, CPI-adjusted benefits may not fully compensate for increased prices.

The income of the elderly from social security and many of the in-kind benefit programs is largely insulated from decline due to inflation. Questions remain over whether the current adjustment mechanism employing the consumer price index is sufficient (Borzilleri, 1978); however, most evidence indicates that this is not a major problem in maintaining the income of the elderly. Also, an index based solely on the aged may be more inequitable for some older persons than the use of the current CPI (Michael, 1979).

Pension benefits are the source of income of the elderly that is most vulnerable to inflation. Few private pension plans automatically increase benefits with inflation (Hodgens, 1975; Tilove, 1976). Thus, inflation can significantly erode the real value of these benefits (Thompson, 1978). Future research is needed to determine the extent of the sensitivity of the various income sources of the elderly to fluctuations in the rate of inflation. For example, have ad hoc pension adjustments been sufficient to maintain the real value of retirement benefits or have the assets of the elderly risen in value enough to offset the effects of inflation?

## RETIREMENT

This review summarizes the current state of the economic literature in three interrelated areas. Earlier, it was shown that the economic security of the elderly through public transfer programs is affected by population aging and by the age of transition from work to retirement. Table 11–5 illustrates significant income differences among older families depending on their employment status. Thus, the early withdrawal from the labor force is associated with lower incomes for the elderly and greater support costs on the working population. This section reviews the factors that influence the decision to withdraw from the labor force. The available evidence indicates that efforts to raise retirement income through pensions and other transfer methods directly affect the retirement decision, thus exacerbating the cost of these programs. Therefore, the reader should recognize the clear linkage across these three topics in the economics of aging.

### A Framework for Retirement

The decision to terminate one's career and withdraw from the labor force is an important life-cycle decision that is influenced by social, economic, psychological, and physiologic factors. The economic literature identifies the existence and magnitude of pension benefits along with individual health as being the most important factors determining the probability of retirement. This review examines the recent research attempting to explain retirement decisions. Most of these studies employ labor force participation as the measure of labor supply or retirement; however, some use hours of work or receipt of pension benefits. The format of this review is to examine separately the evidence relating to factors that influence the retirement decision and then to integrate them into an overall assessment of the retirement process.

### Social Security

The magnitude of social security benefits has consistently been found to be an important and significant factor influencing the retirement decision. Using the Panel Study of Income Dynamics, Boskin (1977) concludes that a rise in annual social security benefits from $3,000 to $4,000 for a couple increases the annual probability of retirement from 7.5 to 16 percent. Quinn (1977) employed the Longitudinal Retirement History Study (RHS) conducted by the Social Security Administration to determine the

Table 11–5
Median Income in 1977 by Age, Sex, and Work Status

| | *55–59* | *60–64* | *65–69* | *70 and over* |
|---|---|---|---|---|
| Males | | | | |
| All | $13,612 | $10,511 | $6,516 | $5,007 |
| Year round full-time workers | 15,981 | 15,200 | 14,536 | 11,722 |
| Females | | | | |
| All | 5,398 | 3,769 | 3,040 | 3,108 |
| Year round full-time workers | 8,990 | 8,556 | 8,107 | 7,257 |

Source: U.S. Bureau of the Census. "Money Income and Poverty Status of Families and Persons in the United States: 1977," *Current Population Reports*, Series P-60 No. 116 (advanced report). Washington, D.C.: U.S. Government Printing Office, 1978, p. 16.

effect of current eligibility for benefits on labor force participation. He argues that individuals who are currently eligible for social security benefits are 15–20 percent less likely to be in the labor force than those who are not currently eligible.

The expansion in coverage of social security, the liberalization of benefits, and the significant lifetime income transfers to past retirees has probably been one of the principal factors causing the decline in the labor force participation of older men. Burkhauser (1976) argues for the use of the present value of social security benefits as the most appropriate measure of the effect of the anticipated benefit stream. He reports that social security variables account for 8.8 percentage points of the 15 percentage point decline in the participation rate of men aged 60–64 years since 1957.

The earnings test combined with payroll and income taxes may result in a substantial marginal tax rate for older persons (Blinder et al., 1979; Tolley and Burkhauser, 1977). For example, Tolley and Burkhauser (1977) estimate that a married worker earning the median wage would face a tax rate of 73 percent on earnings. Boskin (1977) finds that a decrease in the earnings test from 50 percent to one-third would lower the annual probability of retirement for the typical worker by one-half. The liberalization of the tax over time should have moderated its effect in the labor market. Burkhauser and Turner (1978, 1980) indicate that the alteration of market wage rates late in life can influence work decisions earlier in life.

### Private Pensions

In order to receive a pension benefit, a worker must leave a particular employer. While this does not necessitate the withdrawal from the labor force, the wage offered by other employers may be below the previous wage and the worker will have lost any seniority protection. These factors and other difficulties involved in finding new employment encourage individuals from leaving the labor market. Burkhauser (1979) finds that members of the United Automobile Workers Union responded to changes in the value of their pensions. Quinn (1977) finds that the effect of private pensions is to reduce participation; however, this effect is less than that of social security and falls mostly on those with health limitations.

### Mandatory Retirement

Mandatory retirement requires that workers terminate their employment with a particular firm at a specified age. By forcing relocation, this institution could be expected to reduce labor force participation. The extent of this effect has not been clearly identified. In a review of survey data, Schulz (1980) and Halpern (1978) find that the use of mandatory retirement at age 65 may have lowered the participation of a group of male workers by four to ten percentage points (also see Reno, 1976). Several current studies are attempting to estimate the effect of the 1978 Amendments to the Age Discrimination in Employment Act which raised the minimum permissible age of mandatory retirement from 65 to 70.

### Health

Health impairments may reduce a worker's productive potential and thus lower the wage offers he receives. In addition, such ailments may make work more onerous and increase the desire of the individual to remain at home. Virtually all studies have found health to be an important determinant in individual retirement decisions. The RHS data show that 65 percent of those males who had withdrawn from the labor force responded that health was the primary reason for leaving their last job (Schwab, 1974) and that health is also a principal cause of early retirement for women (Sherman, 1974).

Parnes and co-workers (1975) found that among men in the National Longitudinal Survey, those who had health problems in 1966 were twice as likely to have retired between 1966 and 1971 as men who had no health impairments. Analysis of the same data indicated that health-related problems were a primary determinant of retirement prior to age 65 (Bixby, 1976). Quinn (1977) supports these findings and concludes that the effect of pensions and social security falls mostly on those with health limitations.

### Wages

The evidence concerning the effect of wages on the retirement decision is less certain. Quinn (1977) finds no significant correlation between labor force participation and the wage of the worker; however, he finds a negative effect on the hours of work. Parnes and co-workers (1975) also fail to find a significant correlation between wages and retirement. Contradictory evidence is found by Boskin (1977), who reports a large positive result, and by Burkhauser (1979) and Clark, Johnson, and McDermed (1980).

Few studies have included the earnings of the spouse in a labor supply equation. Boskin (1977) finds a negative effect of the wife's earnings on the probability of the husband retiring. Clark, Johnson, and McDermed (1980) estimate a model of simultaneous labor force participation of a married couple. They find that increases in the husband's wage lowers the probability of his wife remaining in the labor force. However, the presence of a wife in the labor force raises the probability of the husband's being in the work force.

### The Retirement Decision

Current knowledge indicates that pension characteristics and health are the primary factors governing retirement. Quinn (1977) suggests strong interactive effects, with the social security effect being five times greater for those with a health limitation. It has also been suggested that early retirees can be divided into two groups: (1) retirees who are characterized by good health, sufficient financial resources, and a desire for increased leisure and (2) retirees with health problems sufficient to restrict their market activity (Parnes et al., 1975). A final observation is that the causes of retirement may change as a cohort ages, with health declining as a reason for leaving the job and pension-related factors increasing in importance (Bixby, 1976; Reno, 1976).

### References

Aaron, H. Demographic effects on the equity of social security benefits. In M. Feldstein and R. Inman (Eds.), *The Economics of Public Services*. London: Macmillan Press, 1977, pp. 151–173.

Barro, R. *The Impact of Social Security on Private Savings*. Washington, D.C.: American Enterprise Institute Studies, 1978.

Bixby, L. Retirement patterns in the United States: research and policy interactions. *Social Security Bulletin*, August 1976, *39*, pp. 3–19.

Blinder, A., Gordon, R., and Rise, D. Reconsidering the work disincentive effects on social security. Unpublished paper, May 1979.

Board of Trustees of the Federal Old-Age and Survivors Insurance and Disability Insurance Trust Funds. *1979 Annual Report.*

Borzilleri, T. The need for a separate consumer index for older persons. *The Gerontologists,* June 1978, *18,* pp. 230–236.

Boskin, M. Social Security and retirement decisions. *Economic Inquiry,* January 1977, *15,* pp. 1–25.

Brotman, H. Income and poverty in the older population in 1975. *The Gerontologist,* June 1977, *17, 23–26.*

Burkhauser, R. The early pension decision and its effect on exit from the labor market. Unpublished Ph.D. dissertation, University of Chicago, Chicago, Illinois, 1976.

Burkhauser, R. The pension acceptance decision of older workers. *Journal of Human Resources,* Winter 1979, *14,* pp. 63–75.

Burkhauser, R. and Turner, J. A time series analysis on social security and its effect on the market work of men at younger ages. *Journal of Political Economy,* August 1978, *86,* pp. 701–716.

Burkhauser, R. and Turner, J. The effects of pension policy across life. In R. L. Clark (Ed.), *Retirement Policy in an Aging Society.* Durham, North Carolina: Duke University Press, 1980.

Califano, J. The aging of america: questions for the four generation society. *Annals of the American Academy of Political and Social Science,* July 1978, *438,* pp. 96–107.

Campbell, C. *Over-indexed Benefits: The Decoupling Proposals for Social Security.* Washington, D.C.: American Enterprise Institute, 1976.

Cantrell, S. and Clark, R. Implications for retirement age policy and population change on individual promotional prospects. Unpublished paper, North Carolina State University, Raleigh, North Carolina, 1979.

Cantrell, S. and Clark, R. Retirement policy and promotional prospects. *The Gerontologist,* October 1980, *20,* pp. 575–580.

Clark, R. Increasing income transfers to the elderly implied by zero population growth. *Review of Social Economics,* April 1977, *35,* pp. 37–54.

Clark, R. and McDermed, A.A. Inflation, pension benefits and retirement. Unpublished paper, North Carolina State University, Raleigh, North Carolina, 1979.

Clark, R. and Spengler, J. Changing demography and dependency costs. In B. Herzog (Ed.), *Income and Aging.* New York: Human Science Press, 1978.

Clark, R. and Spengler, J. *Economics of Individual and Population Aging.* New York: Cambridge University Press, 1980a.

Clark, R. and Spengler, J. Economic responses to population aging with special emphasis on retirement policy. In R. L. Clark (Ed.), *Retirement Policy in An Aging Society.* Durham, North Carolina: Duke University Press, 1980b.

Clark, R. Johnson, T. and McDermed, A.A. Allocation of time by married couples approaching retirement. *Social Security Bulletin,* April 1980, *43,* pp. 3–17.

Diamond, P. A framework for social security analysis. *Journal of Public Economics,* December 1977, *8,* pp. 275–298.

Espenshade, T. How a trend toward a stationary population affects consumer demand. *Population Studies,* March 1978a, *32,* pp. 147–158.

Espenshade, T. Zero population growth and the economies of developed nations. *Population and Development Review*, December 1978b, *4*, pp. 645–680.

Esposito, L. Effect of social security on savings: review of studies using U.S. time series data. *Social Security Bulletin*, May 1978, *41*, pp. 9–17.

Feldstein, M. Social security induced retirement, and aggregate capital accumulation. *Journal of Political Economy*, October 1974, *82*, pp. 905–926.

Feldstein, M. Facing the social security crisis. *The Public Interest*, Spring 1977, *47*, pp. 88–100.

Flaim, P., and Fullerton, H. Labor force projections to 1990: three possible paths. *Monthly Labor Review*, December 1978, *101*.

Fox, A. Earnings replacement of retired couples: findings from the retirement history study. *Social Security Bulletin*, January 1979, *42*, pp. 17–39.

Freidman, M. Payroll taxes, no; general revenues, yes. In M. Boskin (Eds.), *The Crisis in Social Security*. San Francisco: Institute of Contemporary Studies, 1977, pp. 25–30.

Gordon, J. and Schoeplein, R. Tax impact from repeal of the retirement test. *Social Security Bulletin*, September 1979, *42*, pp. 22–32.

Grad, S. *Income of the Population Aged 60 and Older, 1971*, SSA, Office of Research and Statistics, Publication No. (SSA) 77-11851, Staff Paper No. 26. Washington, D.C.: U.S. Government Printing Office, 1977.

Grad, S. and Foster, K. Income of the population aged 55 and older, 1976. *Social Security Bulletin*, July 1979, *42*, pp. 16–32.

Greenough, W. and King, F. *Pension Plans and Public Policy*, New York: Columbia University Press, 1976.

Halpern, J. Raising the mandatory retirement age: its effect on the employment of older workers. *New England Economic Review*, May 1978, pp. 23–35.

Hemming, R. State pensions and personal savings. *Scottish Journal of Political Economy*, June 1978, *25*, pp. 135–147.

Henson, M. *Trends in the Income of Families and Persons in the United States: 1947–64*, U.S. Bureau of Census, Technical Paper No. 17, No. NSF/RA-770024. Washington, D.C.: U.S. Government Printing Office, 1967.

Hodgens, E. Key changes in major pension plans. *Monthly Labor Review*, July 1975, *98*, pp. 22–27.

Hudson, R. The "graying" of the federal budget and its consequences for old-age policy. *The Gerontologist*, October 1978, *18*, pp. 428–440.

Keyfitz, N. Individual mobility in a stationary population. *Population Studies*, July 1973, *27*, pp. 335–352.

Kreps, J. Age, work, and income. *Southern Economic Journal*, April 1977, *43*, pp. 1423–1437.

Leimer, D. Projected rates of return to future social security retirees under alternative benefit structures. *Policy Analysis With Social Security Research Files*, U.S. Department of Health, Education, and Welfare. Washington, D.C.: U.S. Government Printing Office, 1978.

Michael, R. Variations across households in the rate of inflation. *Journal of Money, Credit, and Banking*, February 1979, *11*, pp. 32–46.

Moon, M. *The Measurement of Economic Welfare: Its Application to the Aged Poor*. New York: Academic Press, 1977.

Moon, M. The incidence of retirement among the aged. *Journal of Human Resources*, Spring 1979, *14*, pp. 211–221.

Munnell, A. *The Effect of Social Security on Personal Saving*. Cambridge, Massachusetts: Ballinger, 1974.

Munnell, A. *The Future of Social Security*. Washington, D.C.: The Brookings Institution, 1977.

Munnell, A. The impact of inflation on private pensions. In R.L. Clark (Ed.), *Retirement Policy in an Aging Society*. Durham, North Carolina: Duke University Press, 1980.

Okner, B. The social security payroll tax: some alternatives for reform. *Journal of Finance*, May 1975, *30*, pp. 567–578.

Parnes, H., Adams A., Andrisani, P., Kohen, A., and Nestel, G. *The Preretirement Years*, vol. 4. Manpower Research and Development Monograph No. 15, U.S. Department of Labor. Washington D.C.: U.S. Government Printing Office, 1975.

Pechman, J. The social security system: an overview. In M. Boskin (Ed.), *The Crisis in Social Security*. San Francisco: Institute of Contemporary Studies, 1977, pp. 31–39.

Pension Benefit Guaranty Corporation. *Analysis of Single Employer Defined Benefit Plan Terminations, 1976*. Publication No. PBGC505, 1977.

Pogue, T. and Sgontz, L.G. Social security and investment in human capital. *National Tax Journal*, June 1977, pp. 157–170.

Quinn, J. Microeconomic determinants of early retirement: a cross-sectional view of white men. *Journal of Human Resources*, Summer 1977, *12*, pp. 329–346.

Rejda, G. and Shepler, R. The impact of zero population growth on the OASDHI program. *Journal of Risk and Insurance*, September 1973, *40*, pp. 313–325.

Reno, V. Incidence of compulsory retirement policies. *Reaching Retirement Age*, SSA, Research Report No. 47, pp. 53–64. Washington, D.C.: U.S. Government Printing Office, 1976.

Ridker, R. The effects of slowing population growth on long run growth in the U.S. during the next half century. In T. Espenshade and W. Serow (Eds.), *The Economic Consequences of Slowing Population Growth*. New York: Academic Press, 1978.

Robertson, A. H. Financial status of social security programs after the Social Security Amendments of 1977. *Social Security Bulletin*, March 1978, *41* pp. 21–29.

Ryder, N. Notes on stationary populations. *Population Index*, January 1975, *41* pp. 3–28.

Schulz, J. Pension adequacy and pension costs. *Aging*, January 1978a, pp. 14–21.

Schulz, J. Liberalizing the social security retirement test: who would receive the increased pension benefits. *Journal of Gerontology*, March 1978b, *33*, pp. 262–268.

Schulz, J. *The Economics of Aging*. Belmont, California: Wadsworth, 1980.

Schulz, J., Currin, G., Krupp, H., Paschke, M., Sclar, E., and Steenberg, J. *Providing Adequate Retirement Income*. Hanover, New Hampshire: University Press of New England, 1974.

Schwab, K. Early labor force withdrawal of men: participants and nonparticipants aged 58–63. *Social Security Bulletin*, August 1974, *37* pp. 24–38.

Serow, W. Slow population growth and the relative size and productivity of the male labor force. *Atlantic Economic Journal*, Spring 1976, *4*, pp. 61–68.

Serow, W. Return migration of the elderly in the United States: 1955–60 and 1965–70. *Journal of Gerontology*, March 1978, *33*, pp. 288–295.

Serow, W. and Espenshade, T. Economics of declining populations growth. In T. Espenshade and W. Serow (Eds.), *The Economic Consequences of Slowing Population Growth*. New York: Academic Press, 1978.

Sherman, S. Assets on the threshold of retirement. *Social Security Bulletin*, August 1973, *36*, pp. 3–17.

Sherman, S. Labor force status of unmarried women on the threshold of retirement. *Social Security Bulletin*, September 1974, *37*, pp. 3–15.

Spengler, J. Population aging and security of the aged. *Atlantic Economic Journal*, March 1978, *6*, pp. 1–7.

Sweezy, A. and Owens, A. The impact of population growth on employment. *American Economic Review*, May 1974, *64*, pp. 45–50.

Thompson, G. Pension coverage and benefits, 1972. *Social Security Bulletin*, February 1978, *41*, pp. 3–17.

Tilove, R. *Public Employee Pension Funds*. New York: Columbia University Press, 1976.

Tolley, G. and Burkhauser, R. Integrating social security into an incomes policy. In G. Tolley and R. Burkhauser (Eds.), *Income Support Policies for the Aged*. Cambridge, Massachusetts: Ballinger, 1977.

Torda, T. The impact of inflation on the elderly. *Federal Reserve Bank of Cleveland Economic Review*, October 1972, pp. 3–19.

U.S. Bureau of the Census. Money income and poverty status of families and persons in the United States: 1976. *Current Population Reports*, Series P-60, No. 107 (advanced report). Washington, D.C.: U.S. Government Printing Office, 1977.

U.S. Bureau of Census. Money income and poverty status of families and persons in the United States: 1977. *Current Population Reports*, Series P-60, No. 116 (advanced report). Washington, D.C.: U.S. Government Printing Office, 1978.

U.S. Congress, House Select Committee on Aging. *Funding of Federal Programs Benefiting Older Persons: Hearings Held June 15–16, 1976*, 94th Congress, 2nd Session. Washington, D.C.: U.S. Government Printing Office, 1976.

U.S. Congressional Budget Office. *Poverty Status of Families Under Alternative Definitions*, Background paper No. 17, (revised). Washington, D.C.: U.S. Government Printing Office, 1977.

U.S. Department of Labor. *Employment and Training Report of the President*. Washington, D.C.: U.S. Government Printing Office, 1979.

Wachter, M. and Wachter, S. The fiscal policy dilemma. In T. Espenshade and W. Serow (Eds.) *The Economic Consequences of Slowing Population Growth*. New York: Academic Press, 1978.

Yee, W. and van Arsdol, M. Residential mobility, age and the life cycle. *Journal of Gerontology*, March 1977, pp. 211–226.

Yohalem, M. R. Employee-benefit plans, 1975. *Social Security Bulletin*, November 1977, *40*, pp. 19–28.

## CHAPTER 12

# Long-Term Health Care Planning: The State of the Practice

STANLEY J. BRODY, J.D., M.S.W.
SAUL M. SPIVACK, M.S.
DEPARTMENT OF PHYSICAL MEDICINE AND REHABILITATION
SCHOOL OF MEDICINE UNIVERSITY OF PENNSYLVANIA
PHILADELPHIA, PENNSYLVANIA

The current debate on long-term health care and support is divided by provider and consumer preceptions of health and social needs. Planning for long-term care has gone forward within the context of these considerations.

The topic of this chapter is system-level planning for long-term care. Long-term care is defined as:

> . . .those services designed to provide diagnostic, preventive, therapeutic, rehabilitative, supportive and maintenance services for individuals of all age groups who have chronic physical and/or mental impairments, in a variety of institutional and noninstitutional . . . care settings including the home, with the goal of promoting the optimum level of physical, social and psychological functioning [Task Force on the Organization and Delivery of Human Services, 1977, p. 3].

The term *system* is used in the sense of a set of parts coordinated to accomplish a common goal (Churchman, 1968). Systems thinking necessitates a focus upon goals, from which flow consideration of the environment, structure, resources, and service units as well as on the nature of the service units' activities, performance, and interrelationships. Clear articulation of goals has been a critical problem in developing a long-term care system.

*System level* refers to the focus of planning. There are six contexts in which health and social planning are customarily performed: individual (as in treatment planning and case management), organizational, community, regional system, state, and national. The level addressed in this review is planning at the regional-system level, involving a holistic orientation to all elements of the target group, together with delivery and financing systems and their relationship to the environment and other systems. This planning is performed at the scale of either the geographic/economic market area or that of the epidemiologic scale of the health problem (Saward, 1975). Such areas are of a scale to enable effective interventions and significant rationalization of care production and delivery. They generate demand sufficient to support an integrated system of regionally organized primary, secondary, and tertiary resource specialization.

An additional distinction should be made between program (also termed *categorical* or *segmental*) and comprehensive planning. Program planning refers to ends-oriented design of a specified course of action for a prescribed problem. Comprehensive planning is holistic; it begins with broad-based problem analysis and encompasses all program categories.

Planning is defined in Freidmann's terms as "the guidance of change within a social system" (1967, p. 227). To focus on planning as a design process to achieve the system's goals requires the addition of the phrase "toward conceived future states" to the end of his definition. Since a review of planning literature reveals little consensus on definitions, theories, or typologies, the definition is broadly conceived. Conceptions of the purpose, scope, strategy, and elements of planning activity differ across disciplines and among individuals. Since planning is a process directed toward the design and achievement of some future state (Ackoff, 1970), various disciplines have different perceptions as to the content of planning theory. Additionally, planning is an activity which may be performed at all levels of social organization, from the future-anticipating behavior of the individual to the long-range designs of nations.

Planning and policy are symbiotic activities. If policy is seen as "a purposeful course of action" (Anderson, 1975, p. 3), planning both guides and implements policy choices. Indeed, planning and policy analysis are viewed by many as virtually identical (Klarman, 1976). In Freidmann's (1967) perspective, any given planning activity may be characterized on a continuum from adaptive (decisions heavily contingent upon other external entities) to developmental (high degree of autonomy in ends and means determination). Activities at the developmental end resemble policymaking, and those close to the adaptive end, program planning. The degree to which planning resembles policymaking is related to whether it is developmental in nature and to the degree of autonomy the organization has with respect to establishing ends and selecting means. To use Ozbekhan's (1974) hierarchical construct, planning at the normative (designing what "ought" to be) and strategic (goal-setting) levels is essentially policy development. Indeed, some planning agency products are solely "policies plans." Hence, it is difficult and perhaps pointless to establish boundaries between planning and policymaking except to note that planning is more often focused upon operationalizing policy.

## A BRIEF HISTORY OF HEALTH AND SOCIAL PLANNING PROGRAMS AFFECTING LONG-TERM CARE

The traditional separation between health and social care financing and delivery has been reflected in planning programs. While comprehensive, system-level health planning did not begin until the 1960s, categorical health planning is not a new phenomenon. Organized public and private activities aimed at improving some aspect of health have existed for at least a century. These efforts have usually been undertaken within the rubric of public health and focused upon the environment, specific diseases, or certain age groups (Kissick, 1970). Most of the concern has been for the young since the major health problem, infectious disease, primarily affected mortality of that group. Public efforts on behalf of children were initiated at the beginning of this century with maternal and infant care programs and were reaffirmed in 1936 with the enactment of the Social Security Act's Title V programs. These efforts achieved a large degree of success, contributing to increases in life expectancy at birth.

In the 1940s, the orientation toward children was augmented by attempts to improve acute medical care for all age groups and to make it widely available. The initiation of a program of construction grants for hospitals in 1946 under the Hospital Survey and Construction Act (P.L. 79–725, the Hill-Burton program), the creation of the National Institutes of Health, and efforts to stimulate medical practice specialization are examples of such efforts. The purpose of the Hill-Burton program was to support hospital (and in subsequent amendments outpatient facility and nursing home) construction and modernization by providing grants to states for matching funds and loan guarantees. It established state agencies whose principal functions (inventorying resources, determining bed need, priority setting for the use of funds among facilities, and providing technical assistance) were planning and administration.

The 1960s represent a period of legislative activity which radically altered the nature of the American health care system. Health legislation passed in 1965 reiterated the emphasis on acute care. The Medicare and Medicaid programs (Titles XVIII and XIX added to the Social Security Act in 1965, P.L. 89–97) were primarily concerned with making acute medical care available to the elderly and the poor. Medicare represented a reaction to the needs of the increasing proportion of young elderly (age 65–75). The Regional Medical Program (RMP), established by the Heart Disease, Cancer and Stroke Amendments of 1965 (to Title IX of the Public Health Service Act, P.L. 89–239), is often misperceived as a planning effort. In actuality, it was a categorical medical-school-centered technology transfer program responsible for adapting treatment and delivery innovations from major medical centers to practitioners and community hospitals. The legislation charged the RMP with regionalizing and improving services but clearly established it as a research and educational program.

Public comprehensive health planning at the system level was only formalized in 1966. Several localities had evolved voluntary health planning agencies, health facilities councils, or United Way–sponsored planning efforts by the 1950s (Krause, 1977; Thompson, 1975). However, health planning in its modern form was not widespread until implementation of the Comprehensive Health Planning and Public Health Service Amendments Act of 1966 (P.L. 89–749). The Act is also noteworthy as the first attempt to reverse the modus operandi of categorical programming and resultant delivery system fragmentation by integrating autonomous health delivery programs into a block grant (Title XV of the Public Health Service Act). The health planning infrastructure created by the Act consisted of state and regional Comprehensive Health Planning (CHP) agencies under federal supervision. Their purpose was to conduct voluntary (noncompulsory) planning with the health industry toward the goals of developing needed services, organizing delivery, and rationalizing the health care system. The CHP agencies had the mandate to address all aspects of the environment and the delivery system which have an impact on health. They were required to approve the construction of medical facilities (including nursing homes) which requested federal construction grants. This mandate was rhetorical in the sense that the CHP agencies were advisory and had no enforcement powers except for the approval of construction using federal grants.

The CHP program experience could be characterized as the initial step at establishing health planning, as a period of learning, and/or a disappointing experiment in voluntary planning. Since it was the first experience at regionalized health planning, the program was a learning period for program design, planning strategies, and methodologies and for exploring relationships among participants in the planning process. The diverse state and regional instrumentalities provided the structure and experience upon which the succeeding planning system was based.

The CHP program was a disappointment in the sense that the "experiment" in voluntary planning and self-regulation by health care providers with the input of consumers (epitomized by the program's slogan "Partnership for Health") did not prove to be a viable strategy. The experience has been characterized in the literature as "one of frustration coupled with intermittent successes" (West and Stevens, 1976, p. 174). This has been attributed variously to exogenous factors such as inadequate appropriations by Congress, opposition by physicians and health providers (e.g., the hospital and nursing home industries), lack of community support to balance health care providers, jurisdictional conflicts with other governmental bodies, inability to obtain data from providers, inadequate authority, and unenforceable sanctions for implementing plans and regulatory decisions.

The CHP agencies themselves have been criticized on various counts: for overemphasis on medical facilities planning and project review; for failure to set priorities for agency planning; for weak implementation programs; for failure to develop health plans; for inadequate levels of applied research and analysis in support of planning; for deficiencies in technical capabilities; for having few trained middle-management personnel; and for lack of attention to the health status of the population (Attkinsson and Grimes, 1976; General Accounting Office, 1978; Klarman, 1976; Waters, 1976; West and Stevens, 1976).

The CHP agencies were perceived by analysts as unable to overcome the obstacles to effective planning (Ardell, 1974; Attkinsson and Grimes, 1976; General Accounting Office, 1978; Klarman, 1976; West and Stevens, 1976) posed by the degree to which organized medicine and the health industry had influenced the legislation. The purpose section of the legislation (termed the "AMA clause") made the perimeters of the planning effort clear:

> . . . to support the marshalling of all resources—national, state and local—to assure comprehensive health services of high quality for every person, but without interference with existing patterns if private professional practice of medicine, dentistry, and related healing arts [Section 2(a), P.L. 89–749, 1966].

The desire for voluntary cooperation in planning reflected the congruence of physician and health industry desire to escape control. It also expressed society's continued reliance upon medicine and the health industry for self-regulation and attempts by policymakers to employ a market-perfecting strategy instead of a centralized regulatory and prescriptive response.

The CHP program was characterized by great expectations without the means to implement them. Health planning agencies lacked the ability and authority to ensure conformity to its decisions and plans. The implementation of this comprehensive planning venture was based on strategies for eliciting voluntary compliance with plans and recommend actions. Health planning agencies had no official sanctions until 1972, when amendments to Titles XVIII and XIX of the Social Security Act (Section 1122 of P.L. 92–603) gave states power to deny Medicare and Medicaid reimbursement for depreciation and other costs related to construction of an unapproved facility (P.L. 92–603). Some states gave regional CHP agencies a review and comment function in this program. There was no other relationship between planning and reimbursement except for isolated local Blue Cross Association requirements for the compliance of member hospitals with CHP dicta.

Cost became an overriding issue during the 1970s. Annual personal health expenditures had increased from $25.9 billion in 1960 to $106.3 billion in 1974 (Gibson and Fisher, 1978). As part of the congressional effort to control costs, physicians were asked in 1972 to self-regulate through peer review in the form of the Professional Standards Review Organization (PSRO) program (P.L. 92–603). The passage of new planning program legislation in 1974 (P.L. 93–641, The National Health Planning and Resources Development Act, Titles XV and XVI of the Public Health Service Act) recognized the failure of the CHP market-perfecting strategy but retained voluntary cooperation as an integral component of health planning.

Congressional intent for P.L. 93–641 was clear: "increases in the cost of health care, particularly of hospital stays . . ." (P.L. 93–641, Section 1502) were to be controlled. While the preamble of the Act expressed a concern for health care quality and accessibility, the short-term functions established for health-planning agencies were primarily concerned with the cost of medical facilities. Skilled Nursing Facilities (SNFs) and Intermediate Care Facilities (ICFs) were defined within the medical facility category.

The significance of P.L. 93–641 lies in its adoption of the idea that successful planning requires imposition of controls on the health system and that planning agencies must have enforcement powers to achieve significant change. The 1974 law placed all acute medical care planning in a single federal-state-regional structure. The CHP program was terminated and RMP phased out, although some of RMP's features were included in the new Act. Hill-Burton was redesigned and limited mostly to inpatient facility modernization, outpatient facility construction, and conversion of facilities to new uses. Hill-Burton functions were placed within P.L. 93–641's state-level organizations.

In this system, a new federal agency to administer the program, the Bureau of Health Planning, was created in the Health Resources Administration of the Department of Health and Human Services. In each state, a State Health Planning and Development Agency (SHPDA), supervised by a State Health Coordinating Council (SHCC), was to carry out activities for states and work with the Health Systems Agencies (HSAs) of the state. The SHPDA is responsible for development and implementation of a five-year State Health Plan, loosely based upon these of the HSAs. While the federal government was given the authority to designate and monitor HSAs, the SHPDA represented the state as the ultimate authority in the major regulatory programs for capital expenditures review.

At the regional level, one or more HSAs (originally nominated by governors and appointed by the Secretary of Health, Education and Welfare) develop and implement health plans. Their areas range from 200,000 to 3,000,000 population. The U.S. is divided into 204 HSAs. The HSAs assist states in conducting capital expenditures regulatory programs: Certificate of Need (CON) and Section 1122. The initial state of the regulatory process of these programs is an HSA function. The SHPDA conducts an independent process after the HSA has completed its recommendations and intercedes if the provider chooses to appeal the HSA's findings in a process characterized as a combination of "trial de novo and an appeal from the HSA decision" (Bovbjerg, 1978, p. 89). States may also choose to regulate rates for institutional health services. In the Proposed Use Service of Federal Funds program, HSAs and SHCCs approve or disapprove uses of funds from the Public Health Services Act (P.L. 78–410), the Mental Retardation Facilities and Community Mental Health Centers Construction Act (P.L. 88–164), the Comprehensive Drug Abuse Prevention and Control Act (P.L. 91–513), and the Comprehensive Alcohol Abuse and Alcoholism Prevention, Treatment and Rehabilitation Act (P.L. 91–616). The SHCC, using the SHPDA as staff, examines only state-level funds applications and has the power to approve or reject categorical state agency plans for health, mental health, and alcohol/drug abuse services. The HSA examines grants, contracts, loans, and loan guarantees which are to be used for development or support of services in its area.

Health planning agencies' repertoire of coercive powers for realizing planning goals is limited to regulating capital investment in health resources through evaluation of proposed capital expenditures under the CON, Section 1122, and Proposed Use of Federal Funds programs.

Most sanctions of the capital expenditures review programs consist of denial of federal construction money loan guarantees, reimbursement for operations, and/or reimbursement of depreciation. Through such programs, the health planning agencies regulate the creation or termination of services, capital investment in health facilities or expensive medical equipment, and the award of funds for certain federal health programs. Decisions are based upon health plans and the merits of the case.

Health planning agencies also conduct "Appropriateness Review" programs, which assess the appropriateness of institutionally based health services (the degree to which they meet certain criteria relative to health plans) in areas such as performance, cost, inefficiency, duplication, quality, and population need. Appropriateness Review is at present advisory and may make public only findings regarding the appropriateness of services in the aggregate.

The social system has its own history of planning efforts. Under the Social Security Act, social services were governed by state categorical Public Assistance plans and administered at the state and local levels. There were no mechanisms for comprehensive planning. There have been a series of attempts at planning for categorical groups; mental health and retardation, children and youth, juvenile delinquency, and geographic low-income areas (i.e., Model Cities) are but a few examples in addition to the state plans required for each of the Social Security Administration categorical public assistance programs.

The Older Americans Act represents the first attempt at comprehensive planning for older people. Its enactment in 1965 (P.L. 89–73) created federal and state agencies. The Administration of Aging (AOA) was charged with developing special programs as well as conducting research and training activities. State agencies received funds to develop plans which would be the basis for community planning and coordination, providing funds to community agencies for social services specified in the Act, reviewing and coordinating all state-level activities for the aging, and training necessary personnel. State agencies developed short-range plans for the allocation of their funds to service providers.

Amendments in 1973 mandated the states to designate substate "planning and service areas" (Section 305 (a) (1) (E), P.L. 93–29), each administered by an Area Agency on Aging (AAA) for the purposes of advocacy, short-range program planning, coordination, and maximizing the allocation of funds to providers serving the aged. These agencies range in service area size from municipality or single county to several counties. There are 560 such areas, 61 percent of which are part of a public agency and 40 percent private nonprofit organizations (National Association of Area Agencies on Aging, 1978).

The AAA is charged with developing a coordinated service system for purposes of access (transportation, outreach, information and referral, escort, case management), community support (congregate meals, legal services, advocacy, day care), home care (home-delivered meals, homemaking, heavy chore, home maintenance), and assistance to Residential Care Facility clients (casework, counseling, complaint and grievance resolution, placement and relocation assistance). The AAA develops an area plan which assesses need for services, evaluates effectiveness of service providers, and allocates funds among services. It enters into contracts with service providers that are based upon the plan. The AAA is the chief advocate for the elderly at the community level and monitors or comments upon all policies, programs, and activities which affect older persons in its area.

The AAA planning function received heavy emphasis in the 1978 Amendments (P.L. 93–29). The Amendments and their implementation regulations required greater technical sophistication in formulating plans and a higher degree of rationality in the AAA planning process. The Amendments also represent the first formal attempt at coordinating the activities of health planning and aging planning agencies, mandating the aging agencies to develop linkages with their respective health-planning instrumentalities.

Historically, planning of mental health services was left to state governments. The Community Mental Health Center Act of 1963 (P.L. 88–164) initially provided funds for construction of Community Mental Health Centers (CMHCs). Subsequent enactments broadened CMHC functions and the required development of programs specifically for the elderly. The CMHCs are fundamentally service providers; mental health planning is performed at the local level of catchment area, paralleling the aging program, as well as at the state level. State mental health departments are required to develop plans. Recognizing the need to integrate mental health into health planning, the 1979 Amendments to the health planning act (P.L. 96–79) require state mental health plans to be reviewed by a health planning instrumentality, the State Health Coordinating Council.

Any discussion of planning systems for the health of the aged would be incomplete without mention of the Veterans Administration (VA). The VA may be considered the largest autonomous comprehensive health delivery system in the United States, providing income maintenance, inpatient and outpatient medical care, rehabilitation, and most of the elements of a long-term support/care system for veterans. Over 60 percent of all males over age 65 will be veterans during the 1980s and, by VA standards, will be eligible for services (Veterans Administration, 1977). The VA conducts its own planning; other agencies, including the HSAs, have no jurisdiction over VA programs or facilities. Such facilities represented 6.8 percent of all general medical and specialty hospital beds (over 94,000) and 1.4 percent of all skilled and intermediate level nursing home beds (19,700) in the United States during 1977 (Veterans Administration, 1977).

In a strict application of our definition, only health planning agencies and the VA (within its own closed system) engage in system-level comprehensive planning. Area Agencies on Aging (with a few exceptions in

Pennsylvania and Wisconsin) are primarily community program planning organizations for allocating Older Americans Act funds and developing the capacity of service providers. Even within their categorical scope, not all AAAs have hegemony over funds of the Older Americans Act nor those earmarked for the elderly from other sources. One-third of AAAs also allocated Title XX monies for elderly services; some have small amounts of ACTION, Comprehensive Employment Training Act, and Urban Mass Transit Assistance Funds.

When last surveyed in 1978, only 11.1 percent of the AAAs viewed their area plans primarily as planning tools. The remainder perceived them as either primarily compliance documents prepared to meet state and federal requirements or combinations of compliance and planning (National Association of Area Agencies on Aging, 1978).

### Status of Long-Term Health Care Planning

Much of the responsibility for long-term health care planning has accrued to HSAs and SHPDAs because most publically funded long-term health care services are within the medical model. Health planning agencies' frame of reference and chief responsibilities are medical and health services, principally those which are institutionally based. Medicare, Medicaid, and the Health Planning Act all define nursing homes as medical facilities. Health planners view individual services as delivered within a care setting (physical site). They distinguish between medically oriented institutions (hospitals, rehabilitation facilities, nursing homes, and some hospices) and ambulatory care settings (outpatient departments, physicians' offices, health centers, day care/day hospitals), for which they have primary responsibility, as opposed to socially oriented settings. Such social settings include residential environments (semi-institutional facilities below the ICF or personal care level such as boarding or domiciliary care), congregate and other housing arrangements, private homes (which receive in-home services); and organized social programs (social-model day care).

Health planning agencies have no specific directive to plan for long-term health care other than to establish performance standards for regulatory decisions. It was not a congressional priority at the time the health-planning program was enacted or amended, reflecting the severity of cost inflation in the acute-care sector.

The impetus to plan for long-term health care comes from the HSAs' or SHPDAs' consideration of the needs of special population groups during the plan development process. Health Systems Agencies are designed to be responsive to the concerns and needs of their regions. Their governing bodies, standing committees, and ad hoc task forces must be composed of local health care providers and consumers. The law requires HSA governing bodies to have a minimum of 51 percent and a maximum of 60 percent consumer membership, representative of the racial and socioeconomic makeup of the area. These bodies have some latitude in selecting areas for agency activity. The SHPDAs are governed by State Health Coordinating Councils, which also have consumer majorities. Consequently, grassroots initiative has occurred in many agencies.

Health planning agencies' conceptions of models for future long-term systems vary widely. The health planning process within the HSA is political in nature. The provider–consumer decision makers on the HSAs' Boards of Directors reflect a complex of values. Accordingly, each HSA's perception of strategy for health system change reflects judgments as to which planning issues are politically amenable to resolution (Palmer, 1978; Spivack and Ryan, 1979). However, many decisions may be related to the HSA's choice of the medical-model, imposed by federal guidance or a locally perceived medical-social model integration. As a result, many HSAs have avoided articulating models of a future long-term care system. All agencies place substantial emphasis upon Skilled Nursing Facility (SNF), Intermediate Care Facility (ICF), and personal care nursing homes but seldom include lower levels of facility care such as domiciliary care or rest homes. Most address medical-model home health services, the majority plan for them in a highly limited fashion. A minority plan for in-home social support services, adult day care, hospice/terminal care, or congregate living. Medical rehabilitation, a prime concern of elderly who are afflicted with chronic disability, is conspicuously absent from 90 percent of plans (Brody and Woodfin, 1979; Spivack and Ryan, 1979). If the most effective interventions in caring for the elderly and disabled must be sustained over long periods and be preventive in nature, then the maintenance of functional and social independence is a primary goal. Many agencies have missed this goal of long-term health care.

In planning for long-term health care systems, health planning agencies are confronted with phenomena which are outside their experience and beyond their authority. Long-term care requires developmental implementation of comprehensive life support and health care systems. Many of these elements are not perceived as health resources nor as institutionally based delivery systems. A long-term care capability requires a close integration of a diverse range of services which belong to the mental health and social service sectors. This sets the planner against structural phenomena beyond the agency's powers of resolution.

At present, the health care system cannot provide the appropriate mix of services and personnel necessitated by the life support function of long-term care nor can it address all factors which influence health mobility and disability. Long-term care requires attention to concerns which lie outside current models of medical and health delivery: environment, economic resources, social integration, the family, mental health, physical mobility, and instrumental needs.

The resources required to create a long-term health care system are funded at the national level under a variety of autonomous categorical programs. The HSA must integrate services from programs with differing funding, administration, eligibility criteria, and benefits. Housing, social services, transportation, and other programs are not included in the instrumental authority given to the agency. The planning function is divorced from agencies which administer, regulate, and finance the programs which generate use of health resources. Most of the forces shaping long-term health care have not been placed under HSA control and remain fragmented among independent agencies at both state and federal levels.

The SHPDAs and HSAs cannot address the forces causing long-term health care system inadequacies directly. They cannot effect the necessary structural changes in that sector of the health industry primarily concerned with long-term care nor provide financial incentives to alter health industry priorities and stimulate change. Health planning agencies are unable to alter a number of other factors, such as health budgets of state or local governments; behavior of other sectors of the economy which increase health care costs; patterns of demand for care; medical personnel cost consciousness; and physician specialty, location, and referral patterns (Bauer, 1978). Another crucial problem is the health planning agencies' inability to influence state and local regulatory agencies whose independent activities may conflict with overall policy intent and implementation of planned change (Lipkind, 1979).

The strategies available for implementing health plans reflect the indirect means available to HSAs and SHPDAs for achieving change. Such strategies are primarily rational and normative in nature (persuasion advocacy, collaboration, community/provider organization, and the customary range of technocratic approaches) and secondarily directive/coercive (regulation or threat of regulation). The principal directive/coercive tool is capital expenditures review, particularly the Certificate of Need (CON) program. Most CON programs were enacted by states in response to the requirements of P.L. 93–641. Through certificate of need, HSAs and SHPDAs control the creation or termination of services or programs, capital investment in facilities, and purchase of "major" medical equipment. The scope of long-term care coverage of CON programs is inconsistent. All state CON legislation regulates SNF and ICF level nursing home care, chronic disease hospitals, and rehabilitation hospitals, but only 28 included home health services in 1980.

The HSAs also control the award of funds for certain federal health programs. In addition, health planning agencies determine the "appropriateness" of existing services and use these findings in planning. They cannot, however, directly terminate a service found to be "inappropriate." The health planning act also reinforces state authority to establish rate-setting programs for institutional services which are federally reimbursed.

Capital expenditures review and Appropriateness review are essentially reactive as well as coercive; that is, they are designed to respond with approval or disapproval to a change proposed by the providers of care or to the suitability of existing institutional services. Essentially, the primary proactive implementation tool currently available to the health planning agency is the persuasive power it is able to exercise through the legitimacy of its plan and the political support it is able to develop among the provider and consumer communities in its health service area.

The current repertoire of implementation strategies encourages disjointed incrementalism and discourages systems approaches. Indeed, the principal intent of the health planning regulation is cost containment; the control of aggregate program expenditures. Planning is not linked with existing state regulation of provider charges, personnel liscensure, professional performance, institutional quality, or health insurer activities. It must achieve cost control by controlling supply of health services, expensive technologies, and facility beds. Capital expenditures review is the available tool for regulating each.

The underlying rationale for supply regulation is that, operating in the context of open-ended funding for medical services, the most effective strategy for cost containment in a supply-induced demand situation is controlling resource input to the system. The health care market is highly segmented and lacks price as a factor in competition. The supply of resources to be consumed plays the major role in cost escalation. This phenomenon is demonstrated by the experience with hospitals; despite excess beds and underutilized, costly high-technology medical equipment, hospitals are able to recover costs either through the intricacies of cost-based reimbursement by third parties or because bed supply induces further demand. A similar effect holds for physicians in that it is the supply of physicians rather than the health status of the population that determines the amount of care delivered in a given area (Klarman, 1969; McClure, 1976; Roemer and Shain, 1959).

The supply issue is somewhat different in long-term care. Supply-induced demand operates in the same fashion in the nursing home industry since SNF and ICF funding is open-ended. Demand, however, is not governed by medical need, but rather by the availability of funding for institutional care and the concurrent absence of funding for community-based services within the context of the changing demography of the elderly population. Demand is usually greater than supply in most areas. Cost escalation results more from additional elderly being institutionalized and inflation in the general economy (e.g., for labor) than from phenomena intrinsic to the nursing home industry. The principal problem as perceived by state and federal government is to slow the increasing spending for nursing home care by controlling the supply of beds.

The number of SNF/ICF beds may directly affect the availability of funds for other services within the long-term care continuum. If public funding allocated to the long-term care system is finite, then the share of those monies spent for nursing home beds consumes funds available for other services such as home care.

In pursuing their goal of controlling the amount expended for long-term health care, funding agencies look to the control of SNF/ICF beds as the primary means of cost containment. Medicaid has become the chief source of payment for long-term care. Forty-eight percent of all SNF and ICF patients (86.4 percent of whom were aged 65 years and over) relied on Medicaid as their primary or only source of payment, at a cost of $7.2 billion in fiscal year 1978 (General Accounting Office, 1979). This level of fiscal support for long-term care also has a significant impact on state Medicaid budgets. Data from fiscal year 1978 show that 19 states spent more than 50 percent of their Medicaid budgets solely on nursing home per diem charges; another 37 spent more than 40 percent. In most cases long-term care represents more than one-third of total state Medicaid expenditures. Reimbursement for home health services represented only one percent of fiscal 1978 expenditures (General Accounting Office, 1979).

Consequently, planning is focused upon need assessment and supply allocation. Unlike acute care, where need for a service results from a definable onset of a medical condition, the need for nursing home care is relatively ambiguous. Any given individual's "need" to be in a nursing home results from a complex of health, social, and economic factors. Nursing homes are long-term residential environments which maintain persons with permanent functional disabilities. While nursing home patients require medical and nursing care or supervision, patient needs are principally for personal care and mental health services and assistance in instrumental activities and social/recreational pursuits. Thus, an objectively determined calculation of need for beds is not yet a prescribed matter. The variability of even professional perceptions of need has been well documented (Sager, 1978, 1979). The difficulty is also apparent in the range in the numbers of beds per 1,000 elderly deemed necessary by health planning agencies to accommodate their areas. Much of this variation cannot be accounted for solely by differences in population disability levels.

A rational decision-making process in planning entails careful need and resource assessment, development of performance criteria and standards for services and facilities, financial and economic analyses, and optimal resource allocation among geographic areas, population groups, and levels of care. However, the supply issue has become so politicized that bed need determination has moved squarely into the realm of budgetary and political processes. A state seeks to develop supplies tailored to its budget while balancing the contradiction between the two points of objective need and demand. Bed supplies established by objectively determined need criteria can leave many elderly without care if other services in the long-term health care continuum are not provided. Yet accommodating demand is perceived as unacceptably expensive. States also limit long-term care expenditures by restricting eligibility for Medicaid, limiting per diem reimbursement rates, or "capping" total expenditures for long term health care.

Experience to date has been that almost all existing "reasonable" estimations of need are lower than demand. The often arbitrary nature of some states' bed supply targets reflect attempts at achieving a balance between these two points. Final responsibility for decision making lies within SHPDAs. In those states which have a longer history of CON activities, the state agency has adopted uniform statewide criteria for making decisions about expanding the supply of nursing home beds. In some states HSAs have been able to exercise sufficient political pressure to demand a role in developing statewide CON criteria. Where HSAs have not been able to participate effectively in that process, there are often conflicts in CON decisions made by the HSA and the SHPDA. In other states, the methodologies for determining nursing home bed needs are not consistent statewide. The HSA has greater latitude in matching its regulatory decisions to planning policy.

The weak link in both of these situations is the validity and accuracy of the needs-assessment methodology. Inadequate data, poorly developed planning approaches, and analytically unsupportable CON criteria cause HSAs to be uncomfortable with assessments of nursing home bed need.

Adjustments to objectively determined need for beds occur frequently in the HSA deliberations. The analyses of HSA staff are often adjusted by technical committees or governing bodies based upon political judgments as to the degree to which the supply should be reduced, expanded, or replaced. Public opinion is also a force, and existing regional use patterns are resistant to change. There are numerous instances in which bed supply targets were increased above those considered appropriate by HSA staff because of consumer demand for more nursing home beds.

Yet another perceived means of lowering the future level of demand for nursing home care is through the development of noninstitutional care services. It is alleged that pressure for nursing home expansion could be reduced by channeling demand to residential care settings and in-home services without harmful effect. The exact substitutability of noninstitutional care for faculty care has not been established. Health planners' perceptions range in magnitude from 5 percent to 20 percent of SNF patients and 20 percent to 40 percent at the ICF level, dependent upon local conditions and state criteria for level-of-care determinations. Future substitution may occur through use of noninstitutional care to postpone nursing home admission and thus lower total patient days of care demanded in a given area. In an undetermined but relatively small number of cases, community care may completely substitute for nursing home use.

Noninstitutional care is viewed by other health planners as constituting underdeveloped services which would complement institutional care and are essential in their own right in order to create a comprehensive long-term health care system. These services are needed to help many noninstitutionalized people to function at better levels of health and well-being. Definition of these community services, their precise quantities, care capabilities, and relationships within a delivery system are topics of ongoing debate.

Apart from demonstration projects, however, comprehensive care systems do not yet exist. The supply of residential settings is limited or nonexistent in some areas, medical model home care benefits are themselves highly limited, and in-home personal care, housekeeping/homemaking, and social services are grossly inadequate relative to need.

The health planning agencies cannot develop home health care, home-delivered social support services, day care, hospices, or residential settings. Many of existing services are outside health planning control. Noninstitutional care provided through the Older Americans Act and Title XX (Social Security Act) funds are not subject to HSA planning but are part of AAA or other agency resources. Yet these services are, at a minimum, health related and function as health service substitutes, and their absence has an impact upon use of health resources.

## THE TASK OF RESOLVING THE HEALTH-SOCIAL DICHOTOMY

Clearly HSA, SHPDA, and AAA long term care system planning and development activities lie on the adaptive end of the Freidmann's (1967) continuum. The dichotomy between health and social services may well lie at the heart of planning agencies' inability to relate effectively to long-term health care. The health-social polarity is common to developed countries (Pinker, 1980). It is manifested in separate health and social delivery systems, neither of which is capable of the comprehensive response to the chronic-care needs of the elderly.

The major federal health programs have developed separate financing and delivery structures. Financing, control, and administration of these medical delivery systems have, in the main, been centralized. Both Medicare and the British health insurance program, for example, are federally administered and funded, with universal eligibility and benefits. Medicaid programs are state administered but must conform to federal criteria and standards. Social programs, however, are administered by state, province, or municipality, with resultant variability in funding, eligibility, benefits, and administration. Medical services for the aged are universally available while eligibility for social and health-related services is restricted by means tests.

The health/medical system is substantially funded and enjoys a significantly higher acceptance from older people than the minimally funded social service system. The salary structures within each system reflect the public's willingness to pay medically oriented personnel at higher levels than those providing social services. The HSAs, representing the medical system, are designated, funded, and controlled by the federal government. The AAAs, representing the social sector, are designated by states. Their funding, even if partially federal in origin, is routed through state government.

Health in the United States is narrowly defined. Preventive and therapeutic interventions are principally medical in nature by contrast with a broader definition, which places health and long-term care in a social context. Dubos (1959, 1968) reflects this broader approach in equating health with an ability to adapt in terms of level of function acceptable to the individual and his referent group. Evans (1980) describes the British Health and Social Service system's goal for the elderly as enabling

> . . . old people suffering from physical or mental disability to live where they would wish to live if they were not disabled. . . . The aid of assessment, treatment and rehabilitation services is to improve their functioning to a maximum consistent level and if this is still inadequate we must reduce the demands of the environment [p. 1].

Clearly, such a goal requires an integration of primary health and medical care as well as mental health and social services.

Three possible auspices have been proposed for the requisite health–

social model synthesis. One would be an autonomous entity drawing resources from both systems based on the individual's primary need. The other options are to place the long-term health care responsibility within an expanded health system or to lodge it in a remodeled social service structure. There have been a variety of attempts to integrate the health and social services planning efforts in the past eight years. Congress recognized the desire of local communities to plan and develop service delivery systems since the federal government declined to assume responsibility for interdisciplinary planning for health of the aged. Through amendments to Medicare and Medicaid (Sections 222 and 1115 of the Social Security Amendments of 1972, P.L. 92–603, respectively), Congress authorized local demonstration efforts to provide long-term care. Existing requirements for long-term care benefits were waived and payment was permitted for new types of community services. The value of these demonstrations lies in their role of financing and delivery-system experiments. The data they generate can be used in long-term health care planning, and they provide a few localities with an opportunity to develop community-based long-term care systems. A number of other projects have been undertaken and are currently being evaluated.

A number of other demonstration projects are being undertaken, funded by the Health Care Financing Administration (HCFA) and AOA (Benedict, 1980; Fox and Clauser, 1980). The AOA and HCFA collaboration in establishing "channeling" projects is the most notable. Channeling demonstrations are designed to test strategies to coordinate health and social services, to promote appropriate care setting placements through the application of assessment and case management mechanisms, to determine how existing long-term care resources may be effectively managed, to limit inappropriate hospital and nursing home use, and to use in-home and other community care services to the fullest extent.

The eventual adoption of the long-term health care definition quoted at the beginning of this chapter may not create the requisite health–social model synthesis nor an integrated delivery system. Rather, it may serve to expropriate social care into the health system in an analogous fashion to the concept of medicalization developed by Zola (1972) and expanded by Fox (1978). In this process, medical and health personnel "generalize their expertise beyond technical matters" (Zola, 1977, p. 21), and the medical/health sector expands its jurisdiction over a wider domain of life. Health system delivery is feasible by virtue of its existing consumer acceptance and pervasive influence on society's approach to long-term health care. The health system has an established physical plant and delivery system with the financing, administrative, and control structures lacking in the social service sector. Existing efforts at expanding long-term care benefits through Medicare, Medicaid, and the proposed Title XXI are indications of possible health system capture of long-term care functions. It is notable that a health agency, the Health Care Financing Administration, is taking the lead in community-based long-term health care demonstration and research.

As HSAs expanded their role in planning for long-term health care, it became evident to policy analysts that AAAs had a major contribution to make in such planning.

Several studies have indicated that many HSAs were approaching their task of planning for comprehensive long-term care from a systems perspective which required the involvement of social system organizations (Brody and Woodfin, 1979; Spivack and Ryan, 1979; Wall, 1979). The roles and achievements of HSAs have received attention at the 1979 and 1980 annual meetings of the American Health Planning Association, the American Public Health Association, and the Gerontological Society. The Administration on Aging recognized the significance of this potential interface by suggesting to AAAs that they participate in HSA planning efforts. Currently, significant collaboration between HSAs and AAAs in planning occurs only in isolated instances. Recognizing this, the AOA authorized research to examine current practice and make recommendations for developing HSA–AAA relationships.

Equally significant are trends in the hospital industry. The acute care hospital, currently the principal setting for health service delivery in the United States, is becoming involved in long-term health care. Following the lead of many hospitals which have already taken steps to expand their acute medical focus, the American Hospital Association has initiated educational efforts on the role of hospitals in providing health and social services for the elderly. This will reinforce the dominance of the hospital as the principal community organization serving older people.

These health-sector initiatives reaffirm the truism that delivery systems evolve within the context of historical patterns, in this case America's corporate response to social problems (DeTocqueville, 1945). The most universally available entity providing care to the elderly in the United States is the acute care general hospital system consisting of 5,842 non-federal short-term general hospitals (American Hospital Association, 1980), and the 144 Veterans Administration hospitals (Veterans Administration, 1977). In 1979, approximately 5 million persons aged 65 years and over were hospitalized at least once, for a total of over 10 million admissions, comprising 38.8 percent of the inpatient days. Hospital outpatient utilization is also considerable, with almost 25 percent of elderly persons making at least one visit per year, for a total of 10 million visits (Brody, 1979). Clearly, these inpatient and outpatient episodes represent a large proportion of the formal health and social services provided to the elderly.

In light of these events, it appears likely that the direction of future planning for the elderly in the United States will be toward the health model as HSAs, SHPDAs, and AAAs will be unable to resolve the health-social dichotomy. The articulation of a clear federal resolution of long-term care seems delayed by the AOA/HCFA strategy choice of continued demonstration projects. The uncertain future stance of Congress contributes to this sense of impounded policy. However, the adoption of long-term health care goals for maximizing the level of functioning of the disabled depends equally on societal attitudes on the quality and the quantity of the extended life span. In the intervening time, states and localities are left to their own devices in filling the vacuum.

## REFERENCES


Ackoff, R. L. *A Concept of Corporate Planning.* New York: Wiley–Interscience, 1970.

American Hospital Association. *American Hospital Association Guide to the Health Care Field: 1980 Edition.* Chicago: American Hospital Association, 1980.

Anderson, J. E. *Public Policy-Making.* New York: Praeger, 1975.

Ardell, D. B. The demise of CHP and the future of planning. *Inquiry,* 1974, *11* (3), 233–235.

Attkinsson, A. A., and Grimes, R. M. Health planning in the United States: an old idea with a new significance. *Journal of Health Politics, Policy and Law,* 1976, *1,* 295–318.

Bauer, K. *Cost Containment Under P.L. 93–641: Strengthening the Partnership Between Health Planning and Regulation, Final Report* (NTIS Publication No. HRP-0900132). Hyattsville, Maryland: Bureau of Health Planning and Resources Development, 1978.

Benedict, R. AOA's approach to long-term care. Washington, D.C.: Administration on Aging, May 1980.

Bovbjerg, R. Problems and prospects for health planning: the importance of incentives, standards and procedures in certificate of need. *Utah Law Review,* 1978, *83,* 83–121.

Brody, S. J. The greying of america. *Hospitals,* 1979, *54* (10), 63–66, 123–124.

Brody, S. J., and Woodfin, A. B. *Long-term Support Systems: An Analysis of Health Systems Agency Plans.* Philadelphia: National Health Care Management Center, 1979.

Churchman, C. W. *The Systems Approach.* New York: Delta Books, 1968.

DeTocqueville, A. *Democracy in America.* New York: Heritage Books, 1945.

Dubos, R. *Mirage of Health: Utopias, Progress and Biological Change.* New York: Harper and Row, 1959.

Dubos, R. *Man, Medicine and Environment.* New York: Praeger, 1968.

Evans, J. G. Care of the aging in Great Britain: an overview. Paper presented at the Anglo-American Conference on New Patterns of Medical and Social Supports for the Aging, Fordham University, New York, May 12–13, 1980.

Fox, P., and Clauser, S. *Long-term Care for the Aged and Chronically Disabled.* Washington, D.C.: National Commission on Social Security, 1980.

Fox, R. The medicalization and demedicalizations of American society. *Daedalus,* 1978, *106,* 9–22.

Freidmann, J. F. A conceptual model for the analysis of planning behavior. *Administrative Science Quarterly,* 1967, *12,* 225–252.

General Accounting Office, Comptroller General of the United States. *Status of the Implementation of the National Health Planning and Resources Development Act of 1974* (GAO Publication No. HRD–77–157). Washington, D.C.: General Accounting Office, 1978.

General Accounting Office, Comptroller General of the United States. *Entering a Nursing Home—Costly Implications for Medicaid and the Elderly* (GAO Publication No. PAD–80–12). Washington, D.C.: General Accounting Office, 1979.

Gibson, R. M., and Fisher, C. R. National health expenditures, fiscal year 1977. *Social Security Bulletin,* 1978, *41* (7), 3–20.

Kissick, W. Health policy directions for the 1970's. *New England Journal of Medicine,* 1970, *282,* 1343–1354.

Klarman, H. E. Approaches to moderating the increases in medical care cost. *Medical Care,* 1969, *7,* 175–190.

Klarman, H. E. National policies and local planning for health services. *Milbank Memorial Fund Quarterly,* 1976, *54* (1), 1–28.

Krause, E. A. *Power and Illness: The Political Sociology of Health and Medical Care.* New York: Elsevier, 1977.

Lipkind, L. Health systems agency long-term care planning and the regulatory system: cooperation or conflict. In S. Spivack (Ed.), *State of the Practice Review of Health Systems Planning for the Elderly.* Boston: Boston University Center for Health Planning, 1979.

McClure, W. *Reducing Excess Hospital Capacity.* Minneapolis: Interstudy, 1976.

National Association of Area Agencies on Aging, personal communication, 1978.

Ozbekhan, H. Thoughts on the emerging methodology of planning. In R. L. Ackoff et al. (Eds.), *Systems and Management Annual.* New York: Petrocelli, 1974, pp. 1–53.

Palmer, B. Z. Use of quantitative approaches in plan development. *American Journal of Health Planning,* 1978, *3* (2), 43–50.

Pinker, R. Facing up to the eighties: health and welfare needs of British elderly. *The Gerontologist,* 1980, *20* (3), 273–283.

P.L. 79–725. Hospital Survey and Construction Act of 1946, August 13, 1946.

P.L. 78–410. The Public Health Services Act of 1944, July 1, 1944.

P.L. 88–164. Mental Retardation Facilities and Community Mental Health Center Construction Act of 1963, October 31, 1963.

P.L. 89–73. Older Americans Act of 1965, July 14, 1965.

P.L. 89–97. Social Security Amendments of 1965—Grants to States for Medical Assistance Programs and Health Insurance for the Aged, July 30, 1965.

P.L. 89–239. Heart Disease, Cancer and Stroke Amendments of 1965, October 6, 1965.

P.L. 89–749. Comprehensive Health Planning and Public Health Services Amendments of 1966, November 3, 1966.

P.L. 91–513. Comprehensive Drug Abuse Prevention and Control Act of 1970, October 27, 1970.

P.L. 91–616. Comprehensive Alcohol Abuse and Alcoholism Prevention, Treatment and Rehabilitation Act of 1970, December 31, 1970.

P.L. 92–603. Social Security Amendments of 1972, October 30, 1972.

P.L. 93–29. Comprehensive Older Americans Act of 1973, May 3, 1973.

P.L. 93–641. National Health Planning and Resources Development Act of 1974, January 4, 1975.

P.L. 93–647. Social Security Amendments of 1974—Grants to States for Services, January 4, 1975.

P.L. 95–478. Comprehensive Older Americans Act of 1978, October 18, 1978.

P.L. 96–79. Health Planning and Resources Development Amendments of 1979, October 4, 1979.

Roemer, M., and Shain, M. *Hospital Utilization Under Insurance.* Chicago: American Hospital Association, 1959.

Sager, A. Assessing the home care service needs of the elderly: professional prescriptions and patient/family requests. Paper presented at the 31st Annual Meeting of the Gerontological Society, Dallas, November 1978.

Sager, A. Planning home care for the elderly: variations in perceived needs and their costs. Unpublished doctoral dissertation, Massachusetts Institute of Technology, Cambridge, Massachusetts, 1979.

Saward, E. W. (Ed.). *The Regionalization of Personal Health Services.* New York: Prodist, 1975.

Spivack, S., and Ryan, J. *National Review of Health Systems Planning for the Elderly.* Boston: Boston University Center for Health Planning, 1979.

Task Force on the Organization and Delivery of Human Services. *The Future of Long-term Care* (HHS Publication No. HRP-0016874). Washington, D.C.: National Conference on Social Welfare, February, 1977.

Thompson, P. Voluntary regional planning. In E. Ginsberg (Ed.), *Regionalization and Health Policy* [DHEW Publication No. (HRA) 77–623]. Washington, D.C.: U.S. Government Printing Office, 1977.

Veterans Administration. *The Aging Veteran: Present and Future Medical Needs.* Washington, D.C.: Veterans Administration, 1977.

Wall, S. Health systems agency activity in non-traditional health planning areas: the case of congregate housing. In S. Spivack (Ed.), *State of the Practice Review of Health Systems Planning for the Elderly.* Boston: Boston University Center for Life Planning, 1979.

Waters, W. State-level comprehensive health planning: a retrospective.. *American Journal of Public Health,* 1976, *66* (2), 139–144.

West, J. P., and Stevens, M. P. Comprehensive analysis of community health planning: transition from CHPs to HSAs. *Journal of Health Policy, Politics and Law,* 1976, *1,* 173–195.

Zola, I. Medicine as an institution of social control. *Sociological Review,* 1972, *20* (4), 487–504.

Zola, I. Healthism and disabling medicalization. In I. Illich et al. (Eds.), *Disabling Professions.* London: Marion Royars, Inc., 1977.

SECTION V

# Social and Community Services

CHAPTER 13

# Subjective Well-Being: Conceptual and Methodological Issues

LINDA K. GEORGE, PH.D.
CENTER FOR THE STUDY OF AGING AND HUMAN DEVELOPMENT
DUKE UNIVERSITY
DURHAM, NORTH CAROLINA

At first glance, the term *subjective well-being* seems an unlikely candidate for rigorous scientific research. Subjective well-being sounds attractive, it even sounds important, but it seems to lack the precision and objectivity characteristic of conventional scientific terminology. In spite of this, the task of conceptualizing and measuring subjective well-being has intrigued social scientists and absorbed a substantial amount of their efforts.

The history of assessing subjective well-being has suffered its share of conceptual ambiguities and methodological problems. Nonetheless, there are increasing convergences in the conceptualization and measurement of subjective well-being. The purpose of this chapter is to provide an integrated discussion and critical evaluation of the "state of the art" of measuring subjective well-being. Much of the review is devoted to the synthesis of those relevant conceptual and methodological issues for which available evidence provides the foundation for informed resolution. For other issues, solutions are not yet available. In these cases, I have tried to clarify the issue and suggest profitable avenues for future effort. Thus, this review is intended to address both past accomplishments and future challenges in the measurement of subjective well-being.

This review is based upon a broad base of conceptual, methodological, and substantive work involving numerous social scientists and spanning more than 25 years. Two recent efforts merit special recognition, however, in that they represent major contributions to the general topic of subjective well-being. *Measuring Morale: A Guide to Effective Assess-*

*ment,* edited by Corinne Nydegger (1977), is a Gerontological Monograph of the Gerontological Society. This monograph represents a critical and informed consideration of the conceptual and methodological aspects of a concept which has been of major interest to social scientists. As the reader will note by my liberal referencing, the papers in this monograph have been invaluable in the preparation of this review. Second, Lucille Bearon and I recently collaborated in the preparation of *Quality of Life in Older People: Meaning and Measurement* (George and Bearon, 1980). Although we suggest that quality of life includes a broad range of discrete domains, subjective well-being receives considerable attention. This review clearly reflects insights and ideas generated in our previous collaboration. Readers interested in subjective well-being are encouraged to refer to these two compendiums.

## HISTORICAL BACKGROUND

Two broad research traditions inform the conceptualization and measurement of subjective well-being: social epidemiological studies of mental health and gerontological studies of the conditions under which late life is experienced as enriching or debilitating. In both these research traditions, well-being is conceptualized as a subjective phenomenon, related to but distinct from objective life conditions. Further, both research traditions share the concern that well-being captures the richest and most sublime life experiences, as well as the most deleterious and adverse ones. Just as health is viewed as including positive elements beyond the absence of disease and disability, subjective well-being has been conceptualized as having both positive and negative components.

### Social and Epidemiological Surveys

A number of standardized measures of subjective well-being were developed in broad epidemiological studies or social surveys. Earlier studies typically investigated the epidemiology of mental health and illness. More recent studies, with a similar substantive focus, frequently are described as surveys of subjective social indicators. Social indicators have been defined as a social reporting system whereby significant indicators of life quality can be monitored over time, providing an information base for tracing social change and for informed policy planning (cf. Carlisle, 1972; Sheldon and Freeman, 1970). While the choice of a social indicator depends upon the research problem or policy issue under consideration, our concern is subjective indicators of well-being—how individuals' life situations are perceived and evaluated.

The need for standardized, self-report measures of subjective well-being is common to these studies. In epidemiological studies of mental health, communities or other geographical areas are representatively sampled and the distribution and correlates of mental health or illness determined. Although psychiatric diagnosis would undoubtedly yield the most sensitive data about mental illness, the expense of this method for large samples typically precludes its use. The alternative method of case identification has been the development of standardized questionnaires which can be used to order respondents along a continuum of psychological health and impairment. Social indicator surveys of subjective well-being likewise have focused upon the development of valid and sensitive standardized instruments of subjective life quality.

The Midtown Manhattan Study (Srole et al., 1962, 1978; also see Langner and Michael, 1963) was one of the earliest community surveys of mental health and illness. The study sample consisted of 1,660 randomly selected inhabitants of a residential section adjoining Manhattan's central business district. Substantively, the study focused on the prevalence of mental disorder, demographic and social correlates of mental illness, and the relationship between life stress and mental disorder. In terms of measurement, the Midtown Manhattan Study generated a short, standardized screening device to detect mental disorder (Langner, 1962). Items in the instrument are those that best statistically discriminated respondents on the basis of independent psychiatric evaluations. Beyond the impressive contributions of the Midtown Manhattan Study, the Twenty-two Item Screening Scale (Langner, 1962) remains a frequently used measure of subjective well-being.

Another early study of mental health is the Gurin, Veroff, and Feld (1960) survey of attitudes toward mental health. This survey is unique in that it focused upon individuals' perceptions of their mental health, rather than the actual prevalence of mental disorder. The survey was administered to a nationally representative sample of 2,460 American adults in 1957. Gurin and associates defined psychological well-being in terms of self-reported happiness, worries and tensions, fears of a nervous breakdown, self-reports of diagnosed psychiatric disorder, and a checklist of psychophysiologic symptoms. A second survey was administered in 1976 to another nationally representative sample of 2,264 American adults. Comparisons of the two surveys now are becoming available (cf. Kulka et al., 1979). Both surveys included the same measures of subjective well-being, and the measures of Gurin and associates have been used by numerous investigators in other studies.

Although he did not use the term *social indicator*, Hadley Cantril's (1965) study of the subjective manifestations of social and political structure is an illustration of what now is termed the social-indicators perspective. Cantril's measure of subjective well-being is a self-anchoring scale which takes the form of a ladder. Respondents are asked to describe the best and worst possible lives for themselves and to indicate their current life situation relative to those self-defined referents. Cantril's research was cross-national, comparing perceptions of best and worst lives and personal satisfaction across nations and demographic subgroups within nations. The Cantril Self-Anchoring Scale remains a popular survey research instrument, though most investigators report only personal satisfaction ratings, neglecting to describe individual or group variations in perceptions of the best and worst life conditions.

As developed by Bradburn and Caplovitz (1965) and further refined by Bradburn (1969), the Affect Balance Scale was intended as an indicator of mental health suitable for broad social surveys. Bradburn hoped that time series data would be collected, using the instrument to relate subjective states to major social changes. The Affect Balance Scale was standardized on five broad and heterogeneous samples, including approximately 2,800 respondents. This instrument is unique in that it independently taps the quantity, quality, and positive to negative balance of affect within a given time referent. The Affect Balance Scale remains a widely used measure of subjective well-being.

Two recent studies conducted at the University of Michigan have made significant contributions to our understanding of subjective well-being. Both studies were developed from a social-indicators perspective, although their research goals differ somewhat. The first study, *The Quality of American Life* (Campbell et al., 1976), focuses upon Americans' satisfactions with life in general and with specific domains of life experience (e.g., work, community). The focus of the book is substantive, emphasizing (1) the imperfect relationship between objective life conditions and subjective well-being and (2) demographic and social structural variations in subjective well-being. This important work is based upon a nationally representative sample of more than 2,000 respondents. The survey included multiple measures of subjective well-being, including a single-item happiness measure (previously used by Gurin et al., Bradburn, and others), a series of semantic differential scales used to characterize the respondents' perceptions of "life in general," and a single-item global life satisfaction rating.

The second study, *Social Indicators of Well-Being* (Andrews and Withey, 1976), focuses specifically upon the measurement of well-being. Using data from five recent surveys (four national and one regional), including more than 5,000 respondents, Andrews and Withey evaluate the measurement properties of 68 global well-being measures and delineate the domain-specific satisfactions which predict global assessments of subjective well-being. The findings are complex, but the volume is a psychometric delight and constitutes a valuable contribution to our understanding of the measurement of subjective well-being.

**Gerontological Studies**

Maddox and Wiley describe life satisfaction, morale, and other concepts commonly subsumed under the rubric of subjective well-being as "perhaps the oldest, most persistently investigated issue in the social scientific study of aging" (1976, p. 15). Indeed, gerontological researchers have been intensely devoted to describing the subjective well-being of older people and relating perceptions of well-being to older people's current and past life conditions.

Historically, this emphasis upon subjective well-being can be traced to two early and classic gerontological research efforts: the *Five Hundred Over Sixty* survey (Kutner et al., 1956) and the Cornell Study of Occupational Retirement (Streib et al., 1958; Thompson and Streib, 1958; Thompson et al., 1960). In both of these early studies, measures of morale were developed and conceptualized as indicators of personal adjustment. The *Five Hundred Over Sixty* community survey was designed to determine the needs and adjustment of a sample of community residents aged 60 years and older in New York City. The Cornell Study was longitudinal in design and focused specifically upon the impact of retirement on personal adjustment.

The prominence of subjective well-being in gerontological research was further fueled by the heated controversy sparked by the disengagement versus activity theory debate. This debate focused upon alternative hypotheses about the relationship between social involvement and life satisfaction during later life and dominated research in social gerontology for more than a decade. Although it is now widely acknowledged that the disengagement versus activity theory debate is an overly simplistic and specious argument, many gerontological researchers remain actively engaged in studies of the conditions under which later life is subjectively experienced as enriching or debilitating. The major variables suggested as predictors of subjective well-being in later life include health, personal resources, social support and involvement, financial assets, coping capacity, and societal stereotypes about old age. In addition to the influence of historical theoretical allegiances, Rosow (1977) suggests that gerontological attention to issues of subjective well-being reflect an activist and applied orientation characteristic of gerontological investigators. At any rate, it is certain that subjective well-being has enjoyed immense popularity in the social science of aging.

Given the past and continuing significance of subjective well-being in gerontological research, it is not surprising that some gerontological investigators have devoted their energies to the development of measuring instruments specifically designed to assess perceptions of well-being among the elderly. Two major instruments, widely used in aging research, illustrate the research context within which gerontological measures of subjective well-being have developed.

The Life Satisfaction Index (LSI), originated by Neugarten, Havighurst, and Tobin (1961) was developed during the Kansas City Studies of Adult Life and is a direct product of efforts to create a self-report instrument which could replace ratings by observers. Unlike well-being measures developed in epidemiological studies or social surveys of the entire population, the content of several LSI items focuses directly upon old age. Revisions of the LSI—in terms of factor structure and/or the number of items—have been proposed by Adams (1969), Wood, Wylie, and Sheafor (1969), and Edwards and Klemmack (1973).

The Philadelphia Geriatric Center (PGC) Morale Scale (Lawton, 1972; revised in Lawton, 1975) also is a multidimensional instrument designed to measure subjective well-being among older persons. The instrument was developed to fill the void of self-report measures appropriate for use with very old, marginally literate, or institutionalized subjects. Like the LSI, the PGC Morale Scale includes items which focus directly upon the experience of late life.

The LSI and PGC Morale Scales are two of a considerably larger number of well-being measures designed specifically for use with older subjects. They are the most widely used of such measures, as well as the most carefully evaluated in terms of psychometric properties. Many gerontological researchers, however, do not use well-being measures designed specifically for older samples. The Affect Balance Scale, the Cantril Self-Anchoring Ladder, and other instruments developed in epidemiological studies or social surveys have been used in studies of late life. Similarly, the LSI recently was administered to a national sample of adults of all ages (Harris, 1975). Thus, although measures of subjective well-being were developed in two distinct substantive traditions, the research contexts in which these measures have been used are not uniformly separate.

## CONCEPTUAL ISSUES

Although the focus of this review is the measurement of subjective well-being, it is imperative that relevant conceptual issues also be considered. Well-articulated conceptualization is a prerequisite for the development of sensitive and valid measures and serves as a base for the evaluation of existing instruments. In this section of the chapter, four conceptual issues critical to the measurement of subjective well-being are addressed: (1) distinctions among specific concepts, (2) dimensions of well-being, (3) global versus domain-specific measures, and (4) setting the boundaries.

### Distinctions among Specific Concepts

As the previous overview demonstrates, the construct *subjective well-being* encompasses a number of specific concepts, ranging from psychiatric symptoms to happiness. Often these concepts are applied and interpreted as if each is a suitable proxy for the larger construct of subjective well-being or as if they are interchangeable. Neither of these assumptions is theoretically tenable. First, although each concept may comprise an *element* of well-being, no single concept can capture the complexity and scope of subjective well-being. Second, although all of these concepts refer to subjective states, they differ in meaning—especially in terms of cognitive versus affective orientation and temporal referent. In the following paragraphs, four concepts that are commonly used as indicators of subjective well-being are described.

*Life satisfaction* refers to an assessment of the overall conditions of life, as derived from a comparison of one's aspirations to one's actual achievements (Campbell et al., 1976; George, 1979). Life satisfaction is essentially a cognitive assessment of progress toward desired goals—an evaluation of the congruence between ideal and real life circumstances. In that "life in general" or "life as a whole" is the referent, a long-term time perspective and nonspecific life conditions are implied (Andrews and Withey, 1976; Campbell et al., 1976). Existing measures tap life satisfaction along a continuum from dissatisfaction to satisfaction.

In contrast to the cognitive assessments of life satisfaction, *happiness* refers to an affective assessment of subjective life quality (Bradburn, 1969). Happiness is viewed as a transitory, easily changeable phenomenon; consequently, most happiness measures specify a short-term time referent. Like life satisfaction, happiness measures cover the full continuum from highly negative to highly positive experience.

Although it is a frequently used concept, especially in gerontological studies, the definition of *morale* is elusive. The concept originated in social science studies of occupational and military performance. In these studies, morale referred to feelings of social cohesion, motivation, and commitment to group goals. In gerontological studies, morale does not refer to this sense of *esprit de corps*—but it is difficult to determine what the term does represent. In some studies, morale is viewed as a measure of affect; other studies imply that morale is essentially a cognitive assessment of life quality. The time referent is equally unclear. In some cases, morale is conceptualized as a relatively stable personal characteristic; at other times, morale represents transitory mood states. Thus, at this point, there is no consensus about the meaning of morale and it is unclear whether it could differ significantly from happiness or life satisfaction.

*Psychiatric symptom scales* measure the experience of such symptoms as anxiety, tension, worries, headaches, depression, fears, sleeplessness, and delusions. Such measures have a long history as standardized instruments used to identify psychopathology. As indicators of subjective well-being, however, such measures pose conceptual problems. First, psychiatric symptom scales focus exclusively upon negative well-being—an absence of symptoms is the best possible score. Thus, such measures do not tap the full range of subjective experience. Second, it is not clear that such measures in fact tap only subjective experience; there is considerable evidence, for example, that symptom reports may reflect either psychological distress or somatic complaints (cf. Crandall and Dohrenwend, 1967; Norland and Weirath, 1978). Third, both epidemiologists and social scientists increasingly doubt the sensitivity and specificity of symptom scales designed to tap general psychopathology. Instead, measures of specific psychological problems (e.g., anxiety, depression) may be conceptually cleaner and substantively more useful (cf. Houpt et al., 1979, 1980). Finally, the time referent for the experience of such symptoms is often vague and, when specified, varies across studies, ranging from *ever* having experienced the symptom to *current* experience of the symptom.

As these brief descriptions demonstrate, the conceptual clarity of specific concepts related to subjective well-being vary widely. The definitions of life satisfaction and happiness are relatively clear-cut. Further, the two concepts are complementary: life satisfaction refers to relatively long-term assessments of well-being, and happiness refers to more transitory affective feelings about life quality. The concept of morale is especially elusive and indeed there is reason to doubt that its use in gerontological studies is distinct from that of happiness or life satisfaction. The history of psychiatric symptom scales is a long one and the relationships among such measures and other indicators of mental disorder is well established. Nonetheless, psychiatric symptomatology, as typically measured, does not appear to be an attractive indicator of subjective well-being: it is narrow in scope, temporally and conceptually vague, and may reflect either physical or emotional determinants.

The conceptual distinctions among related concepts have important implications for the measurement of well-being. To the extent that life satisfaction, happiness, morale, and psychiatric symptomatology are distinct concepts, equally distinct measuring instruments are needed. Whether these specific concepts can be empirically distinguished is a question of the discriminant validity of available measures (Campbell and Fiske, 1959). The logic of discriminant validity is to determine whether an instrument can discriminate between the phenomenon it is intended to measure and different, but related phenomena. Thus, we might expect a moderate correlation between life satisfaction and happiness, but not so high as to blur the distribution between the two concepts. The essential point is that if our concepts are distinct and well-articulated, then we can develop distinct measures and evaluate the conceptual precision of existing measures.

The conceptual distinction made here between cognitive and affective evaluation is backed by empirical evidence. Andrews and Withey performed a factor analysis based on 12 measures of subjective well-being—some single-item, others multi-item. The analysis generated three distinct factors: cognitive evaluations, positive affect, and negative affect (1976, p. 89). Similarly, the distinction between long- and short-term time referents has been demonstrated to have an impact upon the nature and stability of subjects' self-reports of subjective well-being (Andrews and Withey, 1976).

### Dimensions of Well-Being

Life satisfaction, happiness, morale, and psychiatric symptoms are distinct indicators of the larger construct of subjective well-being, but these concepts may themselves be multidimensional. Typically, the dimensionality of a multi-item measuring instrument is assessed by factor analytic techniques, which determine the number of underlying dimensions in a set of items and their content.

Table 13–1 provides descriptions of the factor structures reported for four multi-item measures commonly used to subjective measure well-being in aging research: the Life Satisfaction Index (developed by Neugarten et al., 1961; factor structure one reported by Adams, 1969; factor structure two reported by Bigot, 1974); the Affect Balance Scale (Bradburn, 1969), an instrument measuring the recent experience of positive and negative affect; the revised version of the Philadelphia Geriatric Center Morale Scale (Lawton, 1975); and the Twenty-Two Item Screening Scale

Table 13–1
Reported Factor Structure[a] for Four Measures of Specific Concepts Related to Subjective Well-Being

Life Satisfaction Index, Factor Structure One:
- Mood tone
- Zest for life
- Congruence between achieved and desired goals
- A residual, unnamed category

Life Satisfaction Index, Factor Structure Two:
- Acceptance-contentment
- Achievement-fulfillment

Philadelphia Geriatric Center Morale Scale (revised version):
- Agitation
- Attitude toward one's own aging
- Lonely dissatisfaction

Twenty-Two Item Screening Scale:
- Psychological distress symptoms
- Physiologic symptoms

Affect Balance Scale:
- Negative affect
- Positive affect

[a] The factor structure of the Twenty-Two Item Screening Scale, reported by Crandall and Dohrenwend (1967), is based on the judgments of internists and psychiatrists rather than statistical evidence. Factor structures of the remaining measures are based upon the results of factor analysis.

(Langner, 1962; factor structure reported by Crandall and Dohrenwend, 1967). The names of the dimensions are those suggested by the investigators who performed the factor analyses. Each of the scales is multidimensional, and the content of the scales can be used to elucidate our understanding of the concept presumably measured by the instrument.

The dimensional structure of the Life Satisfaction Index (LSI) suggests that the instrument measures more than life satisfaction. The first factor structure for the LSI was reported by Adams (1969) and was based on a sample of 508 Missouri residents. The factor "congruence between achieved and desired goals" appears to represent life satisfaction—the items making up the factor tap cognitive assessments of general life quality with a long-term time referent. Both "mood tone" and "zest for life," however, measure affect—the first with a short-term time referent, the latter with a long-term time referent, requiring respondents to compare their current life quality with that of the past. Bigot (1974) reported two factors, based on an analysis of 150 British men's responses to the LSI: "acceptance-contentment" and "achievement-fulfillment." Bigot describes the content of the first factor as an affective assessment of the respondent's current life situation and the content of the second factor as a long-term review of life achievements. Thus, it appears that the LSI includes both happiness and life satisfaction (as they have been defined in this review) and that these separate concepts can be empirically distinguished. Similarly, the Philadelphia Geriatric Center (PGC) Morale Scale does not measure a single concept. The items comprised in the "agitation" subscale appear to be psychiatric symptoms (e.g., the experience of fears and upsets). The second factor, "attitude toward one's own aging," appears to tap a specific aspect of the self rather than a global assessment of life quality. The third factor, "lonely dissatisfaction," was appropriately named—the items in that factor focus on feelings of loneliness and general life satisfaction. Of the three factors, lonely dissatisfaction appears most closely related to an assessment of general life quality.

The Twenty-Two Item Screening Scale reportedly includes two factors—symptoms of psychological distress and physiologic or somatic complaints—based on clinicians' judgments rather than statistical analysis. The items tapping psychological distress appear compatible with the instrument's intended purpose of measuring psychological impairment. The physiologic or somatic items are more troublesome. They may represent psychosomatic symptoms of psychological origin. But it also is possible that they tap objective physical conditions—in which case the measure is not restricted to the measurement of subjective well-being.

What is most bewildering is the fact that this information about the dimensional structures of these three measures has been so consistently ignored in subsequent studies. Researchers continue to calculate simple sums of all the items in these measures and to interpret research results as if the measures are unidimensional. Knapp (1976), addressing this issue in the specific context of the LSI, suggested that the LSI be used *only* as a series of subscales. This suggestion makes indisputable sense and is applicable to the PGC Morale Scale and perhaps the Twenty-Two Item Screening Scale as well as the LSI. Since some dimensions of these scales appear to measure concepts other than subjective life quality and since these discrete dimensions may be differentially related to other variables of interest, the use of subscale scores is heartily recommended.

Psychiatric symptom scales would especially profit from efforts to empirically derive reliable and valid subscales, dimensions, or specific psychological problems. In a recent study, for example, Warheit, Holzer, and Arey (1975) representatively sampled a Southern community in order to examine the relationships among socioeconomic status, race, age, sex, and mental illness. The study included four self-report measures of mental illness—scales measuring general psychopathology, depression, phobia, and anxiety. Results of the study indicated that (1) the measures of specific psychological disorders were more sensitive (i.e., generated higher rates of psychological problems) than the general psychopathology scale and (2) the social status variables—especially age—were differentially related to the four measures of psychological problems. Similarly, in a recent study examining the relationship between housing characteristics and well-being during late life, Lawton and Kleban (1980) found that specific clusters of symptoms representing anxiety and depression were both conceptually and statistically distinct from physical health. Both of these studies illustrate the potential substantive benefits consequent to the conceptualization and measurement of psychological problems or distress in terms of specific dimensions.

The factor structure of the Affect Balance Scale (ABS) suggests that negative and positive affect are independent phenomena. Thus, the ABS contrasts with the other three instruments—in this case both dimensions are relevant to a single indicator of subjective well-being. Building upon this evidence, Bradburn (1969) conceptualizes happiness as the extent to which positive feelings outweigh negative feelings. This conceptualization contrasts sharply with the more common view that affect lies along a single continuum, ranging from the highly negative to the highly positive. Bradburn further demonstrated that the two dimensions of the ABS are related to different variables: positive affect is associated with higher levels of social contact, educational level, and more exposure to new experiences; negative affect is related to anxiety, fears of a nervous breakdown, and symptoms of ill-health. These findings have been replicated by several other investigators (cf. Beiser, 1974; Cherlin and Reeder, 1975; Phillips, 1967; Warr, 1978). The ABS illustrates the conceptual clarity and substantive importance of utilizing information about the dimensional structure of concepts related to subjective well-being.

### Global versus Domain-Specific Measures

Life satisfaction, happiness, morale, and psychiatric symptomatology, as defined above, are global concepts, referring to life as a whole rather than to specific domains of life experience. Domain-specific measures are an alternative to global assessments. In domain-specific measures, the referent is specified (e.g., "your work," "your family life"), rather than phrased in terms of "life in general." In global measures the frame of reference is unspecified and undoubtedly varies across individuals. Domain-specific measures can elucidate "why" and "with what" people are satisfied.

The feasibility of using domain-specific measures varies with the specific concept under consideration. There is considerable evidence that satisfaction with a wide variety of life domains can be meaningfully measured (Andrews and Withey, 1976; Campbell et al., 1976). Domain-specific happiness measures are possible for some life domains. It would be possible, for example, to ask respondents about their happiness with their marriages, their jobs, and so forth. As Campbell and his associates point out, however, such questions are more awkward than questions about the same life domains phrased in terms of satisfaction rather than happiness (e.g., job satisfaction is a more meaningful concept than job happiness). Domain-specific reports of psychological distress are problematic. It would be possible, for example, to ask respondents about their work-related tensions and fears. Nonetheless, the notion of domain-specific mental disorder is conceptually meaningless. Thus, domain-specific assessments are most usefully conceptualized in the framework of satisfaction.

Recent studies by Campbell, Converse, and Rodgers (1976) and Andrews and Withey (1976) focus upon the ability of a discrete set of domain-specific satisfactions to predict global satisfaction ratings. In both studies, domain-specific satisfactions account for 50–60 percent of the variance in diverse measures of global life satisfaction. The regression analyses used in these studies provide information about the specific life domains which significantly influence life satisfaction and the relative importance or weights of the domain-specific satisfactions. The results suggest that global life satisfaction is best predicted by satisfaction with marriage and family life, work and standard of living, leisure activities, friendships, housing, and community. Both studies conclude that global life satisfaction can be viewed as a weighted, linear combination of satisfactions with specific domains of life experience.

The research by Campbell and his associates and by Andrews and Withey is an important contribution to our understanding of the referents individuals use in making global assessments of their life quality. It also should be noted, however, that separate questions about domain-specific satisfactions are but one way of determining the referents individuals use in making global life satisfaction ratings. As described previously, Cantril's Self-Anchoring Ladder (Cantril, 1965) also requires respondents to provide the referents they use in assessing their global satisfaction—specifically, respondents are asked to describe the best and worst possible lives for themselves. These descriptions are viewed as the personal referents used in assessing life satisfaction. Cantril's broad research, performed in 12 countries with a total sample size of nearly 20,000 respondents, suggests that the domains of economic status, family relationships, and health are the primary referents used in global assessments of well-being—regardless of the personal or social characteristics of the respondent (although these factors certainly influence individuals' personal satisfaction ratings).

Beyond the issue of determining the referents people use in making global assessments of well-being, the appropriateness of global versus domain-specific measures depends upon the research question under consideration. There is considerable evidence that global measures of life satisfaction are related to numerous variables, including psychiatric evaluations of mental health (cf. Srole et al., 1962, 1978), financial status (cf. Bigot, 1974; Bull and Aucoin, 1975; Cutler, 1973; Edwards and Klemmack, 1973), health (cf. Bull and Aucoin, 1975; Cutler, 1973; Edwards and Klemmack, 1973), and levels of social activity (cf. Edwards and Klemmack, 1973; Peppers, 1976). On the other hand, domain-specific instruments often comprise more discriminating criterion measures in evaluation studies of focused service interventions (Carp, 1977).

**Setting the Boundaries**

The previous discussion has been intentionally restricted to a relatively narrow range of concepts, posited to represent distinct indicators of subjective well-being. Before leaving the topic of conceptualizing subjective well-being, however, it is important to justify this rather narrow focus.

An alternate approach to the conceptualization of subjective well-being is to include a wider range of social-psychological concepts than those described above. Although the specific configuration of concepts used varies from one study to another, it is not unusual to find assessments of subjective well-being that include such concepts as self-esteem or self-concept, locus of control, feelings of loneliness, self-rated health, and anomie. Indeed, in some research efforts, it appears that virtually any social-psychological concept is viewed as fair game as a measure of subjective well-being.

There are several potential pitfalls in this shotgun approach of making subjective well-being synonomous with the gamut of social psychological states. First, since such a broad definition precludes conceptual clarity and precision, the construct of subjective well-being becomes virtually meaningless: by referring to any- and everything social-psychological, it in effect refers to nothing. Second, the issue of distinctions among concepts becomes even more problematic. The conceptual distinction between life satisfaction and self-esteem, for example, is even greater than that between life satisfaction and happiness. Although they are different, happiness and life satisfaction both refer to global assessments of general life quality; self-esteem, on the other hand, refers to affective evaluations specifically about the self. This is not to say that we would not observe an empirical relationship between life satisfaction and self-esteem—indeed there may be good theoretical reasons to hypothesize such a relationship. But this does not mean that they are both indicators of the same underlying construct. Third, viewing a wide range of distinct social-psychological variables as representing a single underlying construct impedes hypothesis testing. One would expect life satisfaction and self-esteem, for example, to have different antecedents and consequences. To the extent that these distinct concepts are subsumed under a single theoretical label, refinements in our understanding of the causes and consequences of these concepts are less likely. Finally, the indiscriminant use of the label "subjective well-being" hinders our ability to communicate effectively. This is especially relevant to comparisons across studies. If two studies address subjective well-being, but one study focuses on life satisfaction while the other is based on self-esteem, it would not be surprising if the research results were significantly different. In such cases, conceptual differences can be mistaken for contradictory research findings.

For the purposes of this chapter, subjective well-being will be narrowly defined as "subjective perceptions of life quality." The specific concepts of life satisfaction and happiness are best-suited to this focus and are complementary: "life satisfaction" focuses upon the relatively long-term cognitive assessments of life quality, and "happiness" refers to the more transitory affective judgments of well-being. Morale and psychological distress also appear to be indicators of subjective well-being, although their conceptual definitions and temporal referents are less clear. The narrowness of this focus is justified by the increased conceptual clarity it provides.

## CRITERIA FOR EVALUATING THE ADEQUACY OF EXISTING MEASURES

The previous section of this review was both a plea for conceptual purity and a description of the concepts pertinent to this review. Beyond the issue of conceptual clarity, however, is the question of the psychometric or measurement properties of existing instruments. Any type of research is inherently at the mercy of the quality of the measuring instruments. Phrased bluntly, the data, and hence research results, are only as good as the instruments used to gather them. Unless investigators can be confident about the quality of their research measures, it cannot be determined whether negative results (or a lack of significant results) are due to inadequate theory or to the inadequacy of the instruments.

In this section, eight criteria for evaluating the psychometric adequacy of existing measures will be described briefly. These criteria undoubtedly will be familiar and bring back memories of standard academic courses in research methodology. In light of the fact that substantive research findings are frequently reported in the absence of information about the psychometric properties of the instruments used to generate those findings, however, the issue merits explicit attention.

## Normative Data

Ideally, normative data report the distribution of scores, mean value, and amount of variation exhibited by a particular measure in a large, representative, and heterogeneous sample. Normative data are useful in understanding the nature of the samples used in subsequent studies. Typically, investigators wish to use small samples that nonetheless are representative in order to generalize to the larger population. If sample values are not comparable to the normative data, the investigator has two choices: additional subjects may be chosen to yield a representative sample or subjects' responses may be weighted to generate a more representative distribution. The Harris Survey of *The Myth and Reality of Aging in America,* for example, used a weighting procedure to approximate age, race, and sex distributions similar to those of the general United States population (Harris, 1975). In other cases, investigators may use discrepancies between their samples and normative data to identify important subgroups of the population—subgroups that are of theoretical interest or are appropriate "target groups" for specific service interventions.

In addition to population norms, it also is useful to have subgroup norms. Gender, race, and age norms are especially useful.

## Applicability to Heterogeneous Samples

The composition of the samples that have been used in the administration of a particular measure is also important. If an instrument has been administered to subjects who possess heterogeneous social qualities, the instrument is expected to be more applicable than if administration has been limited to homogeneous samples. Lawton and Kleban (1979) refer to this measurement property as *subject versatility.*

The applicability of a given instrument is determined by the concept under consideration and/or item content, as well as by the heterogeneity of the samples used. Some concepts preclude the development of instruments applicable to the general adult population. Questions about retirement, for example, are applicable to only a relatively narrow age range. In most instances, however, concepts are theoretically meaningful across the adult population—as is certainly the case with most measures of subjective well-being. In such cases, the applicability of the instrument to the broader population should be empirically demonstrated.

### Quantification and Discriminability

The best measuring instruments are those that yield quantitative responses and which make fine distinctions among concepts. Quantification is the degree to which response categories can be accurately and meaningfully numbered. The most rigorous methods of data analysis require quantitative data. The ability to discriminate fine differences among respondents is also an important characteristic of the instrument. In general, the finer the distinctions that can be made across subjects, the greater the precision of the instrument. There are limits to subjects' abilities to discriminate accurately, however (e.g., a seven-point continuum would be better than either a dichotomous response or a 100-point continuum). Thus, the desire for fine distinctions must be tempered by the probability that those distinctions will be accurate and meaningful.

### Reliability

Reliability is a standard criterion used to assess the adequacy of measuring instruments. Reliability is most simply defined as the degree to which a measure is free of random error; mathematically, reliability is conceptualized as the correlation between "true scores" (inherently an unknown) and "observed scores" (values obtained by measurement). The consequences of using unreliable measures are profound. Typically, unreliable measurement results in a lack of significant research findings, since random error may blur and mask underlying patterns. More rarely, unreliability will artificially inflate existing patterns, resulting in misleading and inaccurate research findings.

The estimation of reliability is based on a complex body of psychometric theory (cf. Nunnally, 1967), beyond the scope of this review. The three main approaches to reliability assessment, however, will be described briefly.

*Test–Retest.* Using this approach, the instrument is administered twice to the same set of individuals. A correlation is calculated between the two sets of scores. The higher the correlation, the higher the presumed reliability. There are serious threats to the accuracy of test–retest reliability estimates. The general issue is the possibility that an intervening experience may alter the individual's true score on the measure of interest. Consequently, the correlation may be lowered and true change (a property of the individual) interpreted as unreliability (a property of the instrument). Specific examples of factors causing true change include the occurrence of an extraneous event; practice effects, in which the experience of taking a particular instrument alters the individual's score when the measure is taken a second time; and maturational effects, in which some inherent growth or aging process changes the individual's performance on the measure. In general, the longer the interval between the two tests, the less the likelihood of practice effects. Unfortunately, however, the longer the interval between tests, the greater the likelihood of extraneous events or maturational effects having an impact on the individual.

It should be noted that test–retest correlation is the only method of reliability estimation that can be used with single-item instruments.

*Split-Half.* Using this approach, the instrument is divided into two presumably equivalent forms. Both are administered to respondents and a correlation coefficient is calculated between the two forms. The higher the correlation, the higher the presumed reliability. There are two potential problems with this approach. First, the investigator never can be sure that the two forms are actually equivalent. Second, if the correlation is weak or moderate, the investigator has no clue as to which half is the more reliable or which terms incorporate the majority of random error.

*Internal Consistency.* In this approach, the items of a multi-item measure are correlated with each other in all possible combinations. The logic behind internal-consistency reliability estimates is relatively straightforward. If the items are in fact all tapping the same underlying concept, then they should be highly intercorrelated. If the items are not highly intercorrelated, either some items are unreliable or the set of items is tapping more than one underlying dimension. The reliability coefficient—typically Cronbach's alpha (1951)—ranges in value from zero (perfect unreliability) to one (perfect reliability). Reliability coefficients of 0.90 or higher are very high, while coefficients of 0.65 and lower indicate that the instrument is not adequately reliable. Examination of the correlation matrix also can be useful in that it is possible to identify the unreliable items(s).

## Validity

Validity is probably the most important criterion in measurement development and evaluation, and also the most difficult to evaluate. Validity may be defined as the degree to which an instrument measures the phenomenon it is intended to measure (Kerlinger, 1973). Reliability is a necessary but not a sufficient condition for validity. A measure may be perfectly reliable (i.e., contain no random error), and still not measure the intended phenomenon. There is no direct and certain test of validity. Instead, assessment of validity must be conducted by a variety of indirect methods. The four most commonly used approaches to the assessment of validity will be briefly discussed.

*Convergent Validity.* Convergent validity is based on the logic that instruments that measure the same concept should correlate highly (Campbell and Fiske, 1959). Using this approach, measures intended to tap the same underlying phenomenon are administered to the same individuals. The higher the correlations among measures, the greater the inferred validity. The limitation of this approach is that the validity of the other measures also is uncertain. Therefore, low correlations cannot inform the investigator which measures are valid.

*Discriminant Validity.* The logic of this approach, which is virtually the converse of convergent validity, is to determine whether an instrument can discriminate between the phenomenon it is intended to measure and different but related phenomena (Campbell and Fiske, 1959). To the extent that an instrument exhibits this ability to discriminate, there is evidence of discriminant validity.

*Predictive Validity.* If an instrument is valid, then it should predict other variables in a manner and to a degree compatible with theoretical expectations. For example, if high school grades constitute a valid measure of academic promise, we might expect high school grades to predict academic performance in college. This is an empirical proposition that can be tested. To the extent that a measure predicts other variables in a theoretically meaningful manner, there is evidence of predictive validity. The interpretation of negative results is, unfortunately, less straightforward. It also is possible that the prediction is incorrect, in which case invalidity cannot be distinguished from erroneous theory.

*Criterion-Group Validity.* This type of validity assessment can be used in cases where there are known groups that should differ on the phenomenon of interest. For example, if an instrument is intended to measure mental disorder, we might predict that scores on that instrument for a sample of psychiatric patients should significantly differ from scores for a sample of persons not receiving psychiatric services.

The most fruitful approach to validity assessment is to use a variety of methods. In spite of the fact that all the methods are indirect, evidence from a combination of methods is fairly persuasive.

## Scalability

A relatively complex body of psychometric theory guides the assessment of scalability. The details of that theory will not be described (for an excellent review, see Nunnally, 1967), although the criteria will be briefly described. First, the scale must be mathematically unidimensional or comprise a known and specified number of dimensions. Second, each of the items in the scale should significantly contribute to the scale as a whole. Finally, the relative contribution of each item in the scale should be specified. This is typically demonstrated in a weighting procedure, where the different weights assigned to items reflect the differential contributions of individual items.

### Sensitivity to Change

Many questions posed by gerontological investigators concern change over time; in such cases, the measure's sensitivity to change is a critical issue. Two factors determine an instrument's sensitivity to change: the psychometric properties of the instrument and the reactivity or changeability of the underlying phenomenon (George, 1979). If a phenomenon changes, but the measure is not sufficiently precise to detect such change, the instrument is deficient and unsuitable for measuring change. On the other hand, if an investigator unwittingly attempts to measure change in a characteristic which is impervious to change, results will be disappointing. For many concepts, theoretical paradigms are not sufficiently well articulated to decide whether or not the variables should be sensitive to change.

### Ease of Administration

Finally, the best instruments are easy to administer. Although this may seem like a pragmatic rather than a psychometric concern, instruments that are difficult to administer are more likely to generate inaccurate or misleading data. Ease of administration covers a variety of specific characteristics of the measuring instrument, including instrument length (the shorter, the easier to administer, but the greater the threat of unreliability), the simplicity of the language used in both items and instructions, the format of the response categories, and the conceptual complexity or level of abstraction required to understand and respond to items.

## THE PSYCHOMETRIC ADEQUACY OF EXISTING MEASURES OF SUBJECTIVE WELL-BEING

Given this list of criteria, it is possible to evaluate the psychometric adequacy of existing measures of subjective well-being. A detailed examination of the universe of existing measures obviously is beyond the scope of this chapter. An examination of the psychometric properties of selected measures is useful, however, as one way of assessing the current "state of the art" regarding the measurement of subjective well-being.

In this section, the psychometric adequacy of seven commonly used measures of subjective well-being will be assessed. Five of these instruments—the LSI, the PGC Morale Scale, and Cantril Self-Anchoring Ladder, the Twenty-Two Item Screening Scale, and the Affect Balance Scale—have been described previously. Both the original form of the Life Satisfaction Index (LSIA) and a modified version (LSIZ) will be evaluated. The other two instruments are recently developed single-item measures—one of global life satisfaction, the other of global affect. The Seven-Point Satisfaction Rating was the primary measure of global well-being used by Campbell and colleagues in *The Quality of American Life* (1976). This instrument consists of a single question—"How satisfied are you with your life as a whole these days?"—and responses lie along a seven-point continuum, ranging from "completely satisfied" to "completely dissatisfied." The Seven-Point Satisfaction Rating also was one of the global measures of subjective well-being used by Andrews and Withey (1976). The Delighted–Terrible Rating is a single-item measure of global affect used by Andrews and Withey. The instrument consists of a single question—"How do you feel about your life as a whole?"—with labeled responses ranging from "delighted" to "terrible," along a seven-point continuum. The measures included in this review are admittedly selective and were chosen to represent the best and most frequently used instruments available.

Table 13–2 provides an overall evaluation of these measures, using the eight psychometric criteria discussed in the previous section. The symbols used in this table merit careful explanation and cautious interpretation. A minus sign (−) symbolizes either evidence that the measure is deficient on the psychometric criterion *or* the lack of sufficient evidence to evaluate the instrument's adequacy on the specific criterion. A plus sign (+) was assigned in those cases where available evidence suggests that the instrument adequately meets the psychometric criterion. Finally, an asterisk (*) was reserved for those cases in which an instrument can be rated as superb in terms of a given psychometric criterion.

Even a relatively simple coding system such as that used in Table 13–2 is ultimately subjective. In order that the reader can derive his or her own judgments about the validity of the ratings, the psychometric properties of each instrument are evaluated in more detail in the following paragraphs. It is hoped that this review of specific instruments will not only make Table 13–2 more comprehensible but will also serve as a useful reference for those investigators who are searching for a conceptually appropriate and psychometrically sound measure of subjective well-being.

Table 13–2
Evaluations of Psychometric Properties of Commonly Used Measures of Subjective Well-Being

| | *LSIA* | *LSIZ* | *PGC Morale Scale* | *Affect Balance Scale* | *Twenty-Two Item Screening Scale* | *Cantril Ladder* | *Seven-Point Satisfaction Rating* | *Delighted–Terrible Rating* |
|---|---|---|---|---|---|---|---|---|
| Normative data | | | | | | | | |
| Population norms | + | – | – | + | + | * | + | + |
| Subgroups norms | + | – | – | + | + | * | + | + |
| Applicability to heterogeneous samples | + | – | – | + | + | + | + | + |
| Quantification and discriminability | + | + | + | + | + | + | + | + |
| Reliability | – | + | + | + | – | – | – | + |
| Validity | + | + | + | + | + | + | + | + |
| Scalability | + | – | + | + | – | NA | NA | NA |
| Sensitivity to change | – | + | + | + | – | – | + | – |
| Ease of Administration | + | + | * | + | + | + | + | + |

**LSIA and LSIZ**

The Life Satisfaction Index has taken a variety of forms. As originally developed by Neugarten, Havighurst, and Tobin (1961), the LSIA included 20 agree–disagree items and was intended to tap five conceptually derived dimensions: zest for life, resolution and fortitude, congruence between achieved and desired goals, positive self-concept, and mood tone. Adams' subsequent factor analysis of the LSIA (1969) indicated that the instrument tapped four dimensions (previously presented in Table 13–1) and that two items were unrelated to any dimension and should be dropped. One of the confusing aspects of subsequent research is the fact that both the 18-item and the 20-item versions commonly are referred to as the LSIA. The LSIZ is a 13-item modified version of the LSIA developed by Wood, Wylie, and Sheafor (1969) and has been used in several studies.

The 18-item LSIA was administered to a large ($N$ = 4,254), nationally representative sample of adults age 18 years and older in a recent survey of attitudes toward aging (Harris, 1975). This survey provides both population and subgroup norms. Given the frequent use of the LSIA and its administration to a national sample covering the spectrum of adult ages, this measure appears applicable to heterogeneous samples. There is one potential caveat in this regard, however. Several items of the LSIA (and the LSIZ) require respondents to compare current life conditions to conditions in the past. Although the Harris Survey demonstrates that young adults will answer such questions, it is unclear whether such age-related items are meaningful for younger adults. Although the LSIZ has been used in several studies, normative data are not available, and evidence about its applicability to heterogeneous samples is lacking.

Both the LSIA and the LSIZ generate quantitative data, capable of making fine distinctions among subjects. The items in both instruments are dichotomous (agree-disagree), although some investigators add an intermediate, "don't know" response. Total scale or subscale scores, however, permit adequate quantification and discrimination.

I have been unable to locate any information about the reliability of the LSIA. Wood, Wylie, and Sheafor (1969) report an internal consistency reliability coefficient of 0.79 for the LSIZ. Both instruments merit further assessment of reliability.

Both the LSIA and the LSIZ have been examined in terms of validity, with ambiguous results. Neugarten and colleagues (1961) reported that the LSIA correlated 0.55 with independent, interview-based ratings of respondents. The correlation between the LSIA and the PGC Morale Scale has been reported as 0.57 by Lawton (1972) and as 0.76 by Lohmann (1977). Lohmann also reports that the LSIZ and the PGC Morale

Scale are correlated at the 0.79 level. Wood, Wylie, and Sheafor (1969) report that the LSIZ is correlated 0.57 with independent, interview-based ratings. In Lohmann's study, the LSIA and LSIZ correlated at 0.94—as expected in light of their shared content. In terms of convergent validity, then, the LSIA and LSIZ are moderately to strongly correlated with other indicators of subjective well-being.

As noted previously, Adams (1969) demonstrated that the LSIA is multidimensional. Unfortunately, subscale scores and item weights have not been used in subsequent research. The dimensional structure of the LSIZ has not been empirically assessed.

Wylie (1970) used the LSIZ as a criterion measure in an evaluation study and concluded that the instrument is sensitive to change. No information is available concerning the sensitivity to change of the LSIA.

Both the LSIA and the LSIZ are short, easily administered instruments, suitable for interview or paper-and-pencil data collection.

### PGC Morale Scale

The original PGC Morale Scale (Lawton, 1972) included 22 items tapping six empirically derived dimensions: surgency (vigor), attitudes toward own aging, agitation, acceptance of the status quo, optimism, and lonely dissatisfaction. In 1975, Lawton revised the PGC Morale Scale, dropping five items. The three factors comprised in the revised instrument, as previously reported, are agitation, attitude toward one's own aging, and lonely dissatisfaction.

Although the PGC Morale Scale has been used in a number of gerontological studies, broad-based population and subgroup norms (e.g., all ages) are unavailable. Consequently, the limits of applicability are also unknown. Further, in that several items include content specific to late life, it is unclear whether this instrument would be appropriate for younger subjects. One strength of the PGC Morale Scale, however, is its demonstrated appropriateness for use with institutionalized older persons.

Response categories on the PGC Morale Scale are dichotomous. Scale or subscale scores are adequately quantitative, however, and permit distinctions among respondents.

Lawton (1972) reports a split-half reliability coefficient of 0.74, an internal consistency reliability coefficient of 0.81, and test–retest reliability coefficients ranging from 0.75 to 0.91 for the original version of the PGC Morale Scale. Lawton (1975) also reports internal consistency reliability coefficients for the three factors of the revised PGC Morale Scale: 0.85 for agitation, 0.81 for attitude toward one's own aging, and 0.85 for lonely dissatisfaction.

Validity information about the PCG Morale Scale consists of correlations with other measures (i.e., convergent validity). Lawton (1972) reports that the PGC Morale Scale and the LSIA are correlated at the 0.57 level. Lohmann (1977) reports significant correlations between the PGC Morale Scale and the LSIA and LSIZ ($r$ = 0.76 and 0.79, respectively). Lawton (1972) also reports a correlation of 0.47 between the morale scores of a sample of institutionalized patients and the independent ratings of staff members.

The dimensionality of the PGC Morale Scale has been described previously. Lawton has confirmed the three dimensions of the revised PGC Morale Scale on multiple samples (1975). Unfortunately, the use of subscale scores and item weights has been neglected in subsequent research by other investigators employing this instrument.

Kalson (1976) used the original PGC Morale Scale as an outcome measure in an experiment designed to determine the impact of volunteer work upon the well-being of older participants. His results suggest that the PGC Morale Scale is able to detect changes in subjective well-being.

Ease of administration is a strength of the PGC Morale Scale as it was developed to be appropriate for very old, marginally literate, or institutionalized respondents. The instrument is suitable for interview or questionnaire administration.

### Affect Balance Scale

The Affect Balance Scale consists of ten items (five positive, five negative) and generates three scores for each respondent: quantity of positive affect, quantity of negative affect, and affect balance (positive minus negative affect).

Bradburn's standardization of the ABS (1969) was based on five heterogeneous samples, totaling approximately 2,800 adults aged 18 to 60 years. In addition, the ABS was used in a number of gerontological studies (cf. Beiser, 1974; Gaitz and Scott, 1972), the Harris survey of *The Myth and Reality of Aging in America* (Harris, 1975) and in two of the national surveys reported by Andrews and Withey (1976). These sources provide normative data for the population and subgroups. Available evidence suggests that the ABS is applicable to broad samples of the population.

The ABS generates quantitative data and permits distinctions among subjects. The fact that the ABS generates independent scores for the quantity of affect as well as the balance of affect is a strength of this instrument.

Bradburn (1969) reports test-retest reliability coefficients ranging from 0.80 to 0.97 when the ABS was administered over various intervals of one week's duration or less.

In terms of validity, most available evidence consists of correlations between the ABS and other measures of subjective well-being. Bradburn (1969) reports that affect balance, and especially negative affect, are significantly correlated with indices of worries, anxiety, and psychosomatic symptoms. In data from three national surveys, Andrews and Withey (1976) report the following correlations between the ABS and (1) the Seven-Point Satisfaction Rating and (2) the Delighted–Terrible Rating:

| | *Seven-point Satisfaction Rating* | *Delighted–Terrible Rating* | |
|---|---|---|---|
| | | NOVEMBER STUDY | JULY STUDY |
| Positive affect | 0.30 | 0.33 | 0.36 |
| Negative affect | −0.31 | −0.29 | −0.32 |
| Affect balance | 0.43 | 0.44 | 0.48 |

In a study specifically designed to assess the validity of the ABS for older samples, Moriwaki (1974) correlated ABS scores with the Rosow Morale Scale, nine items from the Twenty-Two Item Screening Scale, and a single-item happiness item. The correlation coefficients between the ABS and other variables were as follows:

| | *Rosow Morale Scale* | *Psychiatric symptoms* | *Happiness item* |
|---|---|---|---|
| Negative affect | −0.40 | 0.65 | −0.20 |
| Positive affect | 0.62 | −0.36 | 0.49 |
| Affect balance | 0.61 | −0.64 | 0.40 |

Moriwaki's study also included a criterion-group validity assessment, comparing a group of normal community residents and a group of psychiatric outpatients. Both affect balance and the subscales significantly discriminated between the two groups.

As noted earlier, the negative and positive items on the ABS form independent subscales. This distinction has had important substantive implications in subsequent research.

Bradburn (1969) reports that longitudinal administration of the ABS results in changes that are "substantially larger than we would expect simply based on our reliability estimates" (p. 83) and concludes that the instrument is sensitive to change. It should be noted, however, that this evidence of sensitivity to change is less convincing than change which can be directly related to an investigator-induced intervention.

The ABS is brief and easy to administer in either interview or questionnaire form.

### Twenty-Two Item Screening Scale

Although the Twenty-Two Item Screening Scale has not been administered to a nationally representative sample, the instrument has been widely used, and several of the studies include probability samples of entire communities (cf. Langner, 1962; Manis et al., 1963; Markush and Favero, 1974; Meile, 1972). Consequently, normative data are available and the instrument is appropriate for heterogeneous samples.

The Twenty-Two Item Screening Scale generates quantitative data, capable of making fine distinctions among respondents. One of the controversial issues surrounding use of this measure has been the choice of an appropriate cutting point to distinguish "sick" from "well" (Langner, 1962; Manis et al., 1963; Meile, 1972). Although the issue of a threshold between sick and well may be salient to epidemiological generalizations about the prevalence of mental illness, it should be noted that, for many research purposes, the scale scores can be retained in continuous form. A second issue concerning the interpretation of scale scores is whether higher scores represent greater amounts of mental disorder or an increased likelihood of suffering mental disorder (Seiler, 1973).

There is no available evidence concerning the reliability of the Twenty-Two Item Screening Scale.

There is a substantial amount of evidence concerning the validity of the Twenty-Two Item Screening Scale. Langner (1962) and Manis and co-workers (1963) report significant correlations between scale scores and psychiatric ratings. In terms of convergent validity, Shader, Ebert, and Harmatz (1971) report that the Twenty-Two Item Screening Scale is significantly correlated with the Manifest Anxiety Scale ( = 0.77), the Cattell Anxiety Battery ($r$ = 0.43), and a neuroticism scale ($r$ = 0.72). Criterion-group analysis has been the most frequently used method of validity assessment for the Twenty-Two Item Screening Scale. Langner (1962) reported that the instrument discriminated among psychiatric patients and nonpatients in two samples. Similar results are reported by Manis and colleagues (1963). Mixed results are reported by Dohrenwend and Crandall (1970) and Muller (1971); in these studies patients were accurately discriminated from non-patients, but severity of mental disorder (e.g., inpatients versus outpatients) could not be distinguished. In spite of the accumulation of evidence, the validity of the Twenty-Two Item Screening Scale remains a topic of controversy and heated debate (cf. Norland and Weirath, 1978, Seiler, 1973, for highly negative reviews based on theoretical rather than empirical grounds). Langner, too, has revised his evaluation of what the Twenty-Two Item Screening Scale measures. He now suggests that the instrument is essentially a measure of anxiety rather than a measure of global psychiatric impairment (Gersten et al., 1974).

The scalability of the Twenty-Two Item Screening Scale has not been statistically assessed. Several authors hypothesize that the measure includes both psychological and physical symptoms. Crandall and Dohrenwend (1967) posit two factors—psychological stress and physiologic symptoms—based on the judgments of internists and psychiatrists. This issue merits statistical analysis.

There is no evidence concerning this measure's sensitivity to change.

The Twenty-Two Item Screening Scale is easy to administer in either interview or paper-and-pencil form.

### Cantril's Self-Anchoring Ladder

The Cantril Self-Anchoring Ladder has been administered in several national surveys (Andrews and Withey, 1976; Cantril, 1965). Both population norms and detailed subgroups norms are available. This instrument is applicable to broad and heterogeneous samples. Age norms for older samples have been provided by Bortner and Hultsch (1970).

Respondents' personal ratings of their current life experiences are quantitative and permit distinctions among subjects. It should be noted, however, that the number of rungs on the ladder has varied across studies, compromising comparisons of research results. Respondents' descriptions of their "best" and "worst" possible lives, which presumably serve as the referents for their satisfaction ratings, are not quantitative. Cantril (1965) provides a coding scheme for the domains referenced by respondents, but it is a classification system rather than a quantitative metric. Although Cantril devoted considerable attention to the referents individuals use in assessing their levels of personal satisfaction, subsequent investigators typically ignore this issue, focusing solely on personal satisfaction ratings.

Only very limited data are available about the reliability of the Cantril Ladder. Palmore and Kivett (1977) report a test–retest correlation of 0.65 over two years. Given the lengthy interval between tests, however, this correlation appears to reflect the instrument's stability in a sample of individuals rather than its reliability as an instrument.

Two kinds of evidence speak to the validity of the Cantril Ladder. In terms of convergent validity, Andrews and Withey (1976) report that correlations between the Cantril Ladder and the Delighted–Terrible Rating range from 0.50 to 0.54. Using sophisticated structural models designed to generate validity coefficients that range from zero (perfect invalidity) to one (perfect validity). Andrews and Withey calculate a validity coefficient of 0.70 for the Cantril Ladder.

There is very little evidence concerning the Cantril Ladder's sensitivity to change. The correlation over a two-year interval reported by Palmore and Kivett suggests stability, but given that it is a single study comprised of a narrow age range, this evidence is not compelling.

The Cantril Self-Anchoring Ladder is a brief instrument. Andrews and Withey suggest that the unlabeled response values are problematic. Further, in that descriptions of respondents' best and worst possible lives are reported to frequently require probes (Cantril, 1965), this instrument is best suited to an interview format.

### Seven-Point Satisfaction Rating

Campbell and associates (1976) administered the Seven-Point Satisfaction Rating to a national sample of American adults. This instrument was also included in one of the national surveys reported by Andrews and Withey (1976). Both population and subgroups norms are available. The Seven-Point Satisfaction Rating appears applicable to heterogeneous samples. Campbell and co-workers provide specific age norms.

The Seven-Point Satisfaction Rating generates quantitative data, capable of discriminating across subjects. Andrews and Withey argue that the unlabeled response categories of this instrument are problematic for respondents.

No information is available about the reliability of this instrument. Campbell and associates report a correlation of 0.43 between two administrations of the Seven-Point Satisfaction Rating given eight months apart. The authors suggest that this provides evidence of the measure's sensitivity to change rather than unreliability, given the length of the interval between tests.

Andrews and Withey correlated the Seven-Point Satisfaction Rating with both the Delighted–Terrible Rating and the ABS as evidence of convergent validity. The moderate correlations between the ABS and the Seven-Point Satisfaction Rating have been reported previously. Correlations between the Seven-Point Satisfaction Rating and the Delighted–Terrible Rating ranged from 0.56 to 0.70. Using structural equation models, Andrews and Withey calculated validity coefficients of 0.73 and 0.79 for this measure.

The Seven-Point Satisfaction Rating is brief, straightforward, and easy to administer in either interview or paper-and-pencil format.

### Delighted–Terrible Rating

Of the 68 measures of global well-being examined in their surveys, Andrews and Withey (1976) conclude that the single-item Delighted–Terrible Rating has the best psychometric properties. The measure was included in four national surveys, and both population and subgroup norms are reported. The measure appears applicable to heterogeneous samples.

The Delighted–Terrible Rating generates quantitative data along a seven-point continuum.

Andrews and Withey assessed the test–retest reliability of the Delighted–Terrible Rating by administering the same item twice in the same interview, ten to twenty minutes apart. This procedure was followed in all four surveys, generating test–retest reliability estimates of 0.68, 0.61, 0.74, and 0.64. Given the very short interval between tests, these reliability estimates are adequate but not impressive.

Correlations between the Delighted–Terrible Rating and the ABS, the Cantril Ladder, and the Seven-Point Satisfaction Rating have been previously reported and provide estimates of convergent validity. It should be noted that these correlations are of only moderate strength. Using structural models, intended to correct for measurement error, Andrews and Withey report validity coefficients across the four surveys of 0.71, 0.70, 0.76, and 0.82.

There is no evidence about this instrument's sensitivity to change.

The Delighted–Terrible Scale is easy to administer, brief, and appropriate for either interview or questionnaire format.

## AGENDA FOR THE FUTURE

There are a multitude of profitable directions for future research in subjective well-being. The topic is a rich one—conceptually, methodologically, and substantively. Out of this wide range of potentially fruitful issues, this discussion will focus on two topics that I believe are of critical importance: (1) increased attention to the conceptualization and measurement of subjective well-being and (2) clarifying the relationship between age and subjective well-being.

### Putting the Horse before the Cart

In spite of the popularity of the construct in substantive research, the conceptualization and measurement of subjective well-being are critical areas for further effort. In previous research, the cart has too frequently preceded the horse, with sophisticated models receiving empirical testing before we understand the concepts and measures included in the models. Unless we know what these concepts mean and how they can be measured effectively, we are not prepared to use them in rigorous research. Many of the critical issues in this regard have been described, or at least implied, in previous sections of this review. They are sufficiently important, however, to merit explicit enumeration.

The first and foremost issue is the need for conceptual clarity. In order to communicate effectively and to interpret research findings, we must agree upon what subjective well-being is—and what it is not. The position taken here is that subjective well-being is an abstract construct which can be conceptualized only in terms of more specific indicators. Each of these indicators, in turn, must be conceptually clear—having a unique definition, a specified time referent, a known structure (i.e., unidimensional or multidimensional), and theoretical guidance about its expected stability or reactivity in the face of changing external circumstances. Both the development of new measures and the evaluation of existing instruments are dependent upon conceptual clarity.

Second, existing measures of subjective well-being indicators require increased assessment of their psychometric properties. The instruments selected for detailed examination in this review are all promising measures—indeed they were selected to represent the best and most frequently used instruments available. In spite of their strengths, each of those instruments would profit from increased psychometric assessment. It is difficult to believe, for example, that the LSIA , developed in 1961 and used frequently since then, has not been subjected to any reported test–retest reliability estimate. This is one example of a broad range of tasks that confront us as we strive to assess and improve existing measures of subjective well-being.

Finally, increased efforts to refine existing measures of subjective well-being is a better investment of time and effort than the proliferation of new measuring instruments. To the extent that a discrete set of conceptually clear, psychometrically sound measures of subjective well-being are used, comparability across studies and the cumulation of an integrated knowledge base are enhanced. The growth of comparable research results permits generalization to broader segments of the population and refinement of observed patterns, thus contributing to the cumulative nature of scientific evidence.

This is not to say that there need be a complete moratorium on the development of new measures. Both the Seven-Point Satisfaction Rating and the Delighted–Terrible Rating are relatively new measures of life satisfaction and global affect which have been used in substantively profitable ways. The development of these instruments, however, required substantial attention to psychometric issues. Thus, the decision to develop a new measure should be carefully weighed, keeping in mind that substantial resources will be needed to assess its psychometric adequacy. In general, the refinement of existing measures probably is a more profitable route. The continued use of a few standardized measures is routine procedure in many other disciplines and for other substantive topics. In the area of intelligence testing, for example, several standardized IQ tests with known characteristics are continually used; investigators do not expend their energies developing new measures.

### Age and Subjective Well-Being

Although the relationship between age and subjective well-being has received substantial attention, three basic issues remain unresolved—issues that are relevant to the conceptualization and measurement of subjective well-being.

*Is Age-Related Well-Being a Viable Concept?* As well as life satisfaction, happiness, morale, and psychological distress, the gerontological literature reveals the concept of "age-related morale," defined by Lawton as "the balance of positive and negative experiences related to the period of old age, with either an explicit or implied comparison to earlier periods of life" (1977, p. 7). Thus, age-related morale is a global assessment of life quality, comparing current conditions to those at earlier ages.

The important question is whether age-related morale is a theoretically meaningful concept. There are two possible reasons that such a concept might be useful. First, age-related morale may represent an attempt to provide the temporal referent for respondents to use in reporting their life quality. In that measures already exist which specify a long-term time referent, however, the need for the additional concept of age-related morale is unclear. Second, age-related morale may be intended as a particular domain-specific dimension of subjective well-being. Thus, just as individuals can rate their satisfaction with their health or family life, they also may be able to rate their current sense of well-being as compared with earlier life stages. Indeed, there is empirical evidence that age-related morale can be statistically derived in a reliable fashion (cf. Lawton, 1975; Pierce and Clark, 1973). What is needed, however, is increased theoretical attention to the meaning and utility of this concept, as well as its antecedents and consequences.

The concept of age-related morale is troublesome in another way. Items that require the respondent to compare late life to younger ages are applicable only to older respondents—or at least have very different meanings for younger and older respondents. Consequently, it may be

inadvisable to compare older and younger subjects on such items. As noted previously, both the LSI and the PGC Morale Scale contain items with age-related content.

Clarification of the issue of age-related morale should be a priority item for gerontological investigators interested in subjective well-being.

*Age Changes and Age Differences in Subjective Well-Being.* Currently we do not know whether life satisfaction, happiness, morale, and psychological distress exhibit consistent, identifiable age changes over the life course. Theoretically, the issue is complex. If these indicators of subjective well-being are stable characteristics, age changes are unlikely. If, on the other hand, age changes are typical, there are two possible explanations. First, indicators of subjective well-being may represent true developmental phenomena, intrinsically linked to age or underlying biological mechanisms. Or such concepts may be situationally reactive, with age changes observed to the degree that influential situational variables (e.g., work status, health) change with age.

Data reported by Campbell and associates (1976) suggest that this topic could profit from further research. In this cross-sectional study, patterns of responses to global measures of life satisfaction and happiness differed significantly across age groups. In general, younger individuals scored high in happiness but relatively low in life satisfaction. For older persons the pattern was reversed; these individuals scored relatively low in happiness but quite high in life satisfaction. Middle age appears to be the low point of the life cycle; compared to earlier and later life stages, middle-aged respondents scored low in both happiness and life satisfaction. These data suggest that distinct indicators of subjective well-being may exhibit differential patterns of age changes and age differences.

Such distributions have intriguing implications for life-cycle theory. It may be that young adults, who are typically just entering their careers and in the early phases of consolidating their adult identities, face substantial discrepancies between their aspirations and achievements, consequently generating relatively low levels of life satisfaction. The excitement and potential of young adulthood, however, may facilitate reports of happiness. For older individuals, on the other hand, happiness appears less frequent, perhaps reflecting a flattening of affect in late life, as suggested by Neugarten (1964). Life satisfaction may be relatively high in older persons, however, reflecting either fulfillment of cherished goals or a lowering of aspirations to match actual accomplishments. This kind of interpretation is, of course, merely speculation. The age differences may reflect cohort differences instead. Only longitudinal data will permit analysis to unravel the possible explanatory factors. Nonetheless this discussion highlights the potential importance of this issue.

This issue also has important implications for the use of measures of subjective well-being as outcome measures in the study of change. If subjective well-being is developmental, such instruments may be of limited use in the measurement of change, since developmental change could be confounded with change due to external variables. The extent to which subjective well-being exhibits age changes is clearly an area in need of further research.

*Structure versus Levels of Well-Being.* Given that many measures of well-being are multidimensional, it is possible not only to assess age differences in levels of well-being (i.e., scores on a particular instrument) but also to determine whether the dimensional structure of the instrument is consistent across age groups. The implication of this two-pronged assessment of age differences is that if the structure is not the same across age groups, then it is inappropriate to impose a single scoring system upon respondents of various ages.

Cutler (1979) recently reanalyzed the Quality of American Life data (Campbell et al., 1976), examining the factor structure of 12 domain-specific satisfactions across seven age groups (aged 18–24 to 75–90 years). The results indicated that the 12 domain-specific satisfactions formed multiple factors for each age group. Further, both the number of factors and the content of the factors differed across the seven age groups. Cutler concluded that the referents people use to assess the "good life" vary by age (or cohort) and that this should be kept in mind when interpreting global assessments of well-being across age groups.

Cutler's work is an intriguing initial examination of the structure of subjective well-being across age groups. Nonetheless, there are some cautions which should be appended to his conclusions. First, the fact that the factor structure of domain-specific satisfactions varies across age groups does not necessarily imply that age comparisons on global measures of subjective well-being will be problematic. Respondents using very different referents can nonetheless report their personal levels of life satisfaction on a uniform metric which permits comparisons. Although the life experiences which lead older persons to report that they are "completely satisfied" with life may be different from those which lead younger people to report that they are "completely satisfied" with life, it still is possible to compare the responses. Second, Cutler stops short of providing the evidence we need to determine that domain-specific satisfactions are differentially important for global satisfaction ratings, depending upon the age of the respondent. In order to make that conclusion, it would be necessary to demonstrate that various domain-specific satisfactions are differentially related to global assessments of subjective well-being for various age groups. Such evidence would require correlations between domain-specific satisfactions and the global well-being measure at minimum—although multiple regression would be the preferred technique.

The questions of whether the dimensional structures of global measures of well-being (e.g., the LSI and the PGC Morale Scale) differ across age groups has not been examined. If, in fact, the dimensional structures of such measures vary significantly by age, the utility of such instruments for examining age differences in subjective well-being will be severely compromised. This, too, is a critical area for empirical inquiry.

## CONCLUSIONS

Subjective well-being is a meaningful and significant topic for scientific inquiry. The experiential and subjective components of life are a significant aspect of the human condition. Further, in that individuals' actions reflect their subjective perceptions as well as the demands of the external environment, subjective well-being is of relevance to the scientific investigation of human behavior.

Social scientists have made substantial progress in the conceptualization and measurement of subjective well-being. Now that a firm foundation has been laid for future endeavors, the time is ripe for concerted efforts to resolve the critical conceptual and measurement issues which must precede substantive progress.

## REFERENCES

Adams, D.L. Analysis of a life satisfaction index. *Journal of Gerontology*, 1969, *24*, 470–474.

Andrews, F.M., and Withey, S.B. *Social Indicators of Well-Being*. New York: Plenum Press, 1976.

Beiser, M. Components and correlates of mental well-being. *Journal of Health and Social Behavior*, 1974, *15*, 320–327.

Bigot, A. The relevance of American life satisfaction indices for research on British subjects before and after retirement. *Age and Ageing*, 1974, *3*, 113–121.

Bortner, R.W., and Hultsch, D.F. A multivariate analysis of correlates of life satisfaction in adulthood. *Journal of Gerontology*, 1970, *25*, 41–47.

Bradburn, N.M. *The Structure of Psychological Well-Being*. Chicago: Aldine, 1969.

Bradburn, N.M., and Caplovitz, D. *Reports on Happiness: A Pilot Study of Behavior Related to Mental Health*. Chicago: Aldine, 1965.

Bull, C.N. and Aucoin, J.B. Voluntary association participation and life satisfaction: a replication note. *Journal of Gerontology*, 1975, *30*, 73–76.

Campbell, A., Converse, P.E., and Rodgers, W.L. *The Quality of American Life*. New York: Russell Sage Foundation, 1976.

Campbell, D.T., and Fiske, D.W. Convergent and discriminant validation by the multitrait-multimethod matrix. *Psychological Bulletin,* 1959, *56,* 81–105.

Cantril, H. *The Pattern of Human Concerns.* New Brunswick, New Jersey: Rutgers University Press, 1965.

Carlisle, E. The conceptual structure of social indicators. In A. Shonfield and S. Shaw (Eds.), *Social Indicators and Social Policy.* London: Heinemann Educational Brooks, 1972.

Carp, F.M. Morale: what questions are we asking of whom? In C.N. Nydegger (Ed.), *Measuring Morale: A Guide to Effective Assessment.* Washington, D.C.: Gerontological Society, 1977.

Cherlin, A., and Reeder, L.G. The dimensions of psychological well-being: a critical review. *Sociological Methods and Research,* 1975, *4,* 189–214.

Crandall, D.L., and Dohrenwend, B.P. Some relations among psychiatric symptoms, organic illness and social class. *American Journal of Psychiatry,* 1967, *123,* 1527–1537.

Cronbach, L.J. Coefficient alpha and the internal structure of tests. *Psychometrika,* 1951, *16,* 297–334.

Cutler, N.E. Age variations in the dimensionality of life satisfaction. *Journal of Gerontology,* 1979, *34,* 573–578.

Cutler, S.J. Voluntary association participation and life satisfaction: a cautionary research note. *Journal of Gerontology,* 1973, *28,* 96–100.

Dohrenwend, B.P., and Crandall, D.L. Psychiatric symptoms in community, clinic, and mental hospital groups. *American Journal of Psychiatry,* 1970, *126,* 1611–1621.

Edwards, N., and Klemmack, L. Correlates of life satisfaction: a re-examination. *Journal of Gerontology,* 1973, *28,* 497–502.

Gaitz, C.M., and Scott, J. Age and the measurement of mental health. *Journal of Health and Social Behavior,* 1972, *13,* 55–67.

George, L.K. The happiness syndrome: methodological and substantive issues in the study of social-psychological well-being in adulthood. *Gerontologist,* 1979, *19,* 210–216.

George, L.K., and Bearon, L.B. *Quality of Life in Older Persons: Meaning and Measurement.* New York: Human Sciences Press, 1980.

Gersten, J.C., Langner, T.S., Eisenberg, J.G., and Orzek, L. Child behavior and life events: undesirable change or change per se? In B.S. Dohrenwend and B.P. Dohrenwend (Eds.), *Stressful Life Events: Their Nature and Effects.* New York: John Wiley, 1974.

Gurin, G., Veroff, J., and Feld, S. *Americans View Their Mental Health.* New York: Basic Books, 1960.

Harris, Louis & Associates. *The Myth and Reality of Aging in America.* Washington, D.C.: National Council on the Aging, 1975.

Houpt, J.L., Orleans, C.S., George, L.K., and Brodie, H.K.H. *The Importance of Mental Health Services to General Health Care.* Cambridge, Massachusetts: Ballinger, 1979.

Houpt, J.L., Orleans, C.S., George, L.K., and Brodie, H.K.H. The role of psychiatric and behavioral factors in the practice of medicine. *American Journal of Psychiatry,* 1980, *137,* 37–47.

Kalson, L. M*A*S*H: a program of social interaction between institutionalized aged and adult mentally retarded persons. *Gerontologist,* 1976, *16,* 340–348.

Kerlinger, F.N. *Foundations of Behavioral Research.* New York: Holt, Rinehart and Winston, 1973.

Knapp, M.R.J. Predicting the dimensions of life satisfaction. *Journal of Gerontology,* 1976, *31,* 595–604.
Kulka, R.A., Veroff, J., and Douvan, E. Social class and use of professional help for personal problems: 1957 and 1976. *Journal of Health and Social Behavior,* 1979, *20,* 2–16.
Kutner, B., Fanshel, D., Togo, A., and Langner, T.S. *Five Hundred Over Sixty.* New York: Russell Sage Foundation, 1956.
Langner, T.S. A twenty-two item screening score of psychiatric symptoms indicating impairment. *Journal of Health and Human Behavior,* 1962, *3,* 269–277.
Langner, T.S., and Michael, S.T. *Life Stress and Mental Health.* Glencoe, New York: Free Press, 1963.
Lawton, M.P. The dimensions of morale. In D. Kent, R. Kastenbaum, and S. Sherwood (Eds.), *Research, Planning and Action for the Elderly.* New York: Behavioral Publications, 1972.
Lawton, M.P. The Philadelphia Geriatric Center morale scale: a revision. *Journal of Gerontology,* 1975, *30,* 85–89.
Lawton, M.P. Morale: what are we measuring? In C.N. Nydegger (Ed.), *Measuring Morale: A Guide to Effective Assessment.* Washington, D.C.: Gerontological Society, 1977.
Lawton, M.P., and Kleban, M.H. Assessment: the concept and prospects. Paper prepared for National Institute of Mental Health, 1979.
Lawton, M.P. and Kleban, M.H. *Psychological Well-Being in the Aged.* Final Report of NIMH Grant No. MH30665. Philadelphia: Philadelphia Geriatric Center, 1980.
Lohmann, N. Correlations of life satisfaction, morale, and adjustment measures. *Journal of Gerontology,* 1977, *32,* 73–75.
Maddox, G.L., and Wiley, J. Scope, concepts, and methods in the study of aging. In R. Binstock and E. Shanas (Eds.), *Handbook of Aging and the Social Sciences.* New York: Van Nostrand Reinhold, 1976.
Manis, J.G., Brawer, M.J., Hunt, C.L., and Kercher, L.C. Validating a mental health scale. *American Sociological Review,* 1963, *28,* 108–116.
Markush, R.E., and Favero, R.V. Epidemiologic assessment of stressful life events, depressed mood, and psychophysiological symptoms—a preliminary report. In B.S. Dohrenwend and B.P. Dohrenwend (Eds.), *Stressful Life Events: Their Nature and Effects.* New York: John Wiley, 1974.
Meile, R.L. The twenty-two item index of psychophysiological disorder: psychological or organic symptoms? *Social Science and Medicine,* 1972, *6,* 125–135.
Moriwaki, S.Y. The affect balance scale: A validity study with aged samples. *Journal of Gerontology,* 1974, *29,* 73–78.
Muller, D.J. Discussion of "Langner's Psychiatric Impairment Scale": a short screening device. *American Journal of Psychiatry,* 1971, *128,* 601.
Neugarten, B.L. Summary and implications. In B.L. Neugarten and Associates (Eds.), *Personality in Middle and Late Life.* New York: Atherton, 1964.
Neugarten, B.L., Havighurst, R.J., and Tobin, S.S. Measurement of life satisfaction. *Journal of Gerontology,* 1961, *16,* 134–143.
Norland, S., and Weirath, T. Validating the Langner scale: a critical review. *Social Problems,* 1978, *26, 223–231.*
Nunnally, J.C. *Psychometric Theory.* New York: McGraw Hill, 1967.
Nydegger, C. (Ed.). *Measuring Morale: A Guide to Effective Assessment.* Washington, D.C.: Gerontological Society, 1977.

Palmore, E., and Kivett, V. Change in life satisfaction: a longitudinal study of persons aged 46–70. *Journal of Gerontology,* 1977, *32,* 311–316.

Peppers, L.G. Patterns of leisure and adjustment to retirement. *Gerontologist,* 1976, *16,* 441–446.

Phillips, D.L. Social participation and happiness. *American Journal of Sociology,* 1967, *72,* 479–488.

Pierce, R.C., and Clark, M.M. Measurement of morale in the elderly. *International Journal of Aging and Human Development,* 1973, *4,* 83–101.

Rosow, I. Morale: concept and measurement. In C.N.Nydegger (Ed.), *Measuring Morale: A Guide to Effective Assessment.* Washington, D.C.: Gerontological Society, 1977.

Seiler, L.H. The twenty-two item scale used in field studies of mental illness: a question of method, a question of substance, and a question of theory. *Journal of Health and Social Behavior,* 1973, *14,* 251–264.

Shader, R.I., Ebert, M.H., and Harmatz, J.S. Langner's psychiatric impairment scale: a short screening device. *American Journal of Psychiatry,* 1971, *128,* 88–93.

Sheldon, E.B., and Freeman, H.E. Notes on social indicators: promises and potential. *Policy Sciences,* 1970, *1,* 97–111.

Srole, L., Langner, T.S., Michael, S.T., Opler, M.K., and Rennie, T.A.C. *Mental Health in the Metropolis: The Midtown Manhattan Study.* New York: McGraw Hill, 1962.

Srole, L., Langner, T.S., Michael, S.T., Opler, M.K., and Rennie, T.A.C. *Mental Health in the Metropolis: The Midtown Manhattan Study* (revised edition). New York: McGraw Hill, 1978.

Streib, G. F., Thompson, W.E., and Suchman, E.A. The Cornell study of occupational retirement. *Journal of Social Issues,* 1958, *14,* 3–17.

Thompson, W.E., and Streib, G.F. Situational determinants: health and economic deprivation in retirement. *Journal of Social Issues,* 1958, *14,* 18–34.

Thompson, W.E., Streib, G.F., and Kosa, J. The effect of retirement on personal adjustment: a panel analysis. *Journal of Gerontology,* 1960, *15,* 165–169.

Warheit, G.L., Holzer, C.E., III, and Arey, S.A. Race and mental illness: an epidemiologic update. *Journal of Health and Social Behavior,* 1975, *16,* 243–256.

Warr, P. A study of psychological well-being. *British Journal of Psychology,* 1978, *69,* 111–121.

Wood, V., Wylie, M.L., and Sheafor, B. An analysis of a short self-report measure of life satisfaction: correlation with rater judgment. *Journal of Gerontology,* 1969, *24,* 465–469.

Wylie, M.L. Life satisfaction as a program impact criterion. *Journal of Gerontology,* 1970, *25,* 36–40.

SECTION VI

# Brief Review

CHAPTER 14

# Diagnosis and Treatment of Urinary Incontinence

ROBERT J. KRANE, M.D. MIKE B. SIROKY, M.D.
DEPARTMENT OF UROLOGY
BOSTON UNIVERSITY SCHOOL OF MEDICINE
BOSTON, MASSACHUSETTS

Urinary incontinence, although usually not life threatening, remains one of the most distressing symptoms experienced by the elderly. Approximately 10 percent of the elderly are estimated to experience some degree of urinary incontinence, with an even higher prevalence (30 percent) in hospitalized individuals (Willington, 1976). New evaluation techniques have increased the treatment options for the incontinent patient, with more specific therapies depending upon the underlying vesicourethral dysfunction. Before embarking on a discussion of the evaluation and treatment of the incontinent patient, it is important to review briefly some pertinent neuroanatomic and neurophysiologic aspects of the lower urinary tract.

## NEUROANATOMY OF THE LOWER URINARY TRACT

Voiding dysfunction may be viewed as an alteration of the dynamic interaction among the bladder (or detrusor), the proximal smooth muscle sphincter, and more distal striated muscle sphincter (external sphincter). The bladder, composed of a syncitium of smooth muscle cells under mainly parasympathetic control, receives its neural input from the autonomic fibers which exit from the spinal cord at S2–S4. The proximal smooth muscle sphincter appears to be under alpha-sympathetic control, receiving its neurologic input either via thoracolumbar sympathetic outflow or through short adrenergic fibers (Owman et al., 1971). The striated muscle sphincter is composed of voluntary skeletal musculature and is innervated by somatic motor fibers from S2–S4.

Contraction of the bladder results from a highly coordinated neurologic reflex. The "reflex" is almost certainly not a simple segmental one but rather a long tract spinal reflex which synapses in the pontine micturition center where coordination between the bladder and urethral sphincters occurs (DeGroat, 1975). Descending fibers from the pons coordinate this interaction so that at the time of bladder contraction there is minimal resistance by either sphincter (Figure 14–1). There is a suprapontine influence on the pontine micturitional center which provides the volitional aspects of voiding (Andrew and Nathan, 1964) (see Figure 14–2).

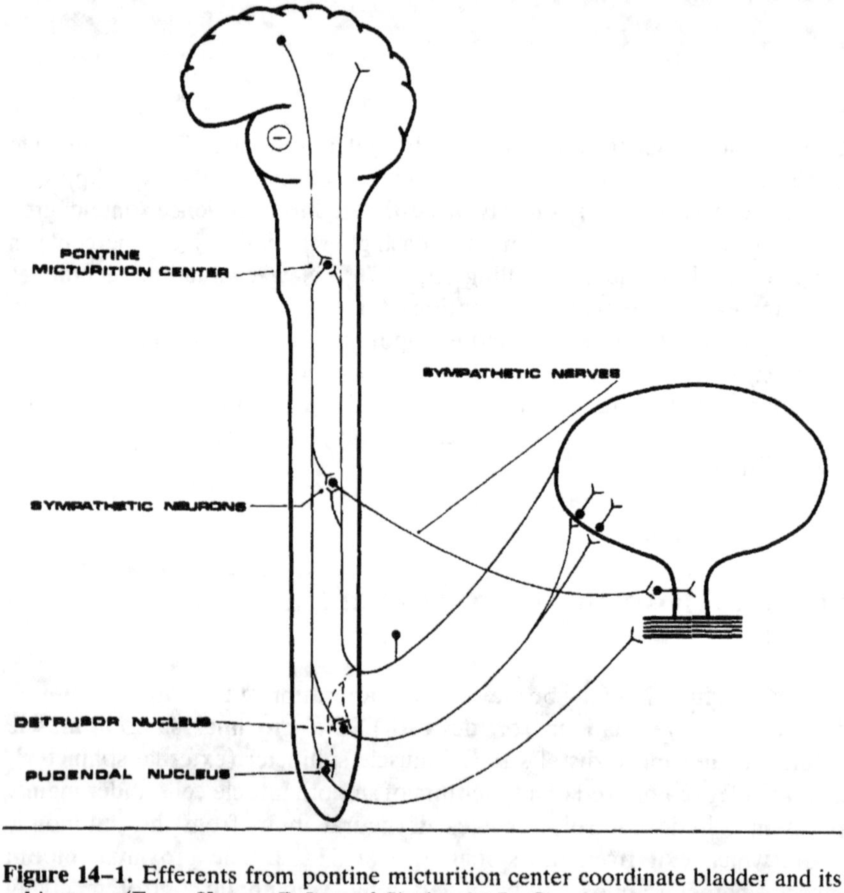


**Figure 14–1.** Efferents from pontine micturition center coordinate bladder and its sphincters. (From Krane, R.J., and Siroky, M.B. Classification and treatment of urinary incontinence. In Krane, R.J., and Siroky, M.B. *Clinical Neuro-Urology*. Boston: Little, Brown and Company, 1979, reprinted with permission.)

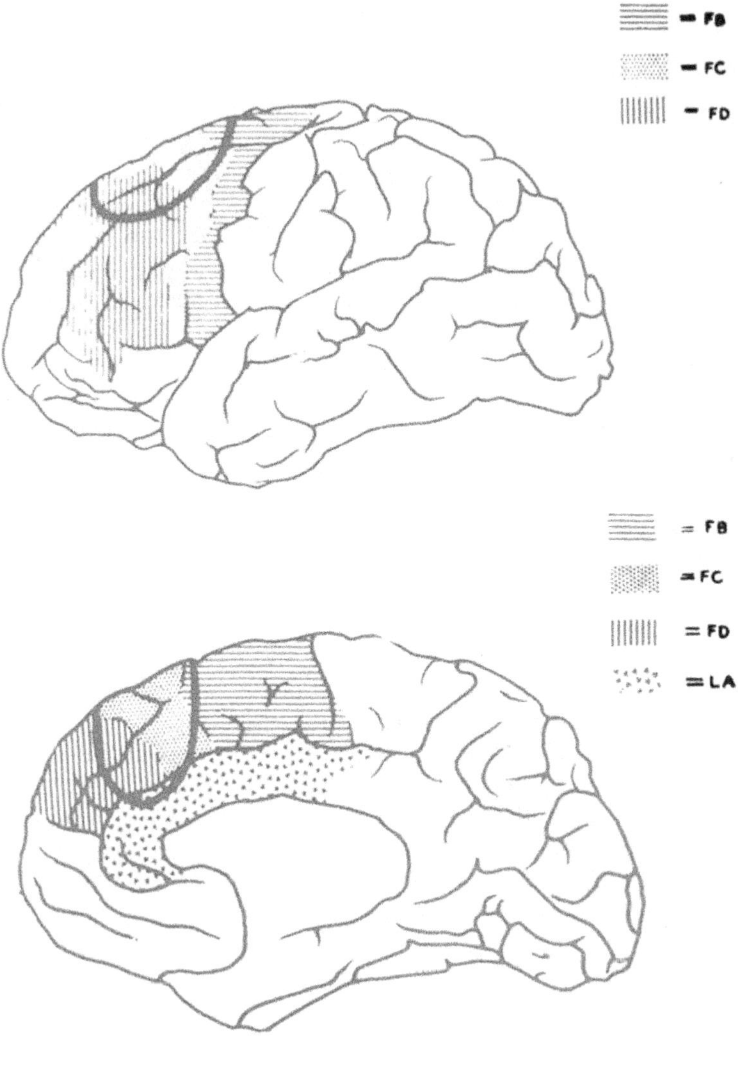


**Figure 14–2.** Areas of human cerebral cortex concerned with micturition (inside heavy black line). Letters refer to areas of Von Economo: FB and FC, premotor cortex, FD prefrontal cortex, LA, Limbic area. (From Andrew, J. and Nathan, P.W. Lesions of the anterior frontal lobes and disturbances of micturition and defecation. *Brain*, 1964, *87*, 233. Courtesy of Oxford University Press.)

## NEUROLOGIC EXAMINATION OF INCONTINENCE

The neurologic examination most appropriate to patients with vesicourethral disorders involves the sacral reflexes and sensation subserved by the sacral nerves. The bulbocavernosus reflex is the usual sacral reflex tested and involves squeezing either the glans penis or clitoris and observing a contraction of the external anal sphincter. Reflex striated muscle activity may also be elicited from the vesicourethral mucosa by tugging on an indwelling catheter (trigonal reflex). Likewise, cutaneous stimulation of the perianal skin will also produce external anal contraction (anal wink). The spinal cord segments subserving these reflexes are primarily S2–S4, but these reflexes involve segments as high as L5. Contraction of the external anal sphincter in response to coughing may also be tested. The afferent limb for this reflex is apparently from muscle receptors in the abdominal wall, and impulses enter the spinal cord from T6–T12 and ascend higher before synapsing. In lesions above T6 this reflex is therefore absent.

A localized loss of sensation in the lateral aspect of the leg suggests the presence of a herniated L4 or L5 disc or nerve root problem. If sensory loss is noted on the lateral border of fifth toe, the S1 and S2 segments are involved. Perineal sensory loss is associated with S2–S4 outflow lesions. Certainly glove or stocking sensory and vibration loss suggests metabolic or toxic neuropathy.

Deep tendon reflexes in the lower extremity, clonus, and plantar responses are all sought. Data derived from urodynamic testing can be considered only within the context of the neurologic examination. If there is complete voluntary control of rectal sphincter, the integrity of the nervous system is preserved from the cerebral cortex through the various spinal tracts out through the pudendal nerves. Therefore vesical areflexia is not necessarily neurogenic and may occasionally be secondary to functional problems due to the testing situation.

### Urodynamic Investigations

Although many types of urodynamic evaluations are possible, only those most applicable to urinary incontinence will be discussed.

*Cystometrography.* A cystometrogram is merely a pressure–volume record obtained during exogenous bladder filling. Fluid (sterile water or saline) or carbon dioxide is instilled via a urethral or suprapubic catheter into the bladder. A typical curve (see Figure 14–3) in which pressure is plotted against volume will show little or no increase in pressure during

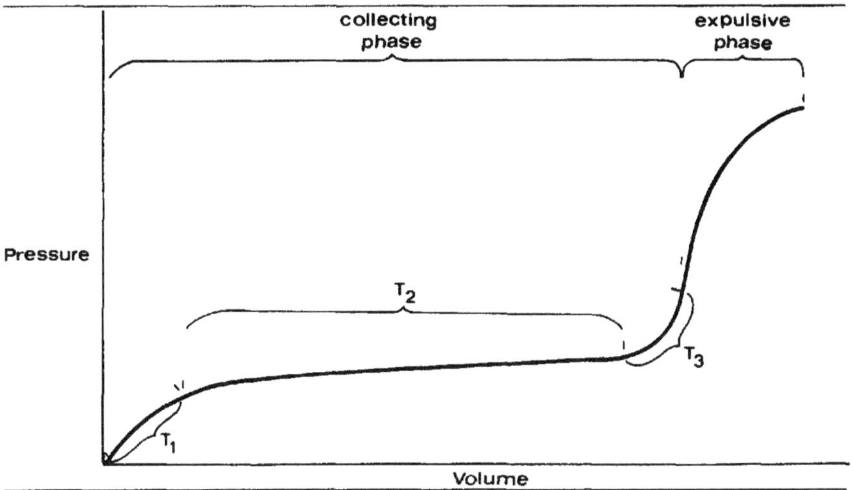


**Figure 14–3.** Diagrammatic rendering of a cystometrogram. (From Blaivas, J.G. A critical appraisal of specific diagnostic techniques. In Krane, R.J., and Siroky, M.B. *Clinical Neuro-Urology*. Boston: Little, Brown and Company, 1979, reprinted with permission.)

bladder filling until "bladder capacity" is reached. A voluntary detrusor contraction (expulsive phase of Figure 14–3) is usually seen after 300–500 ml are instilled in the bladder.

In contrast to the normal situation described above, two abnormal bladder states can be diagnosed by cystometrography. Bladder or *vesical hyperreflexia* may be produced by a neurologic lesion above the suprasacral outflow of the cord (e.g., cerebrovascular disease), or may be due to non-neurogenic causes such as outflow obstruction (unstable bladder). On cystometrography (see Figure 14–4) vesical hyperreflexia is characterized by uninhibited detrusor contractions at a lower than usual volume.

Bladder or *vesical areflexia* can be produced by a neurologic lesion involving the sacral cord (multiple sclerosis), cauda equina roots (herniated intervertebral disc), or peripheral nerves (diabetes mellitus); on occasion there may be functional causes (hysterical retention). It is characterized on cystometrography by a high volume–low pressure state (see Figure 14–5). It is not within the scope of this chapter to present further subtleties of cystometrographic interpretation, and it is most reasonable to consider bladder function in terms of the three categories outlined above; namely, the normal bladder, vesical hyperreflexia, and vesical areflexia.

*External Sphincter Electromyography.* This urodynamic procedure has in the past five years become relatively routine (Blaivas, 1977). It may be performed by placing an electromyographic needle directly into

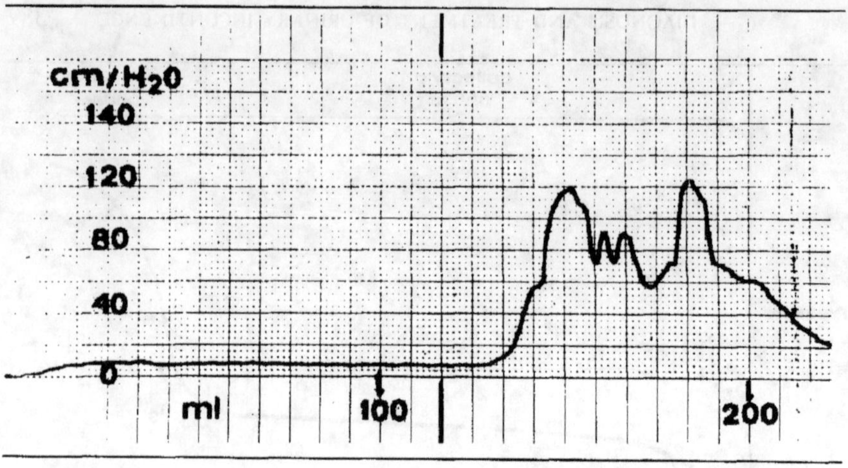


**Figure 14–4.** Cystometrogram showing bladder hyperreflexia with contraction beginning at 130 ml. (From Blaivas, J.G. A critical appraisal of specific diagnostic techniques. In Krane, R.J., and Siroky, M.B. *Clinical Neuro-Urology*. Boston: Little, Brown and Company, 1979, reprinted with permission.)

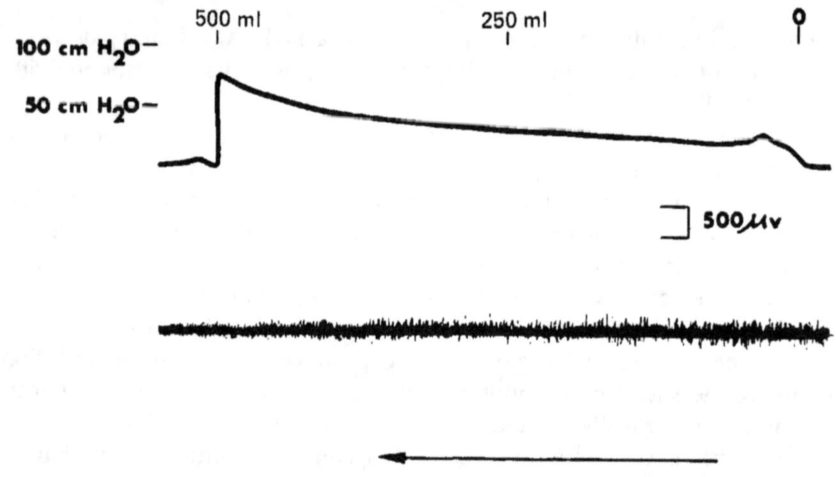


**Figure 14–5.** Cystometrogram (top) and sphincter electromyogram (bottom) showing bladder areflexia with sphincter neuropathy. (From Krane, R.J., and Siroky, M.B. Classification and Treatment of Urinary Incontinence. In Krane, R.J., and Siroky, M.B. *Clinical Neuro-Urology*. Boston: Little, Brown and Company, 1979, reprinted with permission.)

the anal or periurethral sphincter, or with the use of an anal plug electrode. Normally, in the resting state, the external urethral striated sphincter has minimal electrical activity. Increases in bladder volume will produce reflexive increases in electrical activity of this sphincter until maximum bladder capacity is reached. During voluntary voiding, there will be electrical silence of the external sphincter, preceding detrusor contraction (see Figure 14–6). Normal voiding is neurologically coordinated in a complex fashion so that there is minimal flow resistance from the striated sphincter at the time of a detrusor contraction.

Two abnormal striated sphincter states are presently recognizable using sphincter electromyography; namely, sphincter hyperactivity and sphincter neuropathy. As opposed to the normal electrical silence seen during voiding, there may be no decrease, or an increase, in electrical activity during voiding contractions. This is associated with uninhibited neurogenic bladder contractions and is called vesicosphincter dyssynergia (see Figure 14–7). When associated with vesical areflexia, it is more accurately called a nonrelaxing external sphincter. If sphincter silence does not occur during attempted voiding, functional obstruction at the

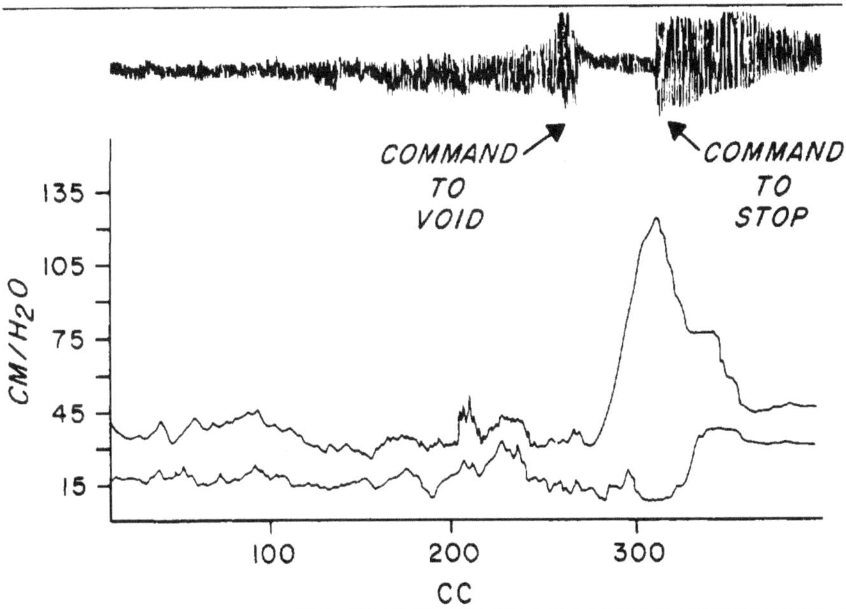


**Figure 14–6.** Cystometrogram (top) and sphincter electromyogram (bottom) in normal individual. (From Blaivas, J.G. A critical appraisal of specific diagnostic techniques. In Krane, R.J., and Siroky, M.B. *Clinical Neuro-Urology*. Boston: Little, Brown and Company, 1979, reprinted with permission.)

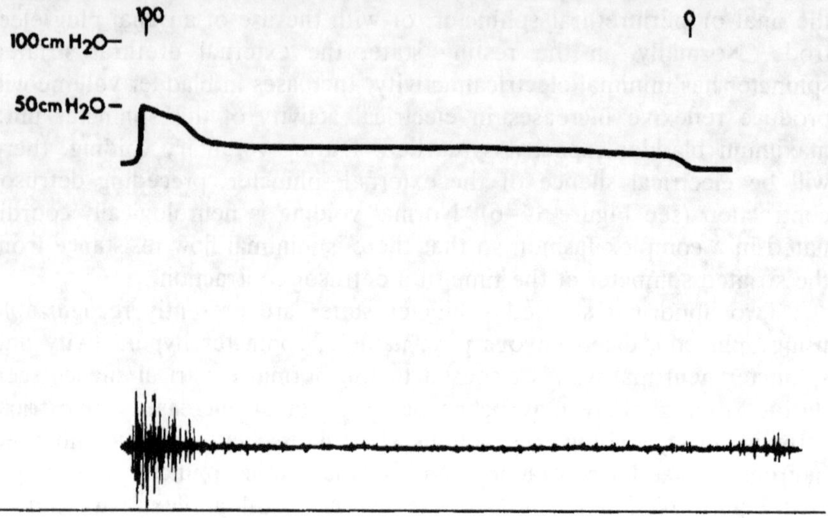


**Figure 14–7.** Cystometrogram (top) and sphincter electromyogram (bottom) showing bladder hyperreflexia and sphincter dyssynergia. (From Krane, R.J., and Siroky, M.B. Classification and Treatment of Urinary Incontinence. In Krane, R.J., and Siroky, M.B. *Clinical Neuro-Urology*. Boston: Little, Brown and Company, 1979, reprinted with permission.)

level of the striated sphincter may be present. In contrast, one may see abnormal potentials on sphincter electromyography which arc consistent with partial or complete denervation (fibrillation potentials, positive sharp waves, etc.). Denervation potentials on sphincter electromyography nearly always indicate a neurologic lesion of the sacral cord, cauda equina, or peripheral nerves.

## Abnormal Voiding States

Neurologic intracranial lesions, causing the majority of neurogenic vesical disturbances in the elderly (e.g., cerebral vascular disorder, Parkinsonism, dementia, brain tumor, etc.), usually produce vesical hyperreflexia associated with a normally relaxing, coordinated, external urethral sphincter. This neurogenic constellation produces frequency, urgency, nocturia, or variable incontinence. Lesions involving the spinal cord above the sacral outflow (conus medullaris) may have vesical hyperreflexia with a normally relaxing external sphincter or with vesicosphincter dyssynergia. The former pattern will usually present with incontinence, although voiding may simultaneously be incomplete. The latter pattern (vesicosphincter dyssynergia) will similarly present with a combined picture of both paradoxical urinary retention and episodes of incontinence. Thus, suspected or known spinal cord disease mandates a complete neurourologic evaluation for accurate diagnosis. Lesions of the conus medullaris or peripheral nerves will produce vesical areflexia, with or without sphincter disturbances, and urinary retention or obstructive voiding symptoms. However, overflow incontinence may coexist.

These urodynamic data in abnormal voiding states introduce the general discussion of incontinence and illustrate the need for a comprehensive urodynamic evaluation in incontinent patients to direct rational therapy. The clinical history rarely clarifies the etiology of incontinence.

## Neuropsychiatry of Urinary Incontinence

*Intracranial Lesions.* The elderly patient with a cerebrovascular accident is often transiently incontinent of urine. In a narrow sense these patients are incontinent because of bladder hyperreflexia secondary to a lesion of the frontal lobes (Andrew and Nathan, 1964). However, other factors must be considered, including impairment of the patient's ability to communicate, decreased sensorium level, and difficulty walking to the toilet. These complicating factors are usually present in the elderly stroke patient. A middle-aged patient with a localized brain tumor is probably a better example of pure frontal lobe incontinence. The dominant clinical characteristic of frontal incontinence is a diminished sensation that micturition is about to occur. The patient with frontal incontinence typically reports that voiding is about to occur when it is actually taking place.

*Parkinson's Disease.* Roughly 30–50 percent of Parkinsonian patients have urinary bladder dysfunction (Anderson and Bradley, 1976). The majority of symptomatic Parkinsonian patients have detrusor hyperreflexia with normal sphincter function. These patients typically complain of frequency of urination, urgency, and occasional urge incontinence. As in the stroke patient, other factors contributing to incontinence should be considered in the Parkinsonian patient, including immobility and dementia. Overflow incontinence secondary to anticholinergic L-dopa therapy should be considered.

*Dementia.* Health professionals providing care to elderly individuals are well aware of the relationship between deterioration of intellectual function and urinary incontinence. There is close correlation between the degree of mental impairment and severity of urinary incontinence (Hodkinson, 1973). Urinary incontinence in demented patients may be secondary to cortical lesions in areas concerned with urinary control, secondary to a general lack of social inhibition and inattention to personal hygiene, or both. Normal pressure hydrocephalus, characterized by the triad of dementia, apraxia of gait, and urinary incontinence, is a reversible cause of the dementia syndrome and should be sought in suggestive clinical situations.

*Spinal Cord Lesions.* In the elderly, myelopathy associated with cervical spondylosis and spinal cord compression due to metastatic tumors are the most common spinal cord lesions leading to urinary dysfunction. Urologic complaints in the patient with cervical spondylosis are typically frequency, urgency, and urge incontinence, and detrusor hyperreflexia is often present. Spinal cord compression by tumor may rapidly produce paraplegia with urinary retention—a surgical emergency in which the bladder difficulty is of minor importance.

Trauma to the spinal cord and multiple sclerosis may cause neurogenic incontinence of urine, although these conditions tend to occur most commonly in middle life. Immediately after an acute insult to the spinal cord, there is urinary retention regardless of the level of the injury, often with overflow incontinence. Within the first three months, however, if the sacral spinal cord is involved, retention and overflow incontinence will persist. With lesions above the sacral segments, bladder hyperreflexia with varying degrees of sphincter dyssynergia is seen. In less complete lesions the patient will complain of frequency of micturition, urgency, and urge incontinence.

*Autonomic and Peripheral Neuropathy.* A large number of conditions commonly seen in the elderly may result in substantial autonomic neuropathy and produce bladder dysfunction, including diabetes mellitus, pelvic surgery, alcoholism, collagen vascular disease, and systemic effects of carcinoma. Diabetic peripheral neuropathy has an insidious onset, producing a symmetrical pattern of sensory loss or dysesthesia, affecting principally the distal portions of the lower extremities. The ankle jerks may be depressed or absent. The onset of bladder dysfunction and diabetic neuropathy is likewise insidious as there are frequently no symptoms until important voiding impairment has occurred. With the accumulation of residual urine, the patient notes difficulty in voiding, overflow incontinence, or urinary retention.

## CLASSIFICATION AND TREATMENT OF URINARY INCONTINENCE

### Urinary Stress Incontinence

This diagnosis implies the loss of urine secondary to increases in intra-abdominal pressure (stress). It usually occurs in aging multiparous women and can be provoked by increases in intra-abdominal pressure, such as coughing, laughing, or rapid change to the standing position. Most women with these symptoms have true stress incontinence (anatomic stress incontinence or urethral incontinence), defined as urine leakage secondary to stress without a detrusor contraction (Table 14–1).

Hypotheses to explain true stress incontinence include: (1) a defect in urethral length; (2) a defect in the vesical-urethral angle; and (3) a defect in transmission of increased abdominal pressure to the proximal urethra. Recent evidence supports inadequate transmission of increased intra-abdominal pressure to the proximal urethra due to urethral displacement into the perineum (Henriksson et al., 1978). This change in anatomic position may explain the differential transmission of intra-abdominal pressure to the bladder and urethra, respectively, resulting in elevated intravesical pressure without a comparable rise in intraurethral pressure, thereby producing periods of incontinence. Many women with stress incontinence are postmenopausal, and deficient hormonal influences on the urethra itself may contribute to the incontinence. Estrogen increases the sensitivity of the urethral smooth muscle to alpha-adrenergic agents; the postmenopausal estrogen deficiency could interfere with the normal continence mechanisms and predispose to stress incontinence (Caine and Raz, 1975).

As mentioned previously, many women with stress urinary incontinence have true stress incontinence. Another important cause of stress incontinence is stress-induced vesical hyperreflexia, in which an increase in intra-abdominal pressure produces a reflex uninhibited bladder contraction producing incontinence. This disorder has been named stress-induced vesical hyperreflexia, vesical instability, detrusor dyssynergia, or detrusor incontinence.

It is important to distinguish patients with detrusor incontinence, since surgery usually does not help them. Patients with detrusor incontinence often give a history indistinguishable from those with true stress incontinence. Mild detrusor incontinence is not necessarily associated with urgency, because these patients usually do not preceive voiding during leakage episodes. In severe detrusor incontinence large volumes leak, compared with the few drops usually associated with urethral incontinence. But history alone cannot determine the etiology of the incontinence.

Women with stress urinary incontinence should be evaluated for other types of incontinence (overflow, etc.), and stress-induced vesical hyperreflexia must not be overlooked. A cystometrogram, with maneuvers which increase intra-abdominal pressure such as coughing and Valsalva (stress cystometrogram), is mandatory in patients with stress urinary incontinence. Most patients with true stress incontinence get symptomatic relief with vesicourethropexy. Patients with stress-induced vesical hyperreflexia should receive a therapeutic trial with anticholinergic drugs (most commonly propantheline hydrochloride or oxybutynin).

Table 14–1
Classification of Urinary Incontinence

| *Clinical type* | *Urodynamic findings* | *Treatment* |
|---|---|---|
| Stress | CMG: Normal<br>Urethral pressure: Normal or low | Vesicourethropexy<br>Alpha-adrenergic agonists |
| Urge | CMG: Detrusor hyperreflexia<br>EMG: Normal | Anticholinergic agents |
| Reflex | CMG: Detrusor hyperreflexia<br>EMG: Normal or dyssynergic | Anticholinergics<br>Condom Drainage<br>Sphincterotomy for obstruction<br>Intermittent self-catheterization |
| Total | Urethral Pressure: Low<br>CMG: Variable<br>EMG: Normal or denervation | Indwelling catheter<br>Anti-incontinence devices<br>Penile clamp<br>Supravesical diversion |
| Overflow | CMG: Normal hyperreflexic or areflexic<br>EMG: Normal or denervation | Bethanecol/phenoxybenzamine<br>Intermittent self-catheterization<br>Surgical treatment of obstruction |

## Urge Incontinence

Urge incontinence patients, unlike stress incontinence patients, usually get a momentary warning before involuntary voidings, which is secondary to vesical hyperreflexia. Urge incontinence may be neurogenic, from a lesion above the sacral outflow, or non-neurogenic secondary to outflow obstruction, urinary tract infection, bladder carcinoma, radiation cystitis, or functional causes (unstable bladder). Patients with urgency incontinence will usually have coexisting irritative voiding symptoms, including frequency of urination, nocturia, and small voidings. Urodynamic assessment will typically show vesical hyperreflexia with appropriate sphincter relaxation, the most common neurogenic incontinence in the elderly. As noted above, lesions above the pontine micturitional center, including cerebral vascular disorders, dementia, brain tumors, and Parkinsonism, will produce vesical hyperreflexia with coordinated sphincter relaxation and the typical clinical picture of urge incontinence. A form of urge incontinence may be present in the postprostatectomy patients and will be discussed later. Anticholinergic treatment is most effective in urge incontinence; and propantheline, 15 mg four times daily, is the starting dose, progressing to 160 mg daily as needed. The major side effect is xerostomia; but it should not prevent increasing the dose to control the distressing incontinence. Most patients, especially those with neurogenically induced incontinence, will require long-term, high-dose anticholinergic medication.

In the elderly male, urge incontinence may occasionally be the initial symptom of increasing benign prostatic hypertrophy. The elderly male with a cerebrovascular accident (CVA) or other suprapontine lesion requires total urodynamic evaluation to determine what role prostatic hypertrophy or neurologically induced vesical hyperreflexia plays in his symptoms. Even urodynamic evaluation may not be able to differentiate these two causes. Conversely, in any male patient with a suprapontine disorder, such as CVA or Parkinson's disease, who is being considered for a prostatectomy, one must clearly demonstrate that obstruction exists and that severe vesical hyperreflexia is not the cause of symptoms. Removing a marginally obstructing prostate in an individual with severe vesical hyperreflexia secondary to a suprapontine lesion may increase the potential for urge incontinence by lowering urethral resistance.

## Reflex Incontinence

Reflex incontinence usually occurs in patients with suprasacral spinal cord disorders such as injury. In the elderly population, transverse myelitis, cervical myelopathy, and vascular myelopathy should be considered.

Urodynamically, the lower urinary tract demonstrates vesical hyperreflexia with appropriate sphincter relaxation. The patient voids in small amounts, but with incomplete bladder emptying. In patients with more complete spinal cord lesions, increased residual urine volumes are secondary to vesicosphincter dyssynergia. Thus, most patients with reflex incontinence on the basis of a suprasacral spinal cord lesion are not treated solely for vesical hyperreflexia, but rather for the combined disorder of vesicosphincter dyssynergia. In males with this disorder, an external collecting device such as a condom catheter will usually suffice if residual urine is not excessive. In females, reflex incontinence is the most difficult to treat, and a chronic indwelling urethral catheter is usually required.

### Total Incontinence

This condition is defined as a constant loss of urine, both nocturnal and diurnal, without any increases in intra-abdominal pressure such as coughing or straining. Rarely is residual urine volume increased. Continence is sometimes improved in the supine position and worsened while standing or walking. In women, total incontinence usually follows multiple anti-incontinence procedures which reduce the urethra to a fibrotic and nonresistant tube. In men, total incontinence sometimes occurs with postprostatectomy incontinence, which will be discussed shortly.

In women, therapeutic choices for total incontinence are few and usually ineffective. Several surgical anti-incontinence devices are useful in men, but are anatomically unsuitable in women. An exception, the Scott sphincter, is a self-contained hydraulic sphincter of medical grade silicone. It can be placed around the urethra and includes a set of inflate/deflate valves which are placed subcutaneously in the vulva and a fluid reservoir which may be placed subcutaneously. Unfortunately, Scott sphincter insertion has usually produced urethral erosion. Thus, these patients generally require chronic Foley catheterization, although incontinence continues for some from leakage around the catheter itself. Reducing bladder contractility with anticholinergic agents and increasing catheter size will sometimes help.

Continued incontinence with urethral Foley catheterization may require urinary diversion at the vesical or supravesical level. The simplest form of diversion is suprapubic tube cystostomy with simultaneous formal operative closure of the bladder neck. Continent vesicostomy, which allows the patients to perform intermittent catheterization through a bladder tube stoma with bladder neck closure, has recently proven successful. Supravesical ileal loop diversion is increasingly rare in this situation, but may on occasion be the only viable option.

**Overflow Incontinence**

This type of incontinence occurs with neurologic lesions of the sacral spinal cord, cauda equina roots, or peripheral nerves causing vesical areflexia, as well as with non-neurogenic conditions producing outlet obstruction. When bladder pressure exceeds sphincter capacity, urine will leak until bladder pressure falls below that of the sphincter. These patients are usually incontinent of small urine volumes at very frequent intervals, and increases in intravesical pressure due to coughing or straining will cause increased leakage, thereby mimicking anatomic or true stress incontinence. Diagnosing overflow incontinence is usually straightforward, based on the clinical history, the physical findings, or an enlarged bladder with elevated residual urine volumes and cystometrographic vescial areflexia.

In women, vesical areflexia commonly is neurogenic, for example, diabetic neuropathy. Neuropharmacologic manipulation and intermittent self-catheterization are the major treatment options. Drugs which decrease the residual urine volume include bethanechol chloride, a cholinergic drug, and phenoxybenzamine, an alpha-sympathetic blocking agent. The rationale for combining these two drugs is that bethanechol may increase vesical contractility, and phenoxybenzamine may decrease smooth muscle sphincteric activity and lower proximal urethral resistance. Unfortunately, most patients with neurogenic vesical areflexia do not respond to neuropharmacologic manipulation alone, and intermittent self-catheterization is the only recourse.

The use of intermittent catheterization predates modern urology, first regaining wide acceptance for acute spinal-cord-injured patients (Guttmann and Frankel, 1966). Recently, its use has been enlarged to include patients with varied urologic disorders. Intermittent catheterization was carried out using aseptic technique for many years, but clean (as opposed to sterile) catheterization has been shown to be a reasonable substitute (Lapides et al., 1976). The advantages of clean self-catheterization are the lack of an indwelling urinary catheter and the ease with which it can be performed in a normal social setting. Intermittent catheterization constitutes a major advance in the modern treatment of vesical disorders. Catheterizations are usually carried out three to five times per day, simulating a normal voiding pattern and preventing prolonged stagnation and over-distention of the bladder. Most patients will not develop clinical urinary tract sepsis using clean intermittent self-catheterization, although some may require long-term low-dose antiseptic or antibiotic therapy. Approximately 35 percent of patients will have bacteriuria using this technique, as compared to nearly universal bacteriuria associated with indwelling catheters.

Men with overflow incontinence should be evaluated for obstruction, usually secondary to prostatic hypertrophy or carcinoma. Overflow incontinence due to prostatic obstruction without neurogenic vesical areflexia will usually respond well to appropriate urologic surgery; but overflow incontinence with a potential cause for neurogenic areflexia (e.g., Miles resection, diabetes) requires careful urodynamic evaluation prior to considering prostatectomy. In these patients, prostatectomy may convert retention and overflow incontinence into total incontinence, which would not benefit the patient.

Urinary continence is primarily a function of the smooth muscle urethral sphincter, though the skeletal or voluntary sphincter can inhibit the urethral stream. In patients with neurogenic vesical areflexia (e.g., diabetes mellitus) and concomitant prostatic hypertrophy, there often is underlying neurogenic loss of proximal urethral smooth muscle function; continence is preserved by the hypertrophied prostate. Removing the prostate surgically may unmask this loss of proximal urethral function and render the patient totally incontinent. Therefore, if neurogenic areflexia and neurogenic loss of proximal urethral smooth muscle activity are suspected in a patient with prostatic hypertrophy, prostatectomy should be avoided in favor of continued intermittent catheterization.

Urinary incontinence is the most distressing long-term complication of a simple prostatectomy; however, the risk of postoperative incontinence usually can be ascertained by a thorough urodynamic evaluation preoperatively. Established postprostatectomy incontinence requires urodynamic evaluation since specific treatment options can often be offered, depending on the etiology of the incontinence.

Outflow obstruction alone, secondary to prostatic hypertrophy, produces bladder wall hypertrophy and vesical hyperreflexia. After prostatectomy, these men, secondary to persistent vesical hyperreflexia, may develop urge incontinence which will slowly disappear with time and may resolve faster with anticholinergics such as propantheline. This non-neurogenic vesical hyperreflexia has been labeled vesicogenic hyperreflexia by some. Neurogenic vesical hyperreflexia, coexisting with bladder outlet obstruction secondary to prostatic hypertrophy, will show, on cystometrogram after intramuscular propantheline, diminished but usually persistent hyperreflexia. In our experience, when intramuscular propantheline can abolish uninhibited detrusor contractions, oral propantheline will usually produce the same effect. In some cases of coexisting neurogenic vesical hyperreflexia and prostatic hypertrophy, we have limited prostatic resection, hoping to preserve some urethral resistance postoperatively.

Unfortunately, some patients without any underlying neurogenic disorder suffer total urinary incontinence after prostatectomy and are unimproved by anticholinergic drugs or time. After approximately one year of persistent incontinence, these patients become candidates for surgical implantation of anti-incontinence devices. The simplest device available is a silicone gel prosthesis placed perineally against the posterior urethral wall that increases urethral resistance (Kaufman and Raz, 1976) and is satisfactory in approximately 40–60 percent of cases. The Rosen prosthesis and the Scott artificial sphincter (Scott et al., 1974) are self-contained hydraulic units which totally surround the urethra so that complete urethral closure is afforded when desired and complete urethral opening likewise is provided during voiding. Unfortunately, these devices share, with most prosthetic devices used for urinary incontinence, the potential for urethral erosion. The Scott artificial sphincter has a high reoperative rate because of either erosion or component failure. Long-term results with large numbers of Rosen prostheses are not yet available. The use of periurethral silicone injection in postprostatectomy incontinence as well as total incontinence in women has provided fairly good results in one large series, but this technique has not gained popularity.

## NEUROPHARMACOLOGIC TREATMENT OF INCONTINENCE

In selected incontinent patients, neuropharmacologic manipulation may be quite effective and should be tried first when possible. In general, drugs which can inhibit detrusor activity or increase proximal urethral activity will permit appropriate storage of urine in the bladder without concomitant incontinence. Therefore, useful drugs include anticholinergics, such as imipramine, propantheline, and oxybutynin; and musculotropic agents such as dicyclomine and flavoxate. These drugs will be most effective in incontinence secondary to vesical hyperreflexia, whether neurogenic or non-neurogenic in origin.

Alpha-sympathetic agonists, increasing proximal urethral smooth muscle activity by stimulating the many alpha-adrenergic receptors, include ephedrine, pseudoephedrine, and phenylpropanolamine. These alpha-sympathomimetic drugs are most useful in stress urinary incontinence from urethral insufficiency in women who are not considered operative candidates, and in postprostatectomy incontinence with impaired proximal urethral smooth muscle activity. Furthermore, beta-adrenergic blocking agents such as propranolol have been used, reasoning that blocking proximal urethral beta-adrenergic receptors allows unopposed alpha-adrenergic activity and better proximal urethral function. Imipramine has both anticholinergic activity and alpha-sympathomimetic activity and may be used adjunctively with alpha agonists and beta blockers.

Overflow incontinence secondary to neurogenic vesical areflexia is presently treated with phenoxybenzamine alone or combined with bethanechol chloride. Phenoxybenzamine is alpha-sympatholytic, decreasing proximal smooth muscle sphincteric function. In addition, perivesical parasympathetic ganglia are modulated by sympathetic nerves under alpha-adrenergic control, and alpha-adrenergic stimulation in the ganglia will decrease parasympathetic impulse transmission to the bladder.

Conversely, by decreasing alpha-adrenergic activity one might theoretically promote parasympathetic stimulation of the bladder and promote voiding. Phenoxybenzamine, while acting at the proximal smooth muscle sphincter area, may also act at the parasympathetic ganglia. Although bethanechol chloride presumably acts at the muscarinic vesical receptor and thus seems the most reasonable choice in neurogenic vesical areflexia, its clinical performance has been variable; nevertheless, it, along with phenoxybenzamine, is the usual initial treatment.

## REFERENCES


Anderson, J.T., and Bradley, W.E. Cystometric sphincter and electromyelographic abnormalities in Parkinson's disease. *Journal of Urology*, 1976. *116*, 75.

Andrew, J., and Nathan, P.W. Lesions of the anterior frontal lobes and disturbances of micturition and defecation. *Brain*, 1964, *87*, 233.

Blaivas, J.G., Labib, K.B., Bauer, S.B., and Retik, A.B. A new approach to electromyography of the external sphincter. *Journal of Urology*, 1977, *117*, 773.

Caine, M., and Raz, S. Some clinical implications of adrenergic receptors in the urinary tract. *Archives of Surgery*, 1975, *100*, 247.

DeGroat, W.C. Nervous control of the urinary bladder of the cat. *Brain Research*, 1975, *87*, 201.

Guttmann, L., and Frankel, H. The value of intermittent catheterization in the early management of traumatic paraplegia and tetraplegia. *Paraplegia*, 1966, *4*, 63.

Henriksson, L., Asmussen, M., Lofgren, O., and Ulmster, U. A urodynamic comparison between abdominal urethrocystopexy and vaginal sling plasty in female stress incontinence. *Urologia Internationalis*, 1978, *33*, 11.

Hodkinson, H.M. Mental impairment in the elderly. *Journal of the Royal College of Physicians*, London, 1973, *4*, 304.

Kaufman, J.J., and Raz, S. Passive urethral compression with a silicone gel prosthesis for the treatment of male urinary incontinence. *Mayo Clinic Proceedings*, 1976, *51*, 373.

Lapides, J., Kiokno, A.C., Gould, F.R., and Lowe, B.S. Further observation on self catheterization. *Journal of Urology*, 1976, *116*, 169.

Owman, C., Owman, T., and Sjoberg, N.O. Short adrenergic neurons innervating the female urethra of the cat. *Experientia*, 1971, *27*, 313.

Scott, F.B., Bradley, W.E., Attia, L.S., and Timm, G.W. The treatment of urinary incontinence by an implantable hydraulic artificial sphincter. *Journal of Urology*, 1974, *112*, 75.

Willington, F.L. *Incontinence in the Elderly*. London: Academic Press, 1976.

# Subject Index

# Author Index

*Note:* Italicized page numbers refer to bibliography pages.

www.ingramcontent.com/pod-product-compliance
Lightning Source LLC
LaVergne TN
LVHW011904200926
848484LV00002B/524